Nutritional Herbology

A Reference Guide to Herbs

Mark Pedersen

Wendell W. Whitman Company
302 E. Winona Avenue
Warsaw, IN 46580
(800) 241-2401

DISCLAIMER:	This book is designed to provide nutritional information on selected herbs. It is not intended for diagnosing ailments or prescribing remedies in any way. It is not meant to be a substitute for professional medical help. Because there is always risk involved, the publisher and author are not responsible for any adverse consequences or effects resulting from the use of any of the information, or suggestions contained in this book. If you are unwilling to assume the risk, please do not use this book.

Library of Congress Cataloging-in-Publication Data

Pedersen, Mark
  Nutritional herbology
  Includes Bibliographical references.
  1. Nutrition–Popular works. 2. Diet therapy–
popular works. 3. Vitamins–Therapeutic use.
4. Herbs–Therapeutic use.
        615.8'54 94-060830
ISBN 1-885653-03-4

Revised and Expanded Edition 1994

Originally Printed 1987

Copyright © 1994 by Wendell W. Whitman Company

Published by: Wendell W. Whitman Company
302 E. Winona Avenue, Warsaw, IN 46580

Printed in the United States of America

94 95 96 97 98 99 00 / 10 9 8 7 6 5 4 3 2 1

Contents

Chapter 1
An Introduction to Nutritional Herbology

Since the dawn of recorded history, plants have been the primary source of medicine for people throughout the world. Even today, plants are the major source of medicine in most countries. Plants which are used as medicines have been referred to as herbs for over 4,000 years by the cultures of Europe and the Mediterranean, the word herb being a derivation of "herbe" and the Latin word "herba."

Anciently, the term herb was applied only to non-woody plants, but today it is also used to refer to any part of any plant used for flavoring or medicine. Although the term herb applies to food spices, we shall use it to refer to any plant or any part of a plant having nutritional and medicinal values. Thus, an herb may be a bark, a flower, a fruit, a leaf or a root, as well as a non-woody plant.

The science and art of using plants for healing is known as herbology. In recent years many people have renewed an interest in the study of medicinal plants because it is based on simple concepts and because herbs are relatively inexpensive. Numerous companies have begun to market herbs and herbal products. Books have been published and distributed on the subject. Consequently, all this has resulted in a dramatic increase in herb use.

Since herbology deals with using plants as medicines, it might seem strange that the title of this book is **Nutritional Herbology**. Aren't medicines and nutrients two separate and distinct things? In western society, we do think of medicines and foods differently. After all, there is a big difference between a bottle of aspirin we buy for our headache and the carrots we put on the dinner table.

But what about something like garlic? You can buy garlic in the produce section of the market right next to onions and celery. Studies have shown that garlic lowers blood cholesterol levels, reduces blood pressure and kills bacteria. These are medicinal qualities. Is garlic a medicine or a food?

According to the medical definition, medicine is anything which enters the body and alters its structure or function. Using that definition, all foods and even water and air could be considered medicines. Of course lay people don't think that way. To a lay person, the term

"medicine" connotes a dangerous and probably toxic substance that must be used with extreme care and only under professional supervision. Lay people associate medicine with substances like valium and aspirin. Garlic is certainly not thought of in these terms.

The simple fact is, garlic is both a food and a medicine. It contains nutrients such as protein, carbohydrates and fats. It also aids the circulatory and immune systems. Garlic, therefore, is a medicinal food.

In the United States, the Food and Drug Administration (FDA) classifies herbs as foods when no claims are made that the herb will cure, treat, mitigate or prevent any disease. When medicinal claims are made for an herb, the herb is regulated as a medicine. Companies selling herbs as food cannot publish any material relating the use of their products to diseases without risking legal prosecution. Hence, herbs are sold as foods, but used as medicines.

This legal issue will be considered later in greater detail. For now, it is important to realize that although herbs are sold as foods there has been very little material available on their nutritional value. Hence, the need for this book. This work details the nutritional content of hundreds of herbs based on research conducted by the author (including certain food herbs like cabbage for comparison purposes). It also breaks their medicinal actions down into five basic categories for discussion of some of their medicinal uses. This is the first book that addresses both the nutritional and medicinal qualities of herbs.

Where does food end and medicine begin?

As we have previously noted, there is a tendency for modern western man to view food and medicine as two completely different things. Such has not always been the case. The oft-quoted maxim of Hippocrates: "Let your food be your medicine and let your medicine be your food," demonstrates that the distinction between food and medicine has not always been that broad.

For example, in the early 1800's, a system of herbal therapy developed by the pioneer herbalist, Samuel Thomson, was very popular. This method of herbal practice, sometimes known as the physiomedical system, considered herbs as an aid to assisting the body's own natural ability to heal itself. Thomson considered his medicinal herbs to be of the same order as foods. In his own words, "I shall now describe the fuel which continues the fire, or life of man. This is contained in two things, food and medicines (herbs): which are in harmony with each other. . ." Thomson's system focused on aiding the eliminative function of the body and regeneration of tissue. These two actions are known to most herbalists as cleansing and toning.

Cleansing the body and building up the health of body systems have been the major goals in much of the world's herbal practice. Herbal therapy is entirely different than drug therapy. In drug therapy, the practitioner seeks to describe specific causes for disease and then seeks to make specific chemical changes in the body to correct the causes. For example, a doctor might view an illness as being caused by the presence of a specific microorganism in the kidney. He would then administer a drug to kill that microorganism.

In herbal therapy, the practitioner views disease as a general imbalance of the body. In the case of the kidney infection, an herbalist would seek to correct this imbalance by administering three types of herbs. These include herbs which would prevent toxins from being absorbed from the bowel, herbs which would tonify and build the kidney and other related organs and herbs which would increase the discharge of toxins through the urinary tract and other eliminative organs. In other words, herbology focuses on assisting the self-healing process of the body. The herbalist's approach is more often nutritional than medicinal.

The difference between herbal therapy and drug therapy is illustrated succinctly in the following quotation from the herbalist, Dr. Edward E. Shook.

> Only an uneducated person would deny the existence of germs. We are prepared to admit that if the human body is in a debilitated condition, and a highly concentrated cluster of pathogenic organisms are placed in contact with a vulnerable portion of the body, certain reactions are apt to occur equivalent to the disease attributed to that type of organism. Right there, however, is the line of demarcation between orthodox medicine and natural healing. Orthodox medicine attempts to effect a cure by killing the infection with powerful inorganic drugs or by the injection of dangerous serums or vaccines. . .The herbalist and natural healer, on the other hand, recognizes that disease, excluding trauma, is the result of

violation, intentional or otherwise, of the laws of nature; that germs cannot exist in harmful numbers for any length of time in or on tissue whose life and vitality is high so that the only way the disease can be overcome is to aid nature in the healing process by the elimination of the poisons and toxins through the body's natural channels and allowing the vitality to return to the body (*Advanced Treatise on Herbology*, page 33).

Dr. Shook maintained that the various elements (especially minerals) in the herbs were their primary virtue. He asserted that herbs supported the natural function of the body by supplying "organic" elements to the organs and systems of the body as illustrated by the following:

> Just as the cells which compose the different organs and tissues select only those elements from the blood which are their natural foods and without which, it would not be possible to constantly maintain their peculiar and particular chemical constitution. . .So, also, do the herbs which supply those particular chemical constituents to the animal or human body select only those elements from the soil which build or maintain their various and peculiar chemical constituents.

Herbalists continue to assert that herbs are foods that build up the health of the various body systems, rather than just being medicines, which correct specific problems. Many of the plants sold as medicinal herbs have been used as food by various groups of people at one time or another. For example, dandelions, marshmallow, comfrey and alfalfa have all been cultivated for food by various peoples. Hawthorne berries, used by today's herbalist as a stimulant for the heart, were originally used by African tribes as a staple flour.

Most traditional schools of medicine do not make clear distinctions between foods and medicines. For example, in Ayurvedic training (schools of traditional medicine in India), they treat pharmacology and nutrition as the science. The use of spices (such as various curry powders) in India was not done solely to provide flavor to food. Spices were and still are used to balance the food medicinally to help prevent illness.

Further, plant substances are classified into three main categories: nutrient, medicinal-nutrient and medicinal. In other words, while some plants may be considered to be foods for normal consumption, there are other plants which are strictly medicinal, and often must be used with caution because they can be toxic. Many of these plants are sources for modern drugs, such as digitalis from the foxglove plant. Western medicine recognizes the existence of these two categories, but frequently fails to recognize the middle category. There are plants, such as garlic, ginger and capsicum, which can be used for both food and medicine.

The Chinese, likewise, use spices and other plants considered of medicinal value in their cooking. Thus, herbs and spices are considered "health foods" in traditional cultures. They are foods consumed for health reasons, but not in the same quantities as regular foods. In other words, they are medicinal foods.

The ancient physician, Avicenna, categorized plants according to their degree of action in speeding up or slowing down the metabolic process. He indicated a plant (or herb) might be heating (meaning it sped up the metabolic process) or cooling (meaning it slowed down the metabolic process). He then subdivided the heating and cooling groups into one of four degrees. A plant might be heating or cooling in the first, second, third or fourth degree. Substances that affect the body in the first degree have no discernable effect on the body; that is, they are totally overwhelmed by the natural forces of the body. The second degree plants have some effect on the body, but in the end are overwhelmed by the body. Third degree substances act on the body and overwhelm the natural forces of the body. Fourth degree substances are poisons, and usually alter the metabolism so far as to cause death. These substances cannot be used as medicines except in very minute quantities and with great skill.

The point is, traditional systems of medicine have not viewed nutrition and medicine as two separate subjects as we do in our modern culture. Instead, they regard them as two ends of a long spectrum of plant substances available to aid the maintenance and restoration of health.

Foods are chemically complex

Because of modern nutritional science, we tend to think of foods as substances containing just fats, proteins, carbohydrates, vitamins and minerals, but the truth is that all natural foods are complex mixtures of chemical substances. For example, a food we think of as relatively simple, the potato, contains over a hundred and fifty known chemical substances and many unknown chemical substances as well. Among other things, potatoes contain the solanine alkaloids, oxalic acid, arsenic, tannins and nitrate, all of which have no recognized nutritional significance to man. Just one of the components of the orange, the orange oil, contains 42 chemicals, including 12 alcohols, 9 aldehydes, 2 esters, 14 hydrocarbons and 4 ketones. All fruits and vegetables and other natural substances are similarly complex.

Many of these substances in isolated form would be toxic. For example, the alkaloid solanine found in potatoes interferes with the transmission of nerve impulses and carrots contain a potent nerve poison called carototoxin. Fortunately, the amount of toxins contained in these foods are extremely small and cause no ill effects when ingested in normal size food portions. Other chemicals found in everyday foods have medicinal qualities. Oats contain an alkaloid which is mildly stimulating and antispasmodic, this explains why an infusion of oats was used in times past as a nerve tonic. Cranberry juice is a New England folk treatment for urinary infections. Researchers found it contains a substance that is converted into a urinary antiseptic in the body, although they concluded that the action wasn't sufficiently strong to be effective.

All natural foods contain substances which affect the structure or function of the body. Most contain about 500 to 1,000 mg of such active compounds per kilogram or about 0.1%. Thus, all natural foods have some medicinal action, however weak it may be. In fact, the only foods which do not contain these substances are refined foods like white flour and white sugar. The herbs we call foods have an abundance of fuel and structural components, while medicinal herbs have a greater abundance of those other chemicals that alter structure or function.

The medicinal value of nutrients

There is still much to learn in nutrition, and it is possible that some of the components now thought of as medicinal, may be considered nutrients in coming years. When one looks back through history and observes how nutritional research has developed, it is evident that cures once thought of as medicinal are now thought of as nutritional. For example, many years ago there was a dreaded disease called scurvy.

In 1753, Dr. James Lind, a physician in the British Royal Navy, published the results of his experiments in determining the cause and prevention of scurvy. Dr. Lind's experiments showed that the introduction of lemon or lime juice into the sailors' diets would prevent and cure this dreaded disease. His proposal was rejected by the Lords of the Admiralty, and after four years of unsuccessfully trying to convince them, Dr. Lind remarked that "there are certain persons who just will not let themselves be convinced that a terrible disease can be cured easily, yes, that it can even be prevented."

It was 42 years before Lind received recognition for his discovery, when lime juice became an optional feature in sailor's diets. It took 88 years before this simple food supplement was made mandatory and another 36 years before vitamin C was isolated. Thus, the chemical substance vitamin C can be thought of as a medicine in that it both cures and prevents scurvy, but as we can see, it took a long time for this fact to become recognized.

Today, a whole new branch of medicine is developing known as orthomolecular medicine which deals with the use of nutrients in the treatment of diseases. The diseases being successfully treated with vitamin and mineral supplements are not necessarily due to deficiencies of these elements. In some cases it may be that the supplements simply act as catalysts to stimulate certain natural functions in the body. Our knowledge of nutrition is really still in its infancy.

Do medicinal components of foods have nutritional value?

In times past, a tea made of rose hips or pine needles was used to treat scurvy. At one time this use of herbs to cure a disease would have been thought of as medicinal, but now, since we know these plants are sources of vitamin C, we would think of the cure as a nutritional one. Similar things are occurring in nutritional research today. In recent years a number of "non-nutritive" substances are becoming recognized as important to good health. A recent example of this is fiber. Fiber is the material in plants that cannot be broken down by the digestive process. Hence, it provides no fuel, no structure-building elements and no nutrients for biochemical reactions.

There is increasing evidence, however, showing that this indigestible fiber in foods has important health benefits. Research has shown that adequate fiber helps protect the body by binding toxic wastes in the bowel to prevent their absorption into the blood stream. Dietary fiber has been shown to lower blood cholesterol levels, slow the release of sugar into the blood, bulk out and lubricate the stool to help maintain "regularity" and most recently, to have a protective effect against certain types of cancer.

Could it be possible that other chemical substances in foods and herbs thought of as "non-nutritional" could be important for good health? It is a question that will require more research to obtain a final answer.

The process of metabolism

Understanding the process of metabolism helps us to see the difference between those compounds thought of as nutrients and those thought of as medicines. In any organism, be it plant or animal, the process of life is sustained by various chemical reactions that take place continually within the cell. Thus, in one aspect, life can be thought of as a series of highly controlled chemical changes. These chemical processes take two basic forms, the building up of tissues (anabolism) and the breaking down of substances to provide fuel and building blocks for anabolism (catabolism). Collectively, these chemical reactions are known as metabolism.

Although both plants and animals carry on similar biochemical processes inside the cells, animals (and man) are different from plants in how they obtain their foods. Plants build up their own food from small molecules whereas animals take large molecules and break them down. All our nutrition and energy comes from plants either directly, by eating the plants themselves, or indirectly, by eating animals which have eaten the plants.

Those substances we think of as ordinary foods contain an abundance of basic nutritional elements, fats, proteins and carbohydrates. These are the essential compounds used to provide fuel for the body and components for building the structure. These plants also contain vitamins and minerals which are needed to catalyze body processes. Other plants contain very little of the basic nutritional elements, although they may contain substantial quantities of trace nutrients.

Herbs are still in use in modern medicine

Many people feel that herbs have no real medicinal value. Herbs do have medicinal value as evidenced by the fact that from 1959-1980 one out of every four prescriptions issued in the United States was derived from an herb. When over-the-counter (OTC) medications are included with prescription drugs, the percentage of drugs derived from or containing an herb rises to well over fifty percent.

For example, the most widely used drug in the world, aspirin, is based on the naturally occurring salicin in white willow bark. The entire class of compounds called amphetamines is based on the alkaloids found in the Chinese ephedra herb. Pseudo-ephedrine and ephedrine, are the basis for most over-the-counter decongestants including Sudafed, Actifed and many others. One can even hear portions of the root word ephedra in many of the brand names. The alkaloids in golden seal root were formerly used to provide the astringent and antiseptic action in eye drop formulas, like Murine. The bark of the cascara sagrada tree is an effective laxative, with so few side effects that to date, no synthetic preparation can match it.

In addition to the plant-based products used in medicine, food and cosmetics, there has been a recent revival of traditional herbal practice. Although modern medicine frequently claims that modern drugs are safer and more effective than herbs, many people find that herbs are safe and effective alternatives to drug medications.

Herbs and the law

In the United States, the legal definition of a drug is anything which affects the structure or function of the body and is sold for the cure, prevention, treatment or mitigation of a disease. Of course, foods may affect the structure and function of the body as well, but they do not become drugs unless they are sold for curing, preventing or treating disease. If this provision were not the law, then all foods would be drugs, since all foods affect the structure or function of the body.

In order for a manufacturer to make claims that a substance will act on the symptoms of a disease, the substance must be put through a series of rigorous tests for safety and efficacy. These tests take many years and costs can run into the millions of dollars. These laws were put into effect mainly because of problems with chemical medicines which proved to have very harmful side effects. These laws do help to protect the public against the introduction of chemical substances which have no proven effect or which may have very toxic side reactions. Unfortunately, they also severely limit the use of natural substances as medicines.

Drug companies rely on patents in order to recover the tremendous cost of proving a new drug. Hence, they are interested in unique chemicals because a specific molecular structure can be patented. However, a natural substance, like garlic, cannot be patented. Therefore, in spite of the fact that garlic has proven antibiotic effects, garlic cannot be marketed for this purpose. In order to sell garlic as an antibiotic, a company would have to pass FDA testing requirements to prove garlic was safe and effective. Among other things, they would have to specify which microorganisms garlic was effective against and at what dosage level.

The major problem is that once a company completed all this research, it would have no way to recover its investment. Anyone could buy garlic at the grocery store for a few cents or grow it in their backyard. No one would buy garlic at the inflated prices the company would have to sell it to pay for the research.

Hence, plant drug researchers look to isolate chemicals which can be modified and patented. As a result, questions like the following have not been adequately researched. Are whole plants safer than laboratory isolated chemicals? Do herbs have ingredients that modify or mitigate the side effects of some of the drug-like chemicals they contain? Is there sometimes a synergistic action in the whole plant such as a combination of a medicinal action and nutritional action?

Several observations surrounding the oral ingestion of whole herbs point toward the as yet unproven concepts of balance and synergy.

Digitalis, for example is a powerful heart stimulant employed widely in conventional medicine. The drug appears today in a purified form but is still extracted from the Digitalis purpurea plant commonly called foxglove.

A doctor is taught to recognize an overdose of Digitalis when the patient begins to experience heart arrhythmias, a potentially serious side effect of the drug. Long before Digitalis was developed, herbalists used foxglove to treat dropsy and what we term today congestive heart failure. The herbalist was alerted to a potential overdose of foxglove when a patient complained of irritation in his stomach which always occurred before the onset of arrhythmias. Nature, it seems, has provided a natural protection against an overdose of foxglove by causing one's stomach to burn, warning him to stop taking the herb or he will get sicker (i.e. have heart arrhythmias).

Lobelia is often criticized as a toxic plant because it contains lobeline and its related alkaloids which, when acting alone, are central nervous system depressants that can cause feeble pulse, coma and death.

In the proper dosage, however, these alkaloids relax the body and especially the respiratory system, making them potentially useful in treating asthma, general tension and a spastic colon. Although the safe dispensing of lobelia alkaloids would require professional supervision, the ingestion of lobelia herb would not. Who is qualified to ingest lobelia safely? Anyone who has vomited before, since nature has built an overdose protection device into lobelia that causes an overdose to be expelled from the body by violent emesis.

Other observations suggest ways in which whole plants can exhibit synergism. There are often correlations between the nutritional value of a plant and its medicinal actions. For example, diuretics cause the kidneys to produce more urine. One of the common side effects of chemical diuretics is that they flush potassium out of the body and often a potassium supplement is required for long-term use of a diuretic. Plant diuretics, on the other hand, often contain potassium in significant amounts, hence avoiding this potentially harmful side effect.

Valerian root is another example of synergy within plants. Valerian is an herb with sedative qualities. It is also high in calcium; in fact, the highest herb tested in that element. High levels of calcium in the blood have a sedative effect on the nervous system. Hence, a warm glass of milk before going to bed has helped many people go to sleep. The nutritional value in valerian root compliments its medicinal action in that area.

The theory of herbology

Herbology, as practiced in Europe and North America, is based on the principle that if the systems (digestive, circulatory, etc.) of the human body are functioning properly, then the body will maintain or achieve optimum health. Herbalists use medicinal plants (herbs) to effect changes in body systems to allow the body to heal itself. The herbs are either ingested orally or applied externally.

Most herbs in common use are mild and require long-term use to affect a change. Using herbs to obtain and maintain health embodies the concepts of preventative medicine, quality of life and increasing longevity, but in practice, this means cleansing and revitalizing body systems.

This reductionist style is dictated by an industrial society that looks upon health practitioners as mechanics that "fix what is broken." Typically, an average person will not consider herbal therapy until traditional allopathy cannot palliate nor placate him anymore. The herbalist then begins to purge the effects of the western diet and sedentary lifestyle from the body by using herbs, exercise, stress management and other lifestyle changes required to help the body heal itself. Ideal health requires a commitment to a complete lifestyle whcrc optimum health is achieved by balancing the body, mind and spirit. The oral ingestion of herbs is only one part of optimal health.

Most negative publicity associated with herbs as alternative medicine comes not from herbal theories, but from superstitions and misunderstandings about alternative medical treatments often associated with herbology, or from persons who have used herbs in a manner that ignores common sense.

However, the recent interest in herbal therapies in the United States has been spawned by a new awareness of our pre-industrial traditions, and a renewed interest in natural sources of food and medicine. More and more people are using herbs to achieve optimal health and to prevent disease conditions than ever before.

The effects of herbs

Ever since Samuel Thompson introduced composition teas over 150 years ago, the focus of modern western herbology has been to eliminate toxins from the various organ systems of the body, thus allowing the body to better heal itself. This purification process is accomplished by the use of aromatic and bitter herbs which stimulate (usually by irritation) the purging mechanism of a particular system. These herbs promote evacuation of the bowel, diuresis, emesis, diaphoresis and expectorant effects that result in the removal of toxins from all body systems.

Once the toxic substances are eliminated from the body, herbalists use astringent, mucilaginous and nutritive herbs to revitalize body systems by soothing, tightening and strengthening inflamed and flaccid tissues.

The purification and revitalizing process achieved by the use of herbs is aimed largely at the digestive system. Herbal therapies also affect the circulatory, urinary, respiratory, skeletal and nervous systems. Organs of the body such as the liver, kidneys, stomach, thyroid and heart are also targeted specifically by combinations of herbs.

Where the herbs come from

Modern herbology as practiced in North America and Europe is a hybrid of health philosophies that are closely related to the immigration patterns of different societies. As each immigrant came to the United States, he brought with him his knowledge of herbs and usually some seeds or plants native to his homeland.

The popularity of an herb used by herbalists often varied with the nationality and traditions of the user and whether the seeds could be cultivated in America.

Based on this scenario, it is little wonder that modern herbology is basically derived from European herbology, especially British, and modified to some extent by Asian, African, Middle Eastern, South American and native American herbs.

European herbs

The Europeans, especially the British, have exerted the greatest influence on western herbology. Fully, one-third of the most popular herbs in America are native to Europe. In addition, the basic philosophy of herbology is European, having been derived from the Greek and Roman civilizations. This is really understandable when one considers the number of European immigrants to the United States. These immigrants were the first and they brought European plants with them which were easily cultivated here. The earliest European colonists (before 1800), brought several food seeds and spices and roughly 10 medicinal herbs. Their spices were also used as aromatic herbs.

With the coming of the 19th century and increased trade, many other herbs from Europe were added to the list of herbs used by North American herbalists. Of the 93 herbs discussed in this work, 31 are of European origin.

South American herbs

When the Spanish explorers conquered and colonized Latin and South America in the 16th and 17th centuries, they brought with them European physicians whose herbology was based on rosemary and rue. Rosemary and rue are aromatic (stimulant) herbs which they introduced to the natives.

The Inca and Aztec Indians, however, were using a humoral (hot-cold) system of medicine that roughly resembled the present Chinese philosophy of humors (yin-yang) with an associated herbology of "hot" and "cold" herbs.

The Latin or South American system of herbology was crude and often inefficient, since superstition played a great role and very little was formally written to provide continuity between generations.

Soon after the arrival of the Spanish, epidemics of fevers killed many of the natives due to new diseases introduced by the explorers. Further, the natives refused treatment by the Spanish physicians because they held tightly to their humoral traditions.

Rosemary and rue were considered "hot" herbs by the natives, since they had stimulant and diaphoretic effects. Their humoral theory held that these herbs were remedies only for "cold" conditions. Meanwhile, most of the diseases introduced in the tropical climate were fevers and other "hot" conditions like dropsy.

Since the Spanish were losing productivity in their mines due to the high mortality rate of the natives, the Spanish evoked sanctions on the natives forbidding the use of their humoral medicine.

This suppression of information accounts in part for the relatively small (in numbers) contribution of native South American plants to the herbalists of North America.

North American herbs

Nearly one-fourth of the most popular herbs are indigenous to North America. One-half of the bitter herbs are also native to North America. This observation is consistent with the few numbers of people who knew how to use bitter herbs. The immigrants to America were not usually specifically trained in herbal medicine, but did have traditions of herb use.

While they did introduce many spices and foods to the West, the colonists didn't usually bring many bitter herbs. In fact, the bitter herbs were largely overlooked as Indian superstition until Thompson and others introduced the physiomedical theory of medicine in the early 1800's.

North American herbalists and Native Americans are largely responsible for bringing the bitter herbs with their unique effects into their current popularity with herbalists.

Herbs from other cultures

The herbs and health philosophies of other cultures of the world migrated to North America through the civilizations of the Mediterranean.

The spice trade routes of Marco Polo's day introduced many herbs and spices from the Asian Continent, although little of the Chinese or Ayurvedic philosophy of health distilled with them at the time. Later, the European colonizers returned several of the herbal traditions of Africa to the civilization centers of Europe.

Chapter 2
Classifying Herbs

The most important part of herbology is the combining of herbs to make effective remedies, yet it is the least understood. Most herbals contain individual herb monographs. They consider herbs individually and mention often, only in passing, the combinations of herbs that complement each other and are most often used.

The reason for this is the lack of an effective classification system for herb use. Many systems have been tried, some classifying by plant part or by humoral theories or by botanical family or by color and morphology.

The Chinese have a complex classification system based on concepts such as "chi" or body energy and hot and cold humors. They have been the most successful at correlating human constitution to herb use, but not herb to herb.

After compiling the known chemical data on the major herbs and completing their nutritional analysis, it became readily apparent that the herbs generally fell into five major categories based on their active constituents. They are: Aromatic (volatile oils), Astringent (tannins), Bitter (phenolic compounds, saponins and alkaloids), Mucilaginous (polysaccharides) and Nutritive (food stuffs).

This classification system simplifies the analysis of herbal combinations and allows one to readily propose useful new ones. It becomes easy to substitute one herb for another. Additionally, the categories are easy to identify using the senses of smell, taste, etc. This means other herbs not yet classified chemically can be more easily singled out for study and use.

Figure 1 gives a general identification scheme for herbs. Remember that herbs often contain constituents from more than one group, but usually have only one or two major effects.

AROMATIC HERBS

These herbs owe their properties mainly to volatile oils. The name aromatic is a reflection of the pleasant odor of many of these herbs. The oils are used therapeutically and as flavorings and perfumes.

The volatile oils vary widely in a chemical sense, but are most often phenolic in nature (i.e. menthol from peppermint), providing the characteristic flavor, odor, analgesic, antiseptic and carminative effects of the herbs. Some volatile oils also contain volatile alkaloids like valerotropes from valerian and capsaicin from capsicum.

The aromatic herbs are divided into two subcategories, the stimulant herbs and the nervine herbs.

Stimulant herbs

The stimulant herbs most often effect the respiratory, digestive and circulatory systems. They are often used as teas. The oils are also extracted and concentrated. They are used in both foods and medicinal preparations. They have a short shelf life since they are often the "soft" part of plants (i.e. flowers, leaves).

Properties of stimulant herbs include analgesic, antipyretic, antiasthmatic, antibiotic, antiseptic, carminative, diaphoretic, expectorant, galactogogue, parasiticide, rubefacient, stimulant and stomachic.

Examples of stimulant herbs include: capsicum, damiana, fennel, garlic, ginger, peppermint, sage, thyme, catnip, feverfew, lemon grass and penny royal.

Nervine herbs

The nervine herbs often effect the respiratory, digestive, circulatory and nervous systems. Their identification as aromatic herbs is not as apparent as the stimulant herbs, since many are roots with a protective covering and must be bruised to release their odor. They are often used as teas or in dried encapsulated form.

Properties of nervine herbs include: analgesic, antipyretic, antiasthmatic, antibiotic, antiseptic, antispasmodic, carminative, nervine, sedative and stomachic.

Examples of nervine herbs are: chamomile, crampbark, dong quai, ginger, hops, lobelia, scullcap, valerian, catnip, lady's slipper and sarsaparilla.

THE CLASSIFICATION OF HERBS

Herbal Type	Active Constituent	Examples	Method of Identification
AROMATIC	volatile oil	Peppermint Valerian	crush the herb and smell carefully (not always pleasant); hot or spicy "pungent" taste
ASTRINGENT	tannins	White Oak Bayberry	astringent taste (often bitter as well); differentiated from bitter herbs by their constipating effect upon ingestion
BITTER	phenolic derivatives (laxative and diuretic) alkaloids and saponins	Cascara Golden Seal	bitter taste; often have laxative or diuretic effects when ingested
MUCILAGINOUS	polysaccharides	Psyllium Slippery Elm	sweet, slippery-mouth feeling; makes slippery solutions and often swells in water
NUTRITIVE	(varies) protein, fats, carbo-hydrates, vitamins, minerals	Alfalfa	mild food stuffs, can be eaten in large quantities

Figure 1

ASTRINGENT HERBS

These herbs owe their properties mainly to their tannins. Formerly tannins were used to produce ink and preserve animal pelts. Systemically, tannins have the ability to precipitate proteins and this "tightens" or tones living tissue. Since tannins are phenolic compounds combined with sugars, these herbs could be classified with the phenolic bitter herbs. However, the properties of astringents are opposite from the bitter laxatives and are classified separately.

Tannins are always found in the "hard" parts of plants (i.e. bark, roots), and sometimes in the leaves. The plant uses the tannin to protect it from parasite, insect and fungal attack.

The astringent herbs effect the digestive, urinary and circulatory systems and large doses are toxic to the liver.

Properties of astringent herbs include: analgesic, antiseptic, antiabortive, astringent, emmenagogue, hemostatic and styptic.

Examples of astringent herbs are: bayberry, comfrey, eyebright, golden seal, pau d'arco, peppermint, red raspberry, slippery elm, white oak, white willow, yarrow, black walnut, crampbark, mullein and penny royal.

BITTER HERBS

These herbs owe their properties to the presence of phenols and phenolic glycosides, alkaloids or saponins. The term "bitter" is derived from the taste of these herbs and was originally limited to an herb's ability to stimulate the production of gastric secretions (i.e. gentain, a bitter tonic). The term here is used in a much broader sense.

The bitter herbs are divided into four subcategories: laxative herbs, diuretic herbs, saponin containing herbs and alkaloid containing herbs.

Laxative herbs

There are three basic types of laxatives. Bulk laxatives (see mucilaginous herbs), lubricant laxatives (mineral oil) and stimulant laxatives (anthraquinone type). The laxative herbs of the bitter category are the contraction stimulating type, often containing the phenolic derivatives called anthraquinones. Purging the digestive tract of toxins is one of the oldest and most common forms of self-medication. These herbs effect only the digestive system and are taken in capsules or as extracts before bed with the purge occurring six to eight hours later.

Properties of laxative herbs include: alterative, anticatarrhal, antipyretic, cholagogue, laxative, purgative, hepatonic, sialagogue, vermifuge and blood purifier.

Examples of laxative herbs are: aloe, cascara, licorice, pumpkin, senna, yellow dock, yucca, barberry, gentain, safflowers and golden seal.

Diuretic herbs

Diuretics are herbs that induce loss of fluid from the body through the urinary tract. The fluids released through the urine eliminate toxins and excess liquid. This is a popular way to cleanse the vascular system and some internal organs such as the kidneys and liver. Herbal diuretics are quite mild when compared to some osmotic diuretics, mercurial compounds, thiaszides and xanthine derivatives (i.e. caffeine). Herbal diuretics exert an irritant action caused by phenolic derivatives called flavonoids.

Flavonoids were discovered long ago for their yellow or orange color and used as dyes. Their therapeutic action was discovered in the early 1900's. They are known to strengthen the capillaries and act as spasmolytics and diuretics. They are often accompanied by the water soluble vitamins, especially vitamin C (See rosehips).

Properties of diuretic herbs include: alterative, antibiotic, anticatarrhal, antipyretic, antiseptic, diuretic, lithotriptic and blood purifier.

Examples of diuretic herbs are: asparagus, blessed thistle, burdock, butcher's broom, buchu, chaparral, chickweed, cornsilk, dandelion, dog grass, grapevine, hawthorn, horsetail, ho shou wu, hydrangea, juniper berries, milk thistle, nettle, parsley, peach bark and uva ursi.

Saponin containing herbs

Plants containing saponins have long been characterized for their ability to produce frothing aqueous solutions. The name "saponin" is derived from the Latin "sapo" meaning soap.

The detergent properties of saponins result in the emulsification of fat soluble molecules in the digestive tract. Saponins are noted for their hemolytic properties. They effectively "dissolve" the cell walls of red blood cells and disrupt them. When taken orally, however, they are comparatively harmless or they are not absorbed at all. For example, saponin rich herbs like yucca and sarsaparilla give the foamy properties to root beer.

Saponins owe their emulsifying properties to the chemicals where either a steroid or triterpene fat-soluble base molecule is joined to a water-soluble sugar molecule.

Saponins' most important property is to accelerate the body's ability to absorb other active compounds. Some saponins are also diuretic and antispasmodic.

Properties of saponin containing herbs include alterative, anticatarrhal, antispasmodic, aphrodisiac, emmenagogue, cardiac stimulant and increased longevity.

Examples of saponin containing herbs are: wild yam root, schizandra, blue cohosh, devil's claw, licorice, alfalfa, black cohosh, yucca, ginseng and gotu kola.

Alkaloid containing herbs

An alkaloid was formerly thought of as a bitter alkaline compound (neutralizing acid) creating the term, alkaloid. Today, however, an alkaloid means any organic compound that contains nitrogen and has physiologic activity. Purified alkaloids are some of the most potent drugs known to man. The central nervous system active drugs from the opium poppy and the coca leaf are some of the most noted alkaloids.

The general definition for alkaloid makes an herb classification difficult since each group of alkaloids has very different physiological effects. Many alkaloid containing herbs are also found under additional classifications (i.e. such as valerian and capsicum).

Properties of alkaloid containing herbs include: emetic, astringent, expectorant, antiseptic, respiratory tonic, stimulant and nervine. Examples of alkaloid containing herbs are: ephedra, golden seal, lobelia, pau d'arco, valerian and capsicum.

MUCILAGINOUS HERBS

Mucilaginous herbs derive their properties from the polysaccharides they contain. These polysaccharides have a slippery, mild taste and swell in water. All plants produce mucilage in some form to store water as hydrates and as a food reserve. Most mucilages are not broken down by the human digestive system but absorb toxins from the bowel and give bulk to the stool. Mucilaginous herbs are most effective topically, as poultices and knitting agents, and internally in the digestive tract. If used as a lozenge or extract, they have a demulcent action effect on the throat.

The major effects of mucilaginous herbs are (1) lower bowel transit time (2) absorb toxins (3) regulate intestinal flora (4) demulcent/vulnerary action.

Properties of mucilaginous herbs include antibiotic, antacid, demulcent, emollient, vulnerary and detoxifier.

Examples of mucilaginous herbs are: althea, aloe, burdock, comfrey, dandelion, echinacea, fenugreek, kelp, psyllium, slippery elm, dulse, glucomannan from Konjak root, Irish moss and mullein.

NUTRITIVE HERBS

These herbs owe their name and classification to the nutritive value they provide to the diet. They are true foods and exert some mild medicinal effects such as fiber, mucilage and diuretic action. Most importantly, they provide the proteins, carbohydrates and fats, along with the vitamins and minerals necessary for good nutrition.

Examples of nutritive herbs are: rosehips, acerola, apple, asparagus, banana, barley grass, bee pollen, bilberry, broccoli, cabbage, carrot, cauliflower, grapefruit, hibiscus, lemon, oatstraw, onion, orange, papaya, pineapple, red clover, spirulina, stevia and wheat germ.

Chapter 3
The Nutrients in Herbs and Foods

ALUMINUM

Aluminum is a space age metal which forms the skin of aircraft and soda pop cans. It is a highly reactive element which readily combines with oxygen. This is responsible for its stability in the metallic state, since it quickly forms a stable oxide coat when it is exposed to air. However, it is infamous when used as a culinary utensil for its incompatibility with tomatoes and other acidic foods, as these foods react strongly with aluminum.

Nutritionally there is no known use for aluminum. Metabolically, aluminum is absorbed in the most minute amounts since it nearly always finds a molecule to react with in the digestive fluids of the stomach.

Disorders of the brain such as Alzheimer's Disease, Parkinson's Disease and Down's Syndrome are thought to be associated with the abnormal absorption of aluminum in specific areas of brain tissue. The presence of aluminum, especially in the brain, blocks the normal reactions that involve the mineral zinc. There is, however, no known relationship between the normal ingestion of aluminum in our diets and these diseases.

The aluminum content of a plant is a good indicator of the cleanliness of an herb sample (especially roots) since aluminum is a major constituent of all soils.

Aluminum Ranges in Descending Order
calculated on a zero moisture
basis per 100 gm

Gotu Kola leaf	206	mg
Chickweed herb	96	mg
Pennyroyal herb	185	mg
Buchu leaf	136	mg
Butcher's Broom root	131	mg
Mullein leaf	109	mg
Grapevine herb	103	mg
Devil's Claw root	93.9	mg
Thyme herb	92.0	mg
Echinacea root	78.6	mg
Blue Cohosh root	76.2	mg
Sarsaparilla root	74.5	mg
Uva Ursi leaf	71.9	mg
Crampbark	70.2	mg
Althea root	68.0	mg
Ginger root	66.3	mg
Dandelion root	65.6	mg
Kelp herb	63.1	mg
Senna leaf	62.0	mg
Dulse herb	61.5	mg

Ranges for Aluminum:

Very High	=	66	-	206	mg
High	=	30	-	66	mg
Average	=	7	-	30	mg
Low	=	2.5	-	7	mg
Very Low	=	0	-	2.5	mg

CALCIUM

Calcium serves a wide variety of purposes in the body. It is the main constituent of bones and teeth and helps to regulate blood pressure, the excitability of nerves and the contractility of the muscles and heart. Acetyl choline, which helps transmit the nerve impulses, is manufactured with the aid of calcium. Also, a number of enzymes cannot function without it.

Calcium helps control blood clotting and is required for the absorption of Vitamin B-12. The National Academy of Science recommends we consume 800-1,200 mg of calcium a day.

The role of calcium in contracting muscles is leading researchers to explore calcium blocking agents in the treatment of migraine headaches. Headaches are often the result of over-constriction in the arteries of the head caused by sodium and calcium replacing magnesium within the muscle cells.

Osteoporosis, a disease of aging where bones are decalcified and weakened, has been attributed to a lack of dietary calcium, but is more probably due to a combination of risk factors of lifestyle such as lack of exercise, smoking, high sodium and phosphate intake and vitamin D imbalances. These day-to-day factors accumulate over the years of life and result in a net loss of calcium. This is because, in spite of its relative insolubility, bone tissue is remarkably active metabolically. There is a continuous exchange between bone tissue and the calcium and phosphate ions circulating in the blood.

Of the 1,200 grams of calcium in an average adult, it is estimated that up to 700 grams of calcium ions are exchanged between bone and blood each day. Women seem especially prone to the decalcification process as a result of pregnancy, lactation and the hormonal changes accompanying menopause.

The relationship between blood pressure and calcium was discovered indirectly by the observation that many hypertensives had low serum calcium levels. Hypertension is now becoming a signal for calcium deficiency, especially in those who decrease their serum calcium levels by a high salt or high fat diet, smoking, not consuming dairy products or consuming large quantities of phosphates found in red meat or canned soda pop.

Cows' milk, a traditional source of calcium has come under fire lately due to a number of reasons. Besides calcium and protein, milk also contains cholesterol and saturated fats. It may also contain antibiotics, steroids and allergens from the feed sources. Many have a genetic intolerence for milk (lactose intolerance) and for others, government intervention and industry advertising claims make the controversy, well, milky.

In favor of drinking milk, however, researchers are finding that patients with colon cancer often drink less than average quantities of milk over their lifetime. You see, calcium can form insoluble soaps with bile acids (potential carcinogens) which are then harmlessly excreted.

In determining the optimum sources of calcium, we must mention a variety of modifiers including sodium, potassium, saturated fat, protein, vitamin D, phosphorus, magnesium, fiber, lactose and heavy metal content. Calcium carbonate sources of calcium like limestone or oyster shells contain the most calcium (up to 40 weight percent), but that doesn't necessarily make them the most useful for our bodies. Nutrient balance is the key to proper absorption and utilization of foods.

Sodium is a calcium antagonist. When looking for a good source of calcium, remember that increased sodium levels will increase calcium and phosphorus excretion through the kidneys, thus lowering serum calcium levels and raising the blood pressure. With time, this can also result in a net loss of bone mass. In the digestive tract sodium can bind with calcium to form insoluble soaps that are excreted, lowering calcium absorption.

Saturated fat is also a calcium antagonist. In the circulatory system, saturated fats contribute to higher low density lipoprotein (LDL) the so called bad cholesterol levels. This bad cholesterol can precipitate with calcium to form atherosclerotic plaque.

Fiber, especially viscous fiber, can also be a calcium antagonist. In much the same way that saturated fat will precipitate calcium, so will fiber. Yet there is an unknown mechanism which allows the digestive system to adapt to a high fiber diet and still maintain a strong, human skeletal system.

Magnesium is a calcium synergist. Chemically, it is very similar to calcium. As nutrients they are complements and opposites. Calcium constipates, magnesium is a laxative. Magnesium assists in the absorption of calcium, and most people find a non-binding, non-laxative balance when calcium and magnesium are consumed in a 2:1 ratio.

Potassium also acts synergistically with calcium. Potassium, like calcium, can help control hypertension. Vegetarians have a low incidence of hypertension and have potassium-rich diets. The very best sources of calcium will also be good sources of potassium.

Vitamin D is the most well-known calcium synergist. This is why milk is supplemented with vitamin D. Vitamin D is the precursor to a hormone which triggers the absorption of calcium chelates (calcium bound to protein, amino acids, etc.) in the intestinal wall.

Lactose, abundant in cows' milk and humans' milk, is an excellent chelating agent for calcium and therefore increases the calcium bioavailability. Lactase, a digestive enzyme for lactose, must also be present for a lactose-calcium chelate to be effective. Otherwise, the bacteria in the colon break down lactose and produce unwanted gas. Lactose intolerance varies by ethnic background. For example, only about 1% of Scandinavians are lactose intolerant, while up to 99% of the population are lactose intolerant in some Oriental races.

Many sources of calcium contain significant quantities of heavy metals such as lead, arsenic, cadmium and mercury. Oyster shells and bone meal are two popular calcium sources that may also contain large quantities of heavy metals.

Phosphorus, in the form of phosphates, combines with calcium to form bones and teeth. The ratio of calcium to phosphorus in the body is very important. The optimum ratio of calcium to phosphorus is approximately 2 parts calcium to one part phosphorus. Variations much above or below this ratio decrease calcium absorption in the digestive tract and the net calcium balance in the bones. Phosphate deficiency is rare in the western society because of the popularity of red meat and phosphate-rich soft drinks. Indeed, most of us run a surplus of phosphates. This surplus, over a lifetime, can deplete our net calcium balance.

The Best Herbal Sources of Calcium
calculated on a zero moisture
basis per 100 gm

Valerian root	4,200	mg
Buchu leaf	3,880	mg
White Oak Bark	3,700	mg
Pau D' Arco bark	3,260	mg
Kelp plant	3,040	mg
Cabbage herb	2,910	mg
Nettle leaf	2,900	mg
Senna leaf	2,630	mg
Crampbark	2,350	mg
Plantain herb	2,340	mg
Bupleurum root	2,000	mg
Barberry bark	1,910	mg
Horsetail herb	1,890	mg
Irish moss herb	1,880	mg
Damiana leaf	1,810	mg
Grapevine herb	1,770	mg
Pennyroyal herb	1,690	mg
Wood Betony herb	1,680	mg
Thyme herb	1,670	mg

Ranges for Calcium:

Very High	=	1,900	-	4,200	mg
High	=	975	-	1,900	mg
Average	=	500	-	975	mg
Low	=	55	-	500	mg
Very Low	=	0	-	55	mg

CHROMIUM

Chromium is essential for the body to produce glucose tolerance factor (GTF) which is necessary for the production and utilization of insulin. Even marginal deficiencies raise the blood sugar level and thus the amount of insulin required to metabolize it. Glucose intolerance is also a risk factor in athersclerosis. Serum high density lipoprotein levels (the cholesterol that protects the heart) are raised by chromium supplementation.

Americans have only one fourth the tissue chromium level found in Asian populations and only one fifth the level compared to Near Eastern populations. These facts are explained by the western diet which is abundant in refined, chromium depleted carbohydrates.

Chromium is used in the process of metabolizing carbohydrates, especially sugars, and since refined sugar contains virtually no chromium, body stores are thus depleted by its use.

The average western diet provides approximately 50-80 mg of chromium per day. Absorption rates average only 5-10% since chromium competes with other metals like zinc for absorption sites. No body organs in humans or animals concentrate this mineral.

No Recommended Daily Allowance (RDA) has been established for chromium, but based on excretion rates and the extremely low toxicity potential, a daily supplement of 200 mcg is in order. Herbs and spices appear to be the best sources.

The Best Herbal Sources of Chromium
calculated on a zero moisture
basis per 100 gm

Hibiscus flower	0.54	mg
Spirulina algae	0.50	mg
Gymnema leaf	0.45	mg
Oatstraw herb	0.39	mg
Nettle leaf	0.39	mg
Red clover flower	0.39	mg
Stevia leaf	0.39	mg
Barley grass	0.37	mg
Lemon grass	0.37	mg
Horseradish root	0.35	mg
Peach bark	0.35	mg
Juniper berry	0.32	mg
Parthenium root	0.32	mg
Pollen	0.32	mg
Red Clover flower	0.32	mg
Damiana leaf	0.31	mg
Safflower	0.31	mg
Buchu leaf	0.29	mg
Ginkgo leaf	0.29	mg
Catnip herb	0.27	mg

Ranges for Chromium:

Very High	=	0.19	-	0.39	mg
High	=	0.13	-	0.19	mg
Average	=	0.07	-	0.13	mg
Low	=	0.03	-	0.07	mg
Very Low	=	0	-	0.03	mg

COBALT

The only known physiological use of cobalt is as a component of vitamin B-12. However, the tissues of plants contain no vitamin B-12. The cobalt present in plants is unrelated to vitamin B-12 and is poorly absorbed by the digestive tract. This is one reason strict vegetarians often need Vitamin B-12 supplements. The cobalt levels in the plants of this study probably give a better indication of soil cobalt concentrations and sample cleanliness than anything else.

The Best Herbal Sources of Cobalt
calculated on a zero moisture
basis per 100 gm

Golden Seal root	1.53	mg
Capsicum fruit	1.51	mg
Dong Quai root	1.51	mg
Pau D' Arco bark	1.51	mg
Dulse herb	1.50	mg
Echinacea root	1.48	mg
Eyebright herb	1.47	mg
Wild Yam root	1.47	mg
Pollen	1.45	mg
Devil's Claw root	1.45	mg
Ho Shou Wu root	1.45	mg
Pumpkin seed	1.43	mg
Sarsparilla root	1.42	mg
Papaya fruit	1.40	mg
Yerba Santa herb	1.40	mg
Nettle leaf	1.32	mg
Damiana leaf	1.29	mg
Comfrey root	1.29	mg
Mullein leaf	1.28	mg
Butcher's Broom root	1.28	mg

Ranges for Cobalt:

Very High	=	1.45	-	1.53	mg
High	=	1.00	-	1.45	mg
Average	=	0.35	-	1.00	mg
Low	=	0.15	-	0.35	mg
Very Low	=	0	-	0.15	mg

COPPER

Copper is a trace mineral essential to the function of several enzymes. Chemically it is related to zinc and iron. In fact, iron and copper deficiency anemias are difficult to differentiate. Sufficient copper is critical in the absorption and transport of iron and the formation of hemoglobin.

Copper deficiency is widespread as it is estimated that only 25% of adult diets supply more than 2 mg per day. It is estimated that 5 mg per day is sufficient and 10 mg are generally safe, although no RDA has been established.

Copper poisoning is rare as it is excreted in the urine. It is also readily detoxified and excreted via the bile and feces.

Deficiency conditions can result in the above mentioned anemia as well as various bone disease, improperly cross-linked collagen and elastin, impaired glucose tolerance and elevated serum cholesterol levels. The latter two being risk factors in atherosclerosis and heart disease.

Copper has many antagonists among the nutrients as it competes for absorption sites. Zinc and copper have an inverse relationship where raising the level of one lowers the level of the other. Those who ingest more than 50 mg of zinc per day probably need to supplement their copper intake as well. A wise rule of thumb is a zinc to copper ratio of 5 to 1.

Other antagonists of copper absorption include fiber, fructose and vitamin C, which are oxidized by copper, thus rendering the copper unabsorbent. Ingestion of non-absorbent antacids can also bind copper and lower its absorption.

Protagonists of copper absorption and utilization include iron and calcium. Calcium supplementation in fact, raises copper stores in the liver.

The best sources of copper are green vegetables, nuts and legumes.

Our study found only trace amounts of copper, except for these eight. So statistical work was not performed.

The Best Herbal Sources of Copper
calculated on a zero moisture
basis per 100 gm

Scullcap herb	0.26	mg
Sage leaf	0.201	mg
White Oak bark	0.13	mg
Horsetail herb	0.11	mg
Yucca root	0.085	mg
Brewer's Yeast	0.082	mg
Pumpkin seed	0.075	mg
Gotu Kola herb	0.035	mg

FATS

Depending on their chemical structure, fatty acids can be classified as saturated, unsaturated, polyunsaturated, fixed fats and oils, waxes, sterols or phospholipids. Along with protein and carbohydrates, fats are a major portion of our food. In the body, they provide the most concentrated form of energy, yielding approximately nine calories per gram compared to four calories per gram for proteins and carbohydrates. Fats generally occur as triglycerides where three fatty acid molecules are bound to glycerine. Fats as triglycerides readily absorb food flavors and delay the gastric emptying which produces a feeling of satiety. Thus, the western palate consumes nearly 40% of its calories as fat in the form of meat, dairy and vegetable products.

Recently, the consumption of fat, and especially the high ratios of saturated fat to polyunsaturated fat in the western diet, has been linked to the high incidence of hypertension, heart disease and atherosclerosis.

Among the many uses of fats by the body, they act as energy storage. Adipose tissue also insulates and cushions the body. Fat is a carrier for fat-soluble vitamins and the essential fatty acids. Unfortunately, fat-soluble drugs like THC from marijuana and LSD can be stored for great lengths of time in adipose tissue and released indiscriminately.

The average adult needs only 15-25 gm of fat per day to maintain the necessary bodily functions provided the S/P ratio is near 1 (one). Fat deficiency is rare, but can lead to dry, flaky skin.

Saturated Fats: Saturated is a term used by chemists to denote the maximum number of hydrogen atoms an organic (carbon bearing) molecule can have. Saturated fats can usually be differentiated from unsaturated fats because they are usually solid at room temperature.

The major source of saturated fats in the diet are animal flesh, coconut and palm oils. Also, many unsaturated vegetable oils are "hardened" by partially saturating them through a process called "hydrogenation." Commercial shortenings are made in this way to help improve shelf life. Overindulging in saturated fats in the diet is indicated as a risk factor in atherosclerosis, hypertension and inflammatory diseases such as arthritis. The ratio of saturated to unsaturated fats in the diet helps regulate blood pressure independent of sodium intake with blood pressure rises being proportional to higher ratios of S/P. Saturated fats are also precursors to certain prostaglandins which produce inflammatory effects that can be a factor in arthritis and eczema.

Saturated fats also raise the levels of low and very low density lipoproteins (LDL, VLDL) in the blood. This in essence means raising blood cholesterol levels, a risk factor in atherosclerosis.

Monounsaturated Fats: Monounsaturated fats contain one unsaturated carbon-carbon double bond. Oleic acid, a major constituent of olive oil is the prime example of a mono unsaturated fatty acid. These oils are usually liquid at room temperature, but freeze readily in the chill of a refrigerator.

Monounsaturates, like polyunsaturates, lower LDL blood levels and lessen the tendency of blood platelets to form clots. But unlike polyunsaturates, monounsaturates raise the blood levels of high density lipoproteins which transport good cholesterol and have been shown to protect the arteries from plaque buildup.

Again, as with saturated fats, the balance of ingested fats is the key to optimum health.

Polyunsaturated Fatty Acids: Polyunsaturated fatty acids are liquids at room temperature which contain multiple unsaturated carbon-carbon double bonds. The richest sources are vegetable and fish oils. Some polyunsaturates which the body cannot manufacture itself, are termed essential fatty acids and include linoleic, linolenic and arachadonic acids.

Two other important polyunsaturates come from fish oils. One is eicosapentanoic acid (EPA) and dodecahexanoic acids (DHA). The polyunsaturates as a group can help to lower blood pressure and prevent unnecessary blood clotting (thrombosis).

Diets deficient in polyunsaturated fats, usually those overloaded with saturated fat, are widespread in western man. Lowering the S/P ratio therefore, can lower total plasma cholesterol and triglyceride levels, prevent unwanted blood clotting, lower blood pressure, relieve skin disorders like eczema and psoriasis, combat inflammatory conditions like arthritis and aid eye and brain development in developing embryos.

Two major mechanisms are responsible for the action of polyunsaturates. First, they are prostaglandin precursors, and specific fat precursors result in the production of specific prostaglandins. Polyunsaturates result in beneficial prostaglindin production. Some prostaglandins help the kidneys slough off sodium and water, while others produce anti-inflammatory and vasodilator effects. The second mechanism results in the regulation of blood lipoprotein levels which are critical to the health of the cardiovascular system.

Linoleic Acid: Linoleic acid is an essential fatty acid found most abundantly in vegetables such as linseed, safflower and wheat germ. It, along with arachadonic acid, is an omega-6-fatty acid. This is a term given by researchers to fatty acids whose last double bond is six carbon atoms from the end of the molecule. Linoleic acid requires niacin, B-6, vitamin C, zinc and magnesium to work efficiently. Saturated fat, alcohol, viral infections, and diabetes inhibit the action of linoleic acid. One can obtain sufficient linoleic acid by ingesting 1-3 tablespoons of vegetable oil per day.

The best sources of this triply unsaturated fatty acid is black currant seed, which contains 16-18 percent of gamma linolenic acid (GLA), and evening primrose seed oil, which contains 7-10 percent of GLA. Supplements of this essential fatty acid have been shown effective in relieving the distress caused by premenstrual syndrome, eczema and multiple sclerosis. Research continues in search of a mechanism of its action, but appears to be centered like other EFA's in prostaglandin synthesis.

Cod Liver Oil: Cod liver oil contains vitamins A and D, sulfur, up to 150 mcg iodine per 100 gm, and the polyunsaturates eicosapentanoic acid (EPA) and dodecahexanoic acid (DHA). The link between the high polyunsaturated fat diets and low incidence of heart disease among fish eating populations, like the Eskimos, lead researchers to the benefits of EPA and DHA. EPA and DHA are omega-3-fatty acids which help lower blood pressure, regulate blood lipoprotein levels and are the precursors to beneficial prostaglandin production. DHA is found in mother's milk and aids eye and brain development in children.

One to three tablespoons of cod liver oil should provide all the EFA's, EPA and DHA an adult needs.

Sterols: Sterols are alcohols which contain a steroid nucleus. The alterative effects of sterols are most prevalent in the bitter herbs. Ergosterol (related to vitamin D) and cholesterol are two important sterols as are certain alkaloids, bile acids, sex hormones and saponins.

These types of compounds appear widely in both plants and animals and usually have regulating or hormonal effects on humans.

Cholesterol is a major building block of other steroids and is transported through the blood with the aid of lipoproteins. Control of the blood sterol levels is important as a risk factor in atherosclerosis and heart disease.

Bile acids, secreted by the digestive tract to aid in fat absorption, can produce potentially harmful byproducts. Diets high in fats also increase the amount of bile acids used by the digestive tract. The toxins produced by the reaction of the fat and bile acids can be absorbed into the intestinal mucosa, but more often pass into the colon to be excreted.

Low fiber, high fat diets slow the passage of waste from the colon and are thus a risk factor for colon cancer because the byproducts of the bile acids have a greater amount of time to form carcinogens in the colon.

Saponins are also sterols. Traditionally, they are those substances that produce foams when mixed with water. Yucca root contains a saponin that has been used in root beer to give it a foaming head!

Sterols are common in plant material. More specifically, steroid precursors are found in abundance in wild yam root, other dioscorea species and fenugreek seeds. Some herbalists use these plants as steroid supplements. However, when ingested orally, many of the sterols are broken down by digestive enzymes and destroyed before the sterols are absorbed.

Phospholipids: Lecithin is the most famous and most important phospholipid. Lecithin assists the absorption of the fat soluble vitamins. It prevents the accumulation of fats on the walls of arteries and, in the brain, transforms to acetyl choline which transmits nerve impulses. It is especially effective in combination with vitamin C.

Diet plans regularly refer to lecithin's ability to dissolve fat. More accurately, it emulsifies fat by keeping fat-soluble and water-soluble substances together, especially in the blood and gastric juices. In its capacity as an emulsifier, it aids in the transportation of fat through the bloodstream.

Volatile oils - or essential oils: These are usually the savory or odorous principles of plants. Volatile oils are liquids at room temperature. They are separated from plant material by pressing, distillation or solvent extraction.

The perfume industry further separates the oils according to melting point. Upon standing in the cold, for example, many oils separate into a solid and liquid phase called respectively, stearoptene and eleoptene. More familiar are the terms bottom note and top note. In a typical perfume, the top notes will overwhelm the olfactory senses, then dissipate while the bottom notes give balance and longevity to the fragrance.

The stimulating effects of volatile oils are one of the five major effects of plant medicine (See aromatic herbs). Just as perfumes stimulate the senses of taste and smell, the aromatic herbs, which usually contain volatile oils, act to stimulate different systems of the body. The overall effect of the stimuli can vary from the sudorific, stimulant effect of capsicum to the relaxing, sedative effect of valerian.

The Best Herbal Sources of Fat
calculated on a zero moisture
basis per 100 gm

Pumpkin seed	52.0	%
Plantain herb	18.0	%
Fennel seed	16.3	%
Sage leaf	13.8	%
Capsicum fruit	12.8	%
Schizandra fruit	11.4	%
Tumeric seed	9.3	%
Passionflower	8.3	%
Yerba Santa herb	8.2	%
Thyme herb	8.0	%
Ginger root	7.2	%
Lemon grass	7.1	%
Celery seed	6.6	%
Fenugreek herb	6.4	%
Safflower	6.3	%
Milk Thistle herb	5.8	%
Gotu Kola herb	5.6	%
Juniper Berry	5.6	%
Peppermint leaf	5.4	%
Black Walnut (fruit rind)	5.2	%

Ranges of Fat:

Very High	=	5.6	-	52.0	%
High	=	3.0	-	5.6	%
Average	=	1.3	-	3.0	%
Low	=	0.5	-	1.3	%
Very Low	=	0	-	0.5	%

FIBER

Fiber has, in recent years, become one of the most popular non-nutrient components of foods. Fiber is a term used to denote a number of indigestible carbohydrates including cellulose, hemicellulose, lignin, pectin and various other gums and mucilages.

Crude fiber includes cellulose, hemicellulose and lignin, the plant material left after hot acid and alkali treatment. This is only a part of dietary fiber which includes crude fiber plus the sum of indigestible carbohydrates and carbohydrate-like components of foods like pectin, algin, glucomannan, carageenen, gums and mucilages.

There is little correlation between the crude fiber and dietary fiber contents of foods. Dietary fiber content can range from 2 to 12 times the amount of crude fiber. The importance of fiber in our diet has come to light because of the correlation between the increase of colonic diseases, like cancer and diverticulosis, and the decrease of fiber consumption in the western diet in the past century. Cereal fiber consumption, for example, has decreased up to 90%. This is due to the shift to refined and processed grains. On the other hand, consumption of other sources of fiber such as legumes, fruits and vegetables has changed very little in the last 100 years.

Nutritional values of crude fiber often give inaccurate accounts of the total fiber in a food. For example, white bread is considered by many to be a poor source of fiber, especially compared to whole wheat bread. If we look only at crude fiber, white bread does, in fact, contain only one-eighth of that found in whole wheat bread. However, if we look at dietary fiber, white bread has one-third of that found in whole wheat bread. In fact, white bread has as much dietary fiber as peaches, lettuce, apples and strawberries.

The physical properties of fiber include water absorption and swelling capacity, cation exchange, absorption of organic constituents and their affinity for certain types of bacteria.

Fiber increases stool frequency and decreases the transit time of materials passing through the large intestine. These effects are due to the water-binding ability of fiber. Cutting the transit time throughout the gut may help protect against colon cancer and diverticulosis, a colon disorder.

Diverticulosis is characterized by small defects which develop as bulges in the wall of the colon. They are similar to the bubble which appears at a weak point on an inflated rubber tire. High fiber diets can relieve the symptoms of diverticulosis.

The swelling ability of fiber to increase the bulk and speed of waste may dilute the carcinogens and leave them less time to do harm.

Dietary fiber also reduces cholesterol by preventing absorption of dietary cholesterol and by increasing the elimination of bile acids and thereby the removal of hepatically synthesized cholesterol. This has the effect of removing a major risk factor of cardiovascular disease (i.e. serum cholesterol).

Pectins have specifically been used with other colloids like clay to treat diarrheal diseases especially in infants and children. They apparently function by changing the intestinal microflora in the colon. The water-soluble pectins are bactericidal, malevolent bacteria like E-coli, while at the same time are encouraging the growth of benevolent bacteria like certain lactobacillus strains.

Pectins are most familiar to us as gelling agents for acids and sugar. Pectin has been an added benefit to diabetics and hypoglycemics. It coats the gastrointestinal wall and delays the stomach emptying time. As a result, sugar absorption is slowed after a meal and is spread over a longer period of time, resulting in a slower rise in blood sugar levels and subsequently a less rapid drop.

Many metals, especially divalent cations, like calcium and magnesium, and the heavy metals, like lead, arsenic and mercury, form insoluble fibrous salts with water-soluble or viscous fiber. This can be of benefit in ridding one's body of toxic metals, but is also of concern to those who may develop calcium deficiency.

Many people complain about the "phlegm" of stringy mucous formed after drinking milk. Much of this is the result of the calcium ions in the milk precipitating natural mucilage in the throat into an insoluble fibrous mass.

Cellulose, which forms the fibers of plants walls, is the most abundant fiber. Hemicellulose and pectin create the matrix in which the cellulose fibers are enmeshed. Plant greens and mucilages also qualify as fiber because of their resistance to digestive enzymes. Young plants have more cellulose than lignin, while mature plants contain more "woody" lignin.

The Best Herbal Sources of Crude Fiber
calculated on a zero moisture
basis per 100 gm

Cascara Sagrada bark	31.0	%
Rose hips	30.0	%
Capsicum fruit	25.8	%
Alfalfa herb	21.0	%
Thyme herb	20.2	%
Horsetail herb	20.2	%
Astragalus root	19.6	%
Sage leaf	19.6	%
Plantain herb	19.0	%
Gotu Kola herb	18.7	%
Aloe Vera	17.7	%
Ho Shou Wu root	17.5	%
Oatstraw herb	17.3	%
Grapefruit	17.2	%
Dong Quai root	17.2	%
Fennel seed	17.2	%
Ginger root	17.1	%
Celery herb	17.1	%
Black Walnut (fruit rind)	16.2	%
Pau D' Arco bark	15.2	%

Ranges of Crude Fiber:

Very High	=	17.5	-	31.0	%
High	=	12.2	-	17.5	%
Average	=	8.8	-	12.2	%
Low	=	5.0	-	8.8	%
Very Low	=	0	-	5.0	%

IRON

Iron is a constituent of hemoglobin and myoglobin and therefore aids in the transportation of oxygen to the cells and carbon dioxide to the lungs. As myoglobin, it provides the oxygen necessary for muscle contraction.

Besides being important biochemically, the affinity of iron for oxygen is widespread in nature. Common rust, an oxide of iron, forms rapidly when iron is exposed to air or water. It is also important in protein synthesis, but 75% occurs in red blood and is stored in bone marrow, the intestinal wall, liver and spleen.

Many enzymes require iron as a cofactor, especially those involved with oxidation reduction reactions. These redox reactions are exemplified by white blood cells which surround invading microbes and disrupt and digest their cell walls with peroxides, the reaction product of iron containing enzymes.

The importance of iron to our immune system is also pointed out by the fact that germs, especially bacteria, chelate iron for their own metabolism and can thus deplete iron stores in the body.

Human iron reserves, unlike many other minerals, are regulated by absorption rather than by the amount excreted. The intestinal mucosa contain ferritin which regulates iron absorption by an unknown mechanism. The body conserves and recycles iron from red blood cells and excretes approximately 1 mg of iron per day in males and 1.5 mg per day from women.

Iron absorption efficiency from the intestinal mucosa is only about 10% because of its reactivity in the alkaline environment of the small intestine.

In the acidic environment of the stomach, iron is freely soluble, but when it gets to the small intestine, the free iron ions look for a partner. Organic acids like vitamin C (ascorbic acid), citric acid, fructose found in honey and amino acids derived from proteins form chelates which aid in the absorption of iron. Meanwhile, most other nutrients like tannic acids, fiber, the phosphates in egg yolks, milk, cheese, and other inorganic phosphates, like carbonated soft drinks, alcohol and aspirin, form insoluble precipitates with iron thus lowering the absorption of iron. In fact, coffee and tea reduce iron absorption 50% because of their tannin content. Many minerals also compete for absorption sites with iron, high intakes of calcium, magnesium, zinc, copper, manganese and cadmium can interfere with iron absorption.

To obtain the most efficient use of iron supplements, one should consume them between meals with a vitamin C source. Even the efficiency of multiple vitamin and mineral preparations containing iron have been questioned because of the reactivity of iron.

The form of iron in our food is also important to the absorption rate. The most bioavailable form of iron is heme iron found in the red blood cells of poultry, fish, meat and other seafood. Up to 23% of heme iron is absorbed. Vegetarians which receive no heme iron should increase their vitamin C intake to compensate for the lower absorption of non-heme iron.

Iron is one nutrient women need more than men. Men are more likely to eat meat more often than women. Women also have higher requirements for iron due to menstruation, pregnancy and lactation.

Women absorb about 6 mg of iron per 1,000 calories of food ingested. They would need to ingest 3,000 calories per day to get enough iron, since the RDA varies from 10-18 mg. Specifically, 18 mg for women generally and up to 60 mg for pregnant women. Few women eat that many calories, so many need iron supplements.

Iron deficiency has been called the most prevalent deficiency state affecting human populations. Iron deficiency anemia caused by lower circulating levels of hemoglobin and red blood cells is characterized by listlessness, tiredness and dizziness upon standing. It lowers one's ability to stay warm when it is cold out.

Since the oxygen carrying capacity is reduced with iron deficiency, fatigue is likely to come on quicker, more often and last longer.

Depression and sleeplessness often accompany iron deficiency. Running has recently been indicted as an antagonist of iron reserves. The pounding action of running apparently causes red blood cells to be destroyed, which in turn, slows the runner's recovery from exercise.

Herbs traditionally used as emmenagogues such as blue cohosh, red raspberry, damiana, dong quai, yellow dock and black cohosh all contain significantly above average quantities of iron.

The Best Herbal Sources of Iron
calculated on a zero moisture
basis per 100 gm

Devil's Claw root	29.0	mg
Chickweed herb	25.3	mg
Mullein leaf	23.6	mg
Pennyroyal herb	23.1	mg
Blue Cohosh root	16.4	mg
Butcher's Broom root	16.4	mg
Kelp herb	15.9	mg
Bilberry	15.1	mg
Burdock root	14.7	mg
Thyme herb	14.7	mg
Barberry root	14.1	mg
Catnip herb	13.8	mg
Horsetail herb	12.3	mg
Celery seed	12.0	mg
Althea root	11.5	mg
Yerba Santa herb	11.0	mg
Milk Thistle seed	10.6	mg
Uva Ursi leaf	10.5	mg
Red Raspberry leaf	10.1	mg
Dandelion root	09.6	mg

Ranges for Iron:

Very High	=	10.0	-	25.3	mg
High	=	4.5	-	10.0	mg
Average	=	0.73	-	4.5	mg
Low	=	0.17	-	0.73	mg
Very Low	=	0	-	0.17	mg

MAGNESIUM

Magnesium is prevalent in bones and is the second most abundant cation in cells, especially the smooth, muscle artery cells. Optimum magnesium levels are vital in the synthesis of RNA, DNA and proteins. It is essential in the metabolism of proteins, carbohydrates and lipids. Over 300 enzymes require the presence of magnesium (more than any other enzyme cofactor) to function including alkaline phosphatase, which is used to activate calcium and phosphorus metabolism.

Magnesium is often called the circulatory mineral because of its vast regulating effect on muscle contraction. It also helps in the utilization of vitamins B-6,C and E.

The Recommended Daily Allowance is 350-450 mg per day, and we get approximately 120 mg per 1,000 calories of food.

The best sources of magnesium are vegetables, especially the chlorophyll-rich greens. Other good sources include nuts, beans, legumes, whole grains, seafood, dairy products and bitter herbs.

Magnesium deficiency plays a key role in all the diseases and conditions that are regulated by constriction of the heart and circulatory system such as arrhythmias, congestive heart failure, angina pain, strokes, hypertension, high LDL cholesterol levels, epilepsy and migraine headaches.

Both calcium and magnesium are present as ions in all cells and particularly heart and artery muscle cells. Calcium stimulates muscle fibers to tense and contract, while magnesium acts as a control mechanism that regulates the amount of calcium that enters the cells.

Without the tempering influence of magnesium, the arteries, especially in the heart and brain, tense up. This constricts blood flow which can lead to high blood pressure, heart attacks, stroke and migraine headaches.

The brain, in fact, stores twice as much magnesium as other body tissues. This safety supply would allow blood to keep flowing to the brain in the event of a drop of magnesium reserves.

It appears that magnesium deficiencies are widespread. Even the type of water we drink can determine whether we maintain magnesium reserves. Recent studies indicate that populations who consume magnesium rich, "hard" water have statistically less cardiovascular disease than those who drink "soft" water. Additionally, those who drink soft water had higher incidences of hypertension than their hard water drinking neighbors.

Magnesium deficiencies can also lead to Kwashiorkor, thrombosis, calcium oxalate kidney stone formation, uncontrollable muscle tics and premenstrual syndrome symptoms such as nervousness and a craving for sweets.

Optimum magnesium serum and cellular levels help to regulate so many body functions that renal magnesium excretion is quickly stopped when either magnesium or calcium intake drops very much.

Chronic magnesium deficiency can be the result of a number of risk factors including the long-term use of diuretics, digitalis, antibiotics, chemotherapy, alcohol and excessive fats or protein intake.

Even living in a hot climate is a risk factor since humans do not acclimatize to magnesium loss through perspiration as we do for potassium and sodium excretion.

The way one's body reacts to stress can also deplete magnesium levels. Type A individuals release more fatty acids into their blood under equal stress than do Type B individuals. This results in a net loss of serum magnesium.

Magnesium toxicity is rare since most of its salts are cathartic. For example, Epsom salts and Milk of Magnesia are two of our modern day laxatives. Magnesium salts also have a diuretic effect and act as depressants. Licorice, senna, burdock and chickweed all contain higher than average quantities of magnesium.

No single nutrient is as important in the absorption and metabolism of magnesium as vitamin D is to calcium. Magnesium behaves much the same as calcium in its relation to other nutrients (See Calcium report).

Calcium and magnesium are mutually antagonistic and compete for absorption sites, but calcium and vitamin D increase magnesium absorption. Again, make sure calcium and magnesium are balanced when ingesting them in about a 2:1 ratio.

Sodium, saturated fat, excess protein and fiber are all magnesium antagonists as discussed in the calcium entry. Calcium, potassium, phosphorus and lactose are all magnesium protagonists as previously discussed.

The Best Herbal Sources of Magnesium
calculated on a zero moisture
basis per 100 gm

Herb	Amount	Unit
Irish Moss herb	1,960	mg
Oatstraw herb	1,200	mg
Tumeric seed	980	mg
Licorice root	965	mg
Kelp herb	867	mg
Nettle leaf	860	mg
Senna leaf	777	mg
Dog grass	757	mg
Elecampane root	750	mg
Peppermint leaf	661	mg
Boneset herb	600	mg
Dulse herb	590	mg
White Willow bark	560	mg
Pennyroyal herb	550	mg
Devil's Claw root	544	mg
Burdock root	537	mg
Chickweed herb	529	mg
Althea root	518	mg
Pumpkin seed	514	mg
Bupleurum root	500	mg
Astragalus root	500	mg
Siberian Ginseng root	500	mg

Ranges for Magnesium:

Very High	=	500	-1,960	mg
High	=	250	- 500	mg
Average	=	140	- 250	mg
Low	=	60	- 140	mg
Very Low	=	0	- 60	mg

MANGANESE

Manganese is a trace mineral required by the body which produces healthy connective tissues like the bone matrix and cartilage. Manganese is present in all plant tissues, but especially in the leaves and seeds.

Manganese is a cofactor in enzymes that transfer phosphate groups and thus an important factor in energy metabolism.

One major concern about adequate manganese intake is that many soils are depleted of this mineral and synthetic fertilizers rarely contain it.

Chemically, it behaves very much like iron and is precipitated in the alkaline environment of the bowel by a variety of substances. Hence its absorption rates are low.

Deficiency and toxicity conditions are extremely low, but no RDA has been established. Because of its importance to the body and relative safety, a daily supplement of 2.5 to 5 mg per day is considered adequate.

Our study found red raspberry leaves to be nearly twice as high in manganese as any other herb. This is probably due to the high manganese soil content of the Willamette Valley where it was grown.

The Best Herbal Sources of Manganese
calculated on a zero moisture
basis per 100 gm

Red Raspberry leaf	14.60	mg
Grapevine herb	9.86	mg
Bilberry	9.10	mg
Yerba Santa herb	9.10	mg
Buchu leaf	6.75	mg
Catnip herb	3.74	mg
Ginger root	3.38	mg
Gotu Kola herb	2.77	mg
White Oak bark	2.53	mg
Blue Cohosh root	2.37	mg
Lady Slipper herb	2.09	mg
Wood Betony herb	1.90	mg
Dog grass	1.88	mg
Hydrangea root	1.87	mg
Uva Ursi leaf	1.65	mg

Spirulina algae	1.60	mg
Mistletoe herb	1.59	mg
Chickweed herb	1.53	mg
Hibiscus flower	1.51	mg
Milk Thistle herb	1.47	mg

Ranges for Manganese:

Very High	=	14.0	-	14.6	mg
High	=	0.63	-	1.40	mg
Average	=	0.40	-	0.63	mg
Low	=	0.15	-	0.40	mg
Very Low	=	0	-	0.15	mg

NIACIN

Niacin is an abbreviation for nicotinic acid vitamin and is used here to denote both nicotinic acid (niacin) and nicotinamide (niacinamide). Both of these forms of niacin can be used by the body. The primary difference in the two forms is that niacin produces a pronounced perfieral vasodilation effect that niacinamide does not.

Niacin functions as an integral part of energy metabolism as niacinamide adenine dinucleotide (NAD) and NAD phosphate (NADP). Niacin is present in all cells and facilitates glucose and fat metabolism. Pellagra, a niacin deficiency disease, is characterized by dermatitis, diarrhea, anxiety, depression and irritability. Its effect on the nervous system has prompted researchers to use it in the treatment of schizophrenics.

The vasodilating ability of niacin makes it popular in stress relief formulas where, by increasing blood flow to the brain, the tension of migraine headaches is mitigated.

Since niacin is a water-soluble vitamin, the potential for toxicity is low and research has shown that large doses of niacin can reduce serum cholesterol levels and prolong blood clotting time, two risk factors in athersclerosis.

Tryptophan, an amino acid present in most food proteins, can be converted into niacin by an oxidation process. Indeed, 1 part in 60 tryptophan units are converted to niacin in the body.

Since niacin is used primarily in the production of energy, the RDA is expressed for adults as 6.6 mg per 1,000 kcal of food. The average diet provides 16-34 mg of niacin. The major populations who are deficient in niacin rely on one primary grain source like unprocessed corn or milled rice.

Niacin is widespread in foods with grain, bran and germ being the most concentrated. It is interesting to note that the top two herbs in niacin are nervines.

The Best Herbal Sources of Niacin
calculated on a zero moisture
basis per 100 gm

Hops flower	43.5	mg
Feverfew herb	38.5	mg
Red Raspberry leaf	38.2	mg
Ginkgo leaf	35.0	mg
Eyebright herb	33.7	mg
Slippery Elm bark	20.0	mg
Asparagus herb	18.1	mg
Spirulina algae	16.0	mg
Cabbage herb	15.1	mg
Chamomile flower	14.9	mg
Hydrangea root	12.5	mg
Red Clover flower	12.5	mg
Black Cohosh root	12.0	mg
Peppermint leaf	11.4	mg
Gotu Kola herb	11.2	mg
Barley Grass	10.6	mg
Damiana leaf	10.2	mg
White Willow bark	9.9	mg
Alfalfa herb	9.7	mg
Mullein leaf	9.5	mg

Ranges for Niacin:

Very High	=	12.5	-	43.5	mg
High	=	6.7	-	12.5	mg
Average	=	3.0	-	6.7	mg
Low	=	0.4	-	3.0	mg
Very Low	=	0	-	0.4	mg

PHOSPHOROUS

Phosphorus is one of the major non-metals in the body. Therefore, as an anion or negatively charged ion, it combines with many of the metals or organic acids to perform a great variety of chemical reactions. With calcium, phosphates make up much of the skeletal system and B-vitamins are only effective when phosphorus is present. Phosphorus is usually combined with four oxygen atoms to form the phosphate ion; as phosphate phosphorus is present in the blood and cells, as phosphorus lipids like lecithin, protein, carbohydrates and as a major part of adenosine triphosphate or ATP, which is an energy transfer catalyst.

Phosphorus is nearly ubiquitous in foods and dietary deficiency is extremely unlikely. Intake of phosphorus is nearly always greater than that of calcium and averages 1,500-1,600 mg per day.

There is only one dietary example of phosphorus and that is through the chronic use of non absorbable antacids like aluminum hydroxide, which can bind phosphorus and prevent its absorption.

Phosphorus occurs with phyticacid as dietary fiber and as such can decrease the absorption of other minerals such as iron, zinc and copper. Adequate calcium and vitamin D ingested with phosphates usually insure adequate supplies of absorbable phosphorus in the body. Over abundance of serum phosphates through the consumption of red meat and carbonated soft drinks causes calcium to be excreted through the urine, which with time can lead to a net loss of calcium and osteoporosis (See Calcium report).

The optimum calcium to phosphorus intake ratio of 1:1 in adults is of more importance than the RDA for phosphorus alone of 800-1,200 mg per day.

Herbs, especially seeds and flowers, contain large quantities of phosphorus. This is expected since the reproductive organs of plants must store great amounts of energy. They do this in the form of fats and oils. Phosphates are used primarily to transfer the energy to the distal parts of the growing plant. The high energy herbs, the aromatics, seeds and flowers generally contain greater than average amounts of phosphorus.

The Best Herbal Sources of Phosphorus
calculated on a zero moisture
basis per 100 gm

Cabbage herb	2,030	mg
Blue Cohosh root	1,560	mg
Bilberry	1,070	mg
Pumpkin seed	1,060	mg
Yerba Santa herb	1,060	mg
Dog grass	951	mg
Soybean	824	mg
Peppermint leaf	772	mg
Cranberry	770	mg
Yellow dock root	757	mg
Asparagus herb	745	mg
Broccoli herb	716	mg
Horseradish root	710	mg
Milk Thistle seed	706	mg
Siberian Ginseng root	700	mg
Buchu leaf	678	mg
Cauliflower herb	622	mg
Ginkgo leaf	600	mg
Fennel seed	596	mg
Barley grass	595	mg

Ranges for Phosphorus:

Very High	=	600	- 2,030	mg
High	=	320	- 600	mg
Average	=	150	- 320	mg
Low	=	50	- 150	mg
Very Low	=	0	- 50	mg

POTASSIUM

Potassium is the second most abundant mineral in plants. Potash, derived from the ashes of burnt wood or other plant material, was used until the advent of synthetic detergents to saponify fats for use as soap. These water-soluble potassium (lye) soaps cleaned by precipitating dirt (calcium and magnesium ions) and thus allowed the soils to be rinsed free.

In the body, potassium plays a crucial role in osmotic equilibrium, the mechanism by which cells are nourished and cleansed. Potassium, in fact, is the principle cation in intracellular fluids and helps cells maintain their volume.

It also assists in carbohydrate metabolism, protein synthesis, muscle contraction and nerve impulse conduction.

Digestive enzyme function and efficiency is proportional to the amount of potassium in the gastric and intestinal fluids. Apparently, the human digestive tract is accustomed to foods rich in potassium like fruits, vegetables and grains. Raw foods, in fact, are the best sources of potassium since processing and cooking leaches potassium from them.

The Recommended Daily Allowance is 2.5 gm per day, but more important is the recommended ratio of potassium to sodium, which should be at least 1:1.

Potassium is a sodium antagonist. When sodium intake increases, it accumulates outside the cells and may pull water from the cells into the extracellular spaces by osmosis. This creates a feeling of puffiness or bloating. Additionally, potassium is excreted through the urine.

When potassium intake increases, potassium accumulates within the cells and forces water, by osmosis, out of the cells and this in turn triggers the kidneys to excrete sodium and water through the urine.

Ideally, the intracellular potassium concentration is less than the extracellular sodium concentration leading to an influx of much osmotically active material. In other words, this is how cells receive nourishment.

If the concentration gradient builds up through excess sodium or depleted potassium, two important actions occur. First, blood pressure increases, and secondly, the active transport cleansing mechanisms of the cells become inefficient and toxic waste material can accumulate which left alone can eventually lead to premature death of individual cells.

Potassium deficiency is quite widespread as many risk factors affect large segments of the population. Roughly 20% of the world's population fight high blood pressure. Recent changes in our Western diet account for most of the hypertension with decreasing potassium to sodium ratios at the top of the list. The body, through evolution, is geared towards getting rid of potassium and conserving sodium which is scarce in a "natural" diet. Vegetarians, which have a low incidence of hypertension, consume large quantities of potassium when compared to sodium.

Potassium deficiency can also occur as the result of climatic changes, diarrhea and long-term use of diuretics.

Dieting, with the intent of quick weight loss, can result in electrolyte imbalances. In the late 1970's, protein powder diets created a scare because the high protein, low calorie diets caused several sudden heart attacks. In more recent years these types of diets have eliminated the problem by supplementing the diet with sufficient potassium to alleviate the potential of electrolyte imbalances.

The Best Herbal Sources of Potassium
calculated on a zero moisture
basis per 100 gm

Celery herb	5,760	mg
Cabbage herb	5,400	mg
Parsley herb	3,810	mg
Broccoli herb	3,500	mg
Asparagus herb	3,350	mg
Cauliflower herb	3,280	mg
Horseradish root	3,000	mg
Blessed Thistle herb	2,600	mg
Barley Grass	2,500	mg
Hydrangea root	2,581	mg
Sage leaves	2,470	mg
Bupleurum root	2,400	mg
Catnip herb	2,350	mg
Hops flowers	2,350	mg
Lemon grass	2,300	mg
Dulse herb	2,270	mg
Peppermint leaf	2,260	mg
Feverfew herb	2,250	mg
Carrot root	2,200	mg
Scullcap herb	2,180	mg

Ranges for Potassium:

Very High	=	2,500	-	5,760	mg
High	=	1,350	-	2,500	mg
Average	=	1,000	-	1,350	mg
Low	=	250	-	1,000	mg
Very Low	=	0	-	250	mg

PROTEIN

All proteins are composed primarily of amino acids, but the proportion in which the twenty or more common amino acids occur differs greatly from one protein to another. Certain amino acids are essential to the diet (i.e., they must be supplied in the diet by food because they cannot be synthesized by the body). Unless the diet supplies protein containing enough of each of these essential amino acids to meet minimum requirements, nutritional deficiency will occur.

Nutritionally, the quality of a protein relates to its amino acid composition, the digestibility of the protein and the ability to supply amino acids in the amounts needed by the species consuming the protein. In the case of human food protein, the essential amino acid requirements of the human are the critical criteria for measuring protein quality.

Nine amino acids–histidine, isoleucine, leucine, lysine, methionine, phenylalanine, threonine, tryptophan and valine–are not synthesized by mammals and are, therefore, indispensable nutrients for man. They are commonly called the essential amino acids.

Except during the first few weeks of life, intact protein is not absorbed directly into the system. Instead, it must be broken down into peptides and amino acids which are then absorbed and used by the body. The health of the digestive system is critical to the efficiency of protein digestion. As humans age, the amount of acid and enzymes in the gastric fluids decrease and protein is less effectively broken into its bioavailable amino acids. Besides producing indigestion and toxins in the bowel, inefficient digestion lowers the absorption of other nutrients, especially certain minerals like iron and calcium, since amino acids are required for their active transport absorption mechanism.

Purified isolated amino acids have recently become popular as nutritional supplements for treating a variety of conditions (Table 1):

Amino Acid	Use
Carnitine	heart disease, hypoglycemia, Reye's Syndrome
Tryptophan	insomnia, pain relief (converted to niacin)
Tyrosine	antidepressant, adaptogen, Parkinson's disease, (converted to norepinephrine)
Lysine	cold sores, shingles, genital herpes (blocks arginine used by viruses)
Glutamine	alcoholism, drug dependence, promotes alertness
Cysteine	antioxidant
Phenylalanine	pain relief, premenstrual syndrome, appetite suppressant
Histidine	rheumatoid arthritis

Amino acids, usually as hydrolyzed vegetable protein, are also used as chelating agents to aid the absorption of minerals from the digestive tract.

Chelates are correctly pronounced "keelates" though you will sometimes hear them called "chellates."

In the process of eating, digestion and absorption, a considerable amount of vital trace elements can be rendered unavailable before they can be fully utilized by the body.

Chelation is a chemical process where the mineral nutrient is protected until it is moved to or carried through the gut wall and can be used in nutritional pathways. The word chelate comes from the Greek "chels" meaning claw, and the chelate can be visualized as surrounding the trace mineral and holding it in at least two places.

True chelates enter the blood as they are ingested. In the bloodstream, amino acids naturally migrate to particular organs and tissue groups according to the dominant amino acid configuration of the organ or tissue. Radioisotope studies have demonstrated the migration of minerals, chelated to specific amino acids, to specific body tissues. This means that one can compound mineral chelates using purified amino acids in which the amino acid will carry the mineral ion to specific body sites.

This property eliminates the need for "shotgun" mineral supplementation where trace minerals are supplied by montmorillonite, bentonite or natural mineral waters.

AMINO ACID CHELATES FOR INCREASING THE BIOAVAILABILITY OF MINERALS

Gland or Tissue	Dominant Amino Acids	Dominant Minerals
Spleen	glutamic leucine lysine	
Testes	arginine threonine lysine	K, Fe
Thymus	arginine lysine threonine	Zn
Thyroid	glutamic leucine proline	Mg
Adrenals	glutamic leucine lysine	Fe, I
Brain	arginine lysine phenylalanine	K
Bone	glutamic leucine serine	K
Heart	glutamic leucine lysine	Mn, Cu Ca, P
Muscle	glutamic lysine isoleucine	K, Fe, Mg
Blood	aspartic acid leucine lysine	Zn, Ca, Mg, P
Liver	glutamic leucine serine	Mn, Cu Fe, Zn
Lung	glutamic leucine threonine	Ca, Fe, Mn
Pancreas	glutamic leucine lysine	Mn
Pituitary	glutamic leucine lysine	Mn
Kidney	glutamic leucine	Ca
	lysine	
Nails	glutamic cystine arginine	Cu, Ca, Mg
Skin	serine glutamic glycine	Zn, Ca, Mg
Prostate	glutamic arginine thronine	Cu
Ovary	glutamic aspartic acid tyrosine	

The Best Herbal Sources of Protein
calculated on a zero moisture basis per 100 gm

Spirulina	71.3	%
Wheat Germ flour	38.0	%
Broccoli herb	33.0	%
Fenugreek herb	30.6	%
Cauliflower herb	30.0	%
Asparagus herb	30.0	%
Pollen	30.0	%
Senna leaf	27.6	%
Cabbage herb	27.5	%
Feverfew herb	26.7	%
Nettle leaf	25.2	%
Horseradish root	25.0	%
Peppermint leaf	24.8	%
Parsley herb	24.6	%
Yellow Dock root	20.3	%
Alfalfa herb	19.9	%
Pumpkin seed	19.2	%
Plantain herb	19.0	%
Juniper Berry	18.2	%

Ranges for Protein:

Very High	=	27.6	-	71.3	%
High	=	15.0	-	27.6	%
Average	=	10.0	-	15.0	%
Low	=	6.0	-	10.0	%
Very Low	=	0	-	6	%

RIBOFLAVIN

Riboflavin helps release energy from carbohydrates, proteins and fats. It is widely distributed in the tissues of plants and animals with beans and green vegetables being the most concentrated plant sources. Dairy products supply nearly one-half the riboflavin in the average American diet.

Besides its function as an energy producer, riboflavin is very important in the manufacture of red blood cells and corticosteroids.

Riboflavin, like thiamine, is not stored to any great extent in body tissues and must be supplied in daily doses since 50-70% of that ingested is excreted within 24 hours. Riboflavin is water-soluble and can be leached from food while cooking.

Deficiency is very rare, but produces symptoms very similar to Beri Beri and indeed riboflavin deficiency is usually indicated in Beri Beri. Others at risk of deficiency include dieters, those who consume unfortified refined grains, no dairy products, sulfa drugs, oral contraceptives or exercise vigorously.

The RDA is based on 0.6 mg of riboflavin per 1,000 kcal of food energy with a minimum of 1.2 mg per day for those on low calorie diets.

The Best Herbal Sources of Riboflavin
calculated on a zero moisture
basis per 100 gm

Spirulina algae	4.60	mg
Peppermint leaf	3.80	mg
Senna leaf	3.50	mg
Barley Grass	2.70	mg
Asparagus herb	2.40	mg
Broccoli herb	2.10	mg
Horseradish root	2.00	mg
Eyebright herb	1.80	mg
Cabbage herb	1.70	mg
Alfalfa herb	1.40	mg
Parsley herb	1.30	mg
Gotu Kola herb	1.30	mg
Echinacea root	1.20	mg
Cauliflower herb	1.10	mg
Ephedra herb	1.10	mg
Yellow Dock root	1.00	mg
Hops flower	1.00	mg
Barberry root	0.94	mg
Blue Cohosh root	0.79	mg
Capsicum fruit	0.75	mg

Ranges for Riboflavin:

Very High	=	1.5	-	4.6	mg
High	=	0.4	-	1.5	mg
Average	=	0.16	-	0.4	mg
Low	=	0.05	-	0.16	mg
Very Low	=	0	-	0.05	mg

SELENIUM

The most beneficial use of selenium in the human body is an antioxidant. When stimulated into action by selenium, the enzyme glutathione peroxidase prevents the conversion of potentially hazardous free radicals to carcinogens by oxidation. The word peroxidase in Glutathione peroxidase is derived from peroxide, an important group of free radicals.

The antioxidant effect of Glutathione peroxidase occurs within the cell protecting DNA structures from damage. Thus as a cofactor of Glutathione peroxidase, selenium is theoretically a cancer preventative.

Apparently selenium performs many of the same antioxidant functions as vitamin E since the selenium deficiency symptoms of irritability, fatigue, nail, hair and teeth damage are mitigated by supplementation with either selenium or vitamin E alone.

Selenium behaves chemically much the same as sulfur and can replace sulfur in certain amino acids and other sulfur containing molecules. The selenium content of our foods, in fact, depends greatly on the soil content of selenium and sulfur where the food is grown.

Selenium is highly concentrated in the pancreas, pituitary gland and the liver. Supplementation with selenium can strengthen the immune system by increasing antibody production in the body.

There is also a correlation between low selenium intakes and high rates of cardiovascular disease, although the role of selenium in its effect on the cardiovascular system are poorly understood.

Selenium is a toxic mineral and daily intake of greater than 1 mg per day should be avoided as sterility and convulsions can result. However, 80% of our population receive less than 100 mcg per day in their diets, which is only one-half of the 200 mcg Recommended Daily Allowance.

Fruits and vegetables are relatively poor sources of selenium. The best sources are grains and fish, especially grains grown in the selenium rich soils of the Northwest plains of the United States.

The Best Herbal Sources of Selenium
calculated on a zero moisture
basis per 100 gm

Hibiscus flower	1.43	mg
Catnip herb	1.23	mg
Yerba Santa herb	1.20	mg

Dog grass	1.02	mg
Ho Shou Wu root	0.74	mg
Milk Thistle seed	0.71	mg
Buchu leaf	0.70	mg
Lemon grass	0.62	mg
Lady Slipper herb	0.49	mg
Yarrow flower	0.45	mg
Valerian root	0.44	mg
Blue Cohosh root	0.35	mg
Barberry root	0.34	mg
Blessed Thistle herb	0.34	mg
Bayberry root	0.34	mg
Althea root	0.33	mg
Dulse herb	0.33	mg
Black Cohosh root	0.32	mg
Pumpkin seed	0.32	mg
Sarsaparilla root	0.31	mg

Ranges for Selenium:

Very High	=	0.30	-	1.43	mg
High	=	0.15	-	0.30	mg
Average	=	0.09	-	0.15	mg
Low	=	0.05	-	0.09	mg
Very Low	=	0	-	0.05	mg

SILICON

Silicon is an abundant inorganic element being the major constituent of sand and glass. It has achieved prominence in the last generation for its value in the semiconductor industry. Silica, or inorganic silicon, is very hard and durable and is not appreciably dissolved in living systems.

However, minute quantities of silicon are dissolved in living tissues of plants and animals. The most important role of silicon in the body is in the skeletal system where silicon gives strength to the bones.

Horsetail herb is known to contain absorbable silicon, but the bioavailability of the silicon in other herbs was not determined by this study.

The Best Herbal Sources of Silicon
calculated on a zero moisture
basis per 100 gm

Horsetail herb	3.86	mg
Dulse herb	3.68	mg
Eyebright herb	3.03	mg
Echinacea root	3.01	mg
Golden Seal root	2.87	mg
Ginger root	2.85	mg
Dog grass	2.53	mg
Cornsilk herb	2.37	mg

Burdock root	2.25	mg
Butcher's Broom root	2.24	mg
Hydrangea root	2.23	mg
Lady Slipper herb	2.22	mg
Thyme herb	2.02	mg
Astragalus root	2.00	mg
Tumeric seed	2.00	mg
Oatstraw herb	1.83	mg
Licorice	1.58	mg
Chickweed	1.57	mg
Gotu Kola	1.40	mg
Lemon grass	1.32	mg

Ranges for Silicon:

Very High	=	1.5	-	3.86	mg
High	=	0.65	-	1.50	mg
Average	=	0.20	-	0.65	mg
Low	=	0.06	-	0.20	mg
Very Low	=	0	-	0.06	mg

SODIUM

Sodium is the principle cation of extra cellular fluids. It is involved with the maintenance of osmotic equilibrium and extra cellular volume. It also plays an important role in the transmission of nerve impulses in its role as an electrolyte. Sodium deficiencies are rare as the daily requirements are low and absorption of sodium is nearly 100% efficient in the digestive tract. Also, one-third of the body's sodium store is in the bones where it acts as a reserve supply.

Sodium concentration is highly regulated as excretion rates are adjusted closely to intake rates. Sudden concentration shocks due to rapid sodium intake are accommodated by a temporary shift of water from within cells thus diluting and maintaining the sodium concentration.

Many kidney patients have been maintained on as little as one-eighth teaspoon of salt per day, yet the daily intake of sodium averages 5-10 grams. More important than total sodium intake is the sodium/potassium intake ratio which should optimally be less than one. Higher ratios can lead to low serum calcium levels and eventually to hypertension and indirectly to osteoporosis (See Calcium and Potassium reports). Also, higher osmotic pressure can lower the effectiveness of the waste removal systems of cells. With time, this can lead to a variety of unhealthy conditions including the premature death of individual cells.

Bananas are traditionally recommended as a source of potassium, not because of an overabundance of potassium, but because of its very low sodium content.

All land plants are traditionally poor sources of sodium. This is exemplified by herbivores like cows, who consume a number of different plants, but must use salt licks to supplement their sodium intake.

The Best Herbal Sources of Sodium
calculated on a zero moisture
basis per 100 gm

Dulse herb	9,917	mg
Irish Moss herb	8,120	mg
Kelp herb	5,610	mg
Rose hips	4,600	mg
Grapefruit	4,300	mg
Celery herb	2,120	mg
Gotu Kola herb	1,040	mg
Licorice root	818	mg
Parsley herb	511	mg
Cabbage herb	451	mg
Oatstraw herb	392	mg
Pennyroyal herb	379	mg
Comfrey root	351	mg
Carrot root	303	mg
Buchu leaf	276	mg
Chamomile flower	258	mg
Safflowers	232	mg
Barley Grass	224	mg
Peppermint leaf	195	mg
Wild Yam root	177	mg

Ranges for Sodium:

Very High	=	300	-	9,917	mg
High	=	60	-	300	mg
Average	=	20	-	60	mg
Low	=	5	-	20	mg
Very Low	=	0	-	5	mg

THIAMINE

Thiamine has a fundamental function in carbohydrate metabolism and is therefore essential to the normal functioning of the body organs and tissues. The vitamin is not stored in the body to any appreciable extent, but deficiencies are rare except in populations where bran and germless grains are consumed with regularity.

Beri Beri, a thiamine and more often a B-complex deficient disease, was widespread when polished rice was introduced into the diets of the populations of the Far East, who relied on this single grain source as the staple of their diet.

Thiamine deficiency mainly effects tissues which utilize large quantities of carbohydrates, like the nerve tissues and the heart muscle.

Thiamine is present in nearly all foods, but is most concentrated in grain germs and brans. Those whose diets include few calories (dieters) or the so-called junk food junkies, who consume large quantities of non-nutritive carbohydrates and alcohol, run the risk of thiamine deficiency. Thiamine is used up in metabolizing carbohydrates; therefore, refined carbohydrates often don't supply enough thiamine. Since it isn't stored in the body appreciably, dieters are also at risk of thiamine deficiency.

Raw fish and tea both contain thiamine inhibitors as well.

Thiamine utilization, like niacin, is related to the metabolism of carbohydrate and energy production. So its RDA is also based on caloric intake; 0.33-0.5 mg per 1,000 kcal of food is recommended for adults and a minimum of 1 mg per day for those on a restricted calorie diet.

The Best Herbal Sources of Thiamine
calculated on a zero moisture
basis per 100 gm

Spirulina algae	5.10	mg
Ephedra herb	4.70	mg
Asparagus herb	2.17	mg
Gotu Kola herb	1.40	mg
Fenugreek seed	1.35	mg
Barley Grass	1.29	mg
Cauliflower herb	1.22	mg
Peppermint leaf	1.21	mg
Wheat Germ flour	1.20	mg
Senna leaf	1.13	mg
Acerola fruit	1.10	mg
Burdock root	1.10	mg
Elecampane herb	1.10	mg
Grapevine herb	1.10	mg
Cabbage herb	1.00	mg
Barberry root	1.00	mg
Blue Cohosh root	0.93	mg
Sage leaf	0.82	mg
Yellow Dock root	0.81	mg
Bilberry	0.78	mg

Ranges for Thiamine:

Very High	=	1.0	-	5.1	mg
High	=	0.4	-	1.0	mg
Average	=	0.2	-	0.4	mg
Low	=	0.05	-	0.2	mg
Very Low	=	0	-	0.05	mg

TIN

Tin is a heavy metal that formerly found use in the canning industry and is still used in the electronics industry as solder.

Nutritionally, there is no known use for tin. The tin present in herbs and food stuffs is a good indicator of heavy metal content (i.e. pollution) in the soil and is included here for that reason.

The ranges for tin content in this study are well below toxic levels.

The Best Herbal Sources of Tin
calculated on a zero moisture
basis per 100 gm

Doggrass	6.7	mg
Juniper Berries	6.3	mg
Bilberry	5.0	mg
Milk thistle seeds	4.2	mg
Dulse herb	3.3	mg
lady Slipper herb	3.3	mg
Althea root	2.9	mg
Valerian root	2.8	mg
Irish moss herb	2.7	mg
nettle leaves	2.7	mg
Barberry root	2.6	mg
Yarrow flowers	2.6	mg
Blessed Thistle herb	2.5	mg
Red Clover tops	2.5	mg
Yellow Dock root	2.4	mg
Licorice root	2.4	mg
Kelp herb	2.4	mg
Senna leaves	2.3	mg
Devil's Claw root	2.4	mg
Pennyroyal herb	2.4	mg

Ranges for Tin:

Very High	=	2.4	-	6.7	mg
High	=	2.0	-	2.4	mg
Average	=	0.9	-	2.0	mg
Low	=	0.4	-	0.9	mg
Very Low	=	0	-	0.4	mg

VITAMIN A AND B-CAROTENE

Vitamin A and its carotene precursors, especially beta-carotene, is most known for its anti-infective and night vision properties. It is also necessary in bone and teeth development where it helps form the connective tissues that make up the framework for skeletal tissue.

Vitamin A is essential to the epithelial cells of the body, a tough sheath of cells that makes up all the covering and linings of the body. The skin for example, is a dry layer of epithelium. The mucous membranes of the digestive, respiratory and reproductive tracts are also lined with epithelial cells. The epithelium uses vitamin A to protect the body from infections and the skin in particular, from harmful radiation. Vitamin A has two major functions in this area. First, vitamin A is fat-soluble and, as a part of cell membranes, sequesters the invasion of bacteria physically and aids in the production of mucous secreting cells. Secondly, vitamin A and the carotenes are antioxidants which react with potential carcinogens to form harmless reaction products.

By acting as a free radical scavenger, it can block the formation of cancer-causing nitrosamines. Nitrosamines, like other free radicals, are oxygen containing compounds that are very reactive (like hydrogen peroxide). They react with other common chemicals in the body to break down cells. B-carotene and vitamin A traps these free radicals.

It is estimated that one-fourth of the population of the U.S. gets less than 70% of the RDA which ranges from 5,000 to 6,000 IU per day in their normal diets. In the developing nations of the world, the problem is even more severe. Deficiencies can cause a greater susceptibility to microbial infections, eye disorders, weight loss, loss of appetite and sterility.

Raw vegetables and animal organs are the best sources of B-carotene and vitamin A respectively. Processing, cooking and even sun drying will oxidize vitamin A by exposing it to oxidation reactions. Alcohol, iron, mineral oil and cortisone all reduce vitamin A absorption.

Zinc and protein are required for vitamin A to be released into the bloodstream by the liver. Vitamin E also protects vitamin A from certain reactions thus making vitamin A more bioavailable. Higher serum levels of vitamin A provide faster production of white blood cells thus strengthening the immune system.

Vitamin A toxicity has been well popularized. It may be concentrated to toxic levels because it is not excreted through the urine to any extent. B-carotene is not toxic because it is formed into vitamin A upon demand at the intestinal absorption sites.

The vegetable sources of vitamin A are in the form of yellow-orange vegetables and root vegetables. Green plants which contain chlorophyll inevitably are rich in B-carotene also.

The Best Herbal Sources of Beta-carotene
as Vitamin A
calculated on a zero moisture
basis per 100 gm

Spirulina algae	79,666	IU
Carrot root	70,943	IU
Gotu Kola herb	61,495	IU
Cabbage herb	54,386	IU
Barley Grass	52,000	IU
Peppermint leaf	39,579	IU
Senna leaf	39,113	IU
Yellow Dock root	37,432	IU
Uva Ursi herb	28,677	IU
Parsley herb	25,648	IU
Horseradish root	25,000	IU
Alfalfa herb	24,800	IU
Chaparral herb	23,000	IU
Broccoli herb	22,917	IU
Blessed Thistle herb	22,200	IU
Red Raspberry leaf	18,963	IU
Yerba Santa herb	16,000	IU
Capsicum fruit	15,798	IU
Nettle leaf	15,700	IU
Safflower	15,000	IU
Dandelion root	14,000	IU
Stevia leaf	12,440	IU
Eyebright herb	12,200	IU

Ranges for Vitamin A:

Very High	=	24,800	-	79,700	IU
High	=	6,200	-	24,800	IU
Average	=	1,000	-	6,200	IU
Low	=	350	-	1,000	IU
Very Low	=	0	-	350	IU

VITAMIN C

Of all the volumes written on the physiological properties of vitamin C, its two most important virtues are its ability to speed wound healing and as an antioxidant.

Supplementation of the diet with vitamin C can make a greater impact between minimum and optimum health than perhaps any other single nutrient.

The RDA of 60 mg is sufficient to prevent scurvy, but to maintain the body pool of 4,000 - 5,000 mg, additional supplementation is essential since cooking and processing of food and inefficiencies in absorption by the gut can, with time, lead to a net loss of vitamin C reserves.

Perhaps more important than its effect on general health, vitamin C supplementation can serve to moderate the severity of the common cold and reduce the intraoccular pressure in glaucoma, the inflammation of periodontal disease and intolerance to heat. Vitamin C supplements can help to concentrate vasodilating prostaglandins to help relieve chest tightness in asthmatics.

Scurvy, a vitamin C deficiency disease, is characterized by severe tension among other things. With sufficient vitamin C, tension is relieved by building vitamin C reserves in the brain, the second largest vitamin C concentration in the body.

The adrenal glands concentrate the most vitamin C in the body where it is used as an ingredient of adrenaline which is essential in the body's reaction to stress.

Serum cholesterol and triglyceride levels, risk factors in heart disease and atherosclerosis, can be reduced significantly by vitamin C supplementation. These reductions occur because vitamin C helps in the transformation of cholesterol to bile acids which can then be more easily excreted by the body.

Vitamin C is also essential for the metabolism of folic acid and certain amino acids like tyrosine. The absorption of iron is increased when chelated to vitamin C.

In wound healing, vitamin C is essential to replace and strengthen the connective tissues of the body. Body stores of vitamin C drop rapidly after surgery and trauma which can lead to weakening and slow healing of collagenous structures like cartilage, bone and blood capillaries.

Vitamin C is an antioxidant which means it will react with a number of substances easily, especially free radicals like nitrosamines. As such, it can reduce the effects of pollution, taking antibiotics, steroids, oral contraceptives and smoking cigarettes.

Vitamin C is a water-soluble antioxidant, unlike the fat soluble antioxidants like vitamin A, B-carotene and vitamin E which work outside of the cell where it is better able to protect DNA and other structures scavenging free radicals. This property makes it unique among the nutrients. The best sources of vitamin C are raw fruits and vegetables since cooking can leach vitamin C.

The Best Herbal Sources of Ascorbic Acid
calculated on a zero moisture
basis per 100 gm

Acerola fruit	14,800	mg
Broccoli herb	1,040	mg
Horseradish root	1,000	mg
Cauliflower herb	867	mg
Rosehips	740	mg
Aloe Vera juice	626	mg
Lemon fruit	557	mg
Senna leaf	557	mg
Papaya fruit	474	mg
Cabbage herb	451	mg
Oranges fruit	406	mg
Yellow Dock root	405	mg
Asparagus herb	398	mg
Red Raspberry leaf	267	mg
Barley Grass	330	mg
Red Clover tops	297	mg
Onion bulb	270	mg
Lobelia leaf	225	mg
Hops flower	178	mg
Pumpkin seed	173	mg

Ranges for Ascorbic Acid:

Very High	= 450	-	14,800	mg
High	= 65	-	450	mg
Average	= 20	-	65	mg
Low	= 5	-	20	mg
Very Low	= 0	-	5	mg

ZINC

Metallic zinc is commonly known for its electro-chemical properties (anti-rusting agent) on galvanized nails. Nutritionally, it is important for healthy skin and nails, proper wound healing, successful pregnancies, male virility and our sense of taste.

The RDA is 15 mg daily, although the average intake is only half this amount. Zinc deficiency in pregnant women can impair the development of the newborn's immune system.

Topical application of zinc on throat infections reduces the length of colds from 10 days to 3 days.

Zinc is most famous nutritionally as the restorer of sexual potency, especially in men. Oysters, also famous for this property, are particulary rich in zinc.

Perhaps most importantly, the onset of certain cancers are being linked to zinc deficiency. This finding makes zinc popular in cancer prevention formulas.

The Best Herbal Sources of Zinc
calculated on a zero moisture
basis per 100 gm

Bilberry	0.87	mg
Mistletoe herb	0.86	mg
Scullcap herb	0.86	mg
Buchu leaf	0.84	mg
Pumpkin seed	0.83	mg
Capsicum fruit	0.77	mg
Lady Slipper herb	0.67	mg
Sage leaf	0.59	mg
Pennyroyal herb	0.56	mg
Wild Yam root	0.56	mg
Spirulina algae	0.53	mg
Chickweed herb	0.52	mg
Echinacea root	0.51	mg
Astragalus root	0.50	mg
Nettle leaf	0.47	mg
Irish moss herb	0.44	mg
Siberian Ginseng root	0.42	mg
Dulse herb	0.39	mg
Elecampane herb	0.39	mg
Parthenium root	0.37	mg

Ranges for Zinc:

Very High	=	0.35	-	0.86	mg
High	=	0.15	-	0.35	mg
Average	=	0.05	-	0.15	mg
Low	=	0.02	-	0.05	mg
Very Low	=	0	-	0.02	mg

Chapter 4
The Single Herbs

INTRODUCTION

The following monographs are the basis for the classification systems presented in chapter two. The chart of each monograph describes the nutritional profile of the herb as completely as possible from the data available. The nutrients in each herb are rated as very high, high, average, low or very low, based on statistical data compiled on 93 herbs. Ranges for the values of each nutrient are provided in Chapter 3. Section two of each entry is the summation of a literature search describing the folk history and use of each herb.

Section three provides a botanical and pharmacological description based on the clinical, nutritional and folk-use profiles of the plant. This description also provides useful information on dosage, method of administration and traditional herbal formulas using the herb. Clinically proven physiological claims from an herb are listed under Definite Actions. While untested, plausible claims are listed as Probable Actions, and uncorrelated or untested folk properties are listed as Possible Actions. Historical uses which are unconfirmed are noted with a (?) after the Action.

NOTE: THE NUTRITIONAL VALUES LISTED IN THIS BOOK ARE BASED ON 100 GRAMS OF HERB FROM WHICH THE MOISTURE HAS BEEN REMOVED. THIS AMOUNT IS APPROXIMATELY EQUIVALENT TO 200 NUMBER "0" GELATIN CAPSULES.

Alfalfa herb

Medicago sativa (Papilionaceae)

Properties: bitter, stomachic, general tonic, antipyretic, alterative, diuretic

Systems Affected: digestive, circulatory, structural

Common Names: lucern, buffalo herb

Folk History and Use

Alfalfa is commonly used throughout the world as an animal feed. In fact, the origin of the term alfalfa has been traced to the Iranian word "aspasti" meaning horsefodder. Currently, over 80 million acres of land worldwide are used to grow alfalfa of which 27 million acres are being cultivated in the United States alone. This "King of Herbs" has been cultivated by man for thousands of years, probably beginning in ancient Armenia about 2,000 B.C. It was introduced to Greece about 490 B.C. Soon afterwards, it spread into the rest of Europe and into northern Africa. Spanish explorers brought it to the New World and gold prospectors carried it from South America into California. It was also introduced to the Eastern shores and central regions of the United States directly from Europe.

Alfalfa is highly esteemed in folk medicine as a cure for all **inflammations** including **arthritis** and **rheumatism**. It is also thought to be **hypocholesterolemic** and **hypoglycemic**. It is most popular as a **blood purifier** and **bitter tonic**.

Alfalfa also makes a popular addition to herb teas. The combination of alfalfa and mint tea has historically been regarded as a soothing beverage to aid the process of **digestion**. This is probably due to the fact that alfalfa contains the digestive enzyme betaine.

Alfalfa contains natural chlorophyllins (the green coloring matter in plants) which degrade rapidly when the plant is cut. For example, compare the green color of uncut alfalfa to the brown color of baled alfalfa hay. This color change is due to oxidation of the chlorophyllins.

Modern technology has developed a way to extract and preserve chlorophyll before it degrades so that we may

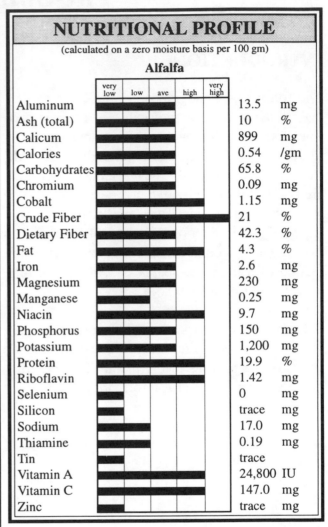

NUTRITIONAL PROFILE
(calculated on a zero moisture basis per 100 gm)

Alfalfa

	very low	low	ave	high	very high		
Aluminum						13.5	mg
Ash (total)						10	%
Calicum						899	mg
Calories						0.54	/gm
Carbohydrates						65.8	%
Chromium						0.09	mg
Cobalt						1.15	mg
Crude Fiber						21	%
Dietary Fiber						42.3	%
Fat						4.3	%
Iron						2.6	mg
Magnesium						230	mg
Manganese						0.25	mg
Niacin						9.7	mg
Phosphorus						150	mg
Potassium						1,200	mg
Protein						19.9	%
Riboflavin						1.42	mg
Selenium						0	mg
Silicon						trace	mg
Sodium						17.0	mg
Thiamine						0.19	mg
Tin						trace	
Vitamin A						24,800	IU
Vitamin C						147.0	mg
Zinc						trace	mg

have its many benefits. The most common starting material is freshly cut alfalfa. The chlorophyllins are extracted before they oxidize and are preserved by removing the fat-soluble phytic acid from the chlorophyll ring. The magnesium atom at the center of the chlorophyll ring is usually replaced by copper and sodium because these minerals make a deeper green color and also render the chlorophyll molecule water soluble and stable. It should be noted that sodium copper chlorophyllin contains nearly 10% copper by weight. This means that 30 mg provide 100% of the U.S.D.A. for copper. One can see from this example why alfalfa is such a rich reservoir of nutrients.

One of the unique characteristics of alfalfa is that it has a deep tap root. It grows in rich soils and sends roots deep into the ground. Ask any farmer who has tried to rotate alfalfa to another crop, and he will tell you about its deep root system.

Cattle ranchers long ago made the observation that cattle were unable to ingest sufficient sodium with a diet of grass-type plants. This is the reason that salt licks are commonly found on grazing land. Our analysis of the sodium content of alfalfa merely confirms what human experience has known for centuries.

Medicinal Properties

Definite action
    Diuretic (flavonoids)
Probable action
    Antithrombotic (coumarin derivatives)
    Antispasmodic to smooth muscles
        (flavonoids)
    Hypocholesterolemic (octacosanol)
    Regulates colonic flora (saponins)
    Hypoglycemic (alkaloids)

The high beta-carotene content of alfalfa acts to strengthen the epithelial cells of the mucous membranes of the stomach and could be responsible for its reported effects on **ulcers**. Its **blood-purifying** properties have been attributed to the chlorophyll content, but is probably due to other factors.

The most popular use of alfalfa in herbology is in arthritis formulas.

How does it work? Primarily as a **detoxifier** of the blood. The high molecular weight alcohols (octacosanol) help to **reduce cholesterol** and serum lipids while the coumarin derivatives provide an antothrombotic effect. The flavonoids relax the smooth muscles and the alkaloids **reduce blood sugar levels**. These systemic effects are accompanied by the regulating effects the saponins have on colonic flora.

Typical Daily Usage

1. Fresh herb: 1/4-1/2 cup
2. Dried herb: 6-12 gm
3. Extract: 9 gm dried herb, 45 ml alcohol, 45
    ml water

Traditional Formulas

Alfalfa and Dandelion combination
Alfalfa and Yucca combination
Marshmallow and Plantain combination

Chemical Constituents

Aromatic compounds
    Volatile oils
        Hexanal and Hexanal (odor principle)
    Fixed oils and resins (0.5-0.8%)
        octacosanol
        triacontanol (hypolipidemic)
    Waxes and fatty acids
        palmitic
        lauric
        myristic
Bitter compounds
    Flavonoids
        tricin
        genistein
        daidzein
        biochanin A
        formononetin (smooth muscle relaxant)
    Coumarin derivatives
        coumestrol
        medicagol
        sativol
        trifoliol
        lucernol
        daphnoretin
Saponins (2-3%)
        soyasapogenols A,B,C,D,E, hederagenin
        medicagenic acid
        beta-sitosterol
        alpha-spinasterol
        stigmasterol
        cycloartenol
        campestrol
Alkaloids
        trigonelline
        stachydrine
        homostachydrine

Nutrients of Note

Water when fresh: 81.2%
Water when air dried: 8.7%
Sugars: 9% (glucose, fructose, arabinose)
Starch: 6%
Vitamins
    biotin
    folic acid
    pantothenic acid
    Vit. B-6
    Vit. E
    Vit. K
Chlorophyllins: 0.21%

Aloe leaf

Aloe spp. (Liliaceae)

Properties: mucilaginous, bitter, vulnerary, laxative, demulcent, emollient, emmenagogue, astringent

Systems Affected: structural, digestive

Common Names: Bombay aloe, Turkey aloe, moka, aloe, Zanzibar aloe

Folk History and Use:

The word aloe is derived from the Arabic "alloeh" meaning bitter and shiny substance. Various species of this member of the lily family have been used for millenia in medical and cosmetic applications. References to aloe are found in Egyptian, Roman, Chinese, Greek, Italian, Algerian, Moroccan, Arabian, Indian and Christian history.

Cleopatra reputedly attributed her irresistible charm to the use of aloe. The New Testament refers (John 19:39) to an embalming mixture of myrrh and aloe. Dioscorides and Columbus both wrote of its healing virtues. Ironically, Aristotle persuaded Alexander the Great to war against the Island of Socotra (East Africa) to obtain aloe and its healing virtues for his soldiers' wounds. Marco Polo found that the Chinese used aloe for stomach ailments and skin disorders. Mixed with rum and sugar, aloe is a cold remedy in Cuba.

Columbians use aloe as an insect repellant. The Spanish conquistadors found Central American Indians using aloe for **burns**, **skin** and **stomach ulcers, dysentery, intestinal disorders, longevity, kidney disorders, prostatitis** and **sexual prowess**.

In Java, aloe juice is massaged into hair and scalp to improve its condition and stimulate growth..

Documented cases of radiation burn victims from the atomic bombs used in Japan show more rapid healing using aloe than any other method of burn treatment.

Today, virtually all societies have access to aloe, as it grows well in the home. Fresh juice is readily obtained from the plant by breaking off a leaf and squeezing the juice out. Prepared juice is also sold at a wide variety of locations. Recently, the market for aloe products has been highly publicized as fortune 500 companies have discovered it and are extolling its virtues in the major advertising media.

Today's consumer should be warned of such marketing fluff since fresh, whole aloe plants are so common and work so simply. Many marketers insist that a product is better because of some extraction, distillation, concentration or flavoring process performed on their aloe product. However, aloe is one medicinal plant where natural is truly best.

Aloe works most effectively when the mucilage is taken from the growing plant as it is sterile and will not contaminate a burn or wound with bacteria. The juice must be refrigerated or treated with a preservative system. However, one good use of processed aloe is freeze-dried aloe capsules that are handy to have in any first aid kit. These capsules can be rehydrated in a glass of water and applied to a sunburn or other wound.

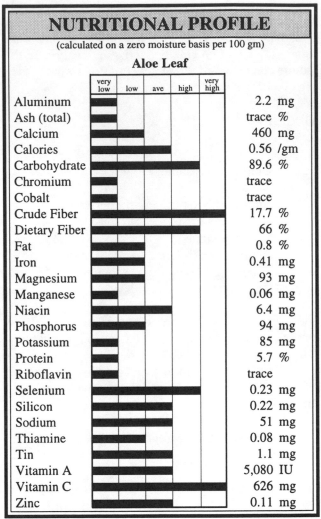

NUTRITIONAL PROFILE
(calculated on a zero moisture basis per 100 gm)

Aloe Leaf

Nutrient	very low	low	ave	high	very high	Value
Aluminum	■					2.2 mg
Ash (total)	■					trace %
Calcium		■				460 mg
Calories			■			0.56 /gm
Carbohydrate				■		89.6 %
Chromium	■					trace
Cobalt	■					trace
Crude Fiber					■	17.7 %
Dietary Fiber				■		66 %
Fat		■				0.8 %
Iron		■				0.41 mg
Magnesium		■				93 mg
Manganese	■					0.06 mg
Niacin			■			6.4 mg
Phosphorus		■				94 mg
Potassium		■				85 mg
Protein		■				5.7 %
Riboflavin	■					trace
Selenium				■		0.23 mg
Silicon				■		0.22 mg
Sodium			■			51 mg
Thiamine		■				0.08 mg
Tin			■			1.1 mg
Vitamin A				■		5,080 IU
Vitamin C					■	626 mg
Zinc		■				0.11 mg

Unrealistic claims are made by aloe marketers such as one company who claims their aloe product is tasteless, odorless and 100 percent aloe. Product literature even describes the distillation process they used to make it odorless and tasteless. This is a clever way of selling purified water since mucilage does not form azeotropes with water.

The quality of aloe juice is easily determined with a simple test to find the concentration of mucilage in the aloe solution. Add a urine sugar test tablet, developed to test for diabetes (manufactured by Ames Co. "Clinitest"), to 1/2 teaspoon of aloe juice. A color is produced that, when matched to a color strip provided in the kit, will give an indication of the mucilage content of the aloe. This color can be compared to the color of fresh aloe juice.

A comparison color can be obtained from fresh leaves by the following procedure: wash the leaves, cut off the ends, remove green rind and take the gel filet out. Grind it in a blender to break up gel structure. Filter to remove the pulp. The juice serves as a standard for comparison. The test indicates the amount of reducing sugars (mucopolysaccharides) present in the sample. Fresh aloe usually contains 0.25 - 0.5 percent mucilage.

Aloe's major properties are as a **cell proliferant**, **healer**, **demulcent** and **allergy reducer**. Therefore, 90% of the treatments using aloe use it alone. For topical application to **skin ulcers**, **burns**, **irritations** and **bites**, no combination of herbs works better than aloe used alone.

However, effective poultices are made using aloe juice mixed with comfrey powder and adding a little golden seal root as an **infection fighter for cuts and scratches**.

Medicinal Properties

    Definite Action
        Cathartic (anthraquinones)
        The benefits of viscous fiber
            Lowers bowel transit time
            Absorbs toxins in the bowel
            Demulcent to digestive tract
        Cell proliferant (mucopolysaccharides)
    Probable Action
        Antibiotic (mucopolysaccharides)

Aloe juice is not complex chemically as many herbs are. The juice itself consists of 99.5% water. The remaining 0.5% of the juice consists of the following:

1. A complex mixture of mucopolysaccharides. This is the mucilage of aloe. Interestingly, the polysaccharides in aloe show action similar to hyaluronic acid.
2. Varying amounts of anthraquinone glucosides consisting mainly of aloin and aloe emodin. These are the bitter gripping cathartic principles. They are easily identified by their yellow-orange color and their presence should be minimized in juice used internally on inflammations.

Typical Daily Usage

External
    Generously cover affected area up to hourly
        with comfrey leaf as a poultice
Internal
    Fresh leaf: 1 tablespoon

Traditional formulas

Comfrey combination

Chemical Constituents

Bitter compounds
    Anthraglycosides (cathartic)
        barbaloin (c-glucoside of aloe emodin)
        aloesin (c-glucoside of aloesone)
    Anthraquinones
        aloe emodin
    Saponins
        Not characterized
Mucilaginous compounds
    Polysaccharides (0.5-1.0%)

Nutrients of note
Water when fresh: 99.5%
Water when air dried: 8.9%
Sugars: 4% (xylose, arabinose, galactose)

Althea root
Althea officinalis (Malvaceae)

Properties: mucilaginous, demulcent, vulnerary, emollient, general, tonic, alterative, diuretic, lithotriptic

Systems Affected: digestive, urinary, respiratory

Common Names: marshmallow

Folk History and Use

Marshmallow root is a member of the mallow family (Malvaceae), a group of a thousand odd species with two common characteristics. They are edible and contain an abundance of mucilage. In fact, mucilage is so common in these plants that the roots of other mallow such as hollyhocks and hibiscus can be readily substituted for marshmallow as they possess similar qualities.

It is hard to pinpoint the earliest use of marshmallow since its first mention in written history refers to its already widespread use as a food. The Old Testament book of Job mentions it being eaten in times of famine. A dish of mallow was considered a delicacy by the ancient Romans and the Chinese also used a species of mallow for food.

The mallow of common use to the European continent and in western herbal medicine is Althea officinalis. The European taxonomists knew of its virtues as a demulcent since its family name, Malvaceae, is derived from the Greek "malake" or soft referring to the soft mucilaginous nature of the herb. The generic name althea is derived from the Greek "althos" meaning to cure.

Althea officinalis grows throughout Europe, where it is native and has been cultivated and now grows wild in America and other temperate climates of the world. It is cultivated as a medicinal plant in Belgium, France and Germany, but is no longer used as a food staple.

Althea inhabits salt marshes, river banks and other moist places. Its habitat and mucilage content accounts in part, for its above average content of sodium (See nutritional profile), since sodium salts of polysaccharides (mucilage) are soluble and are freely transported within the plant. Recently it has been shown that the

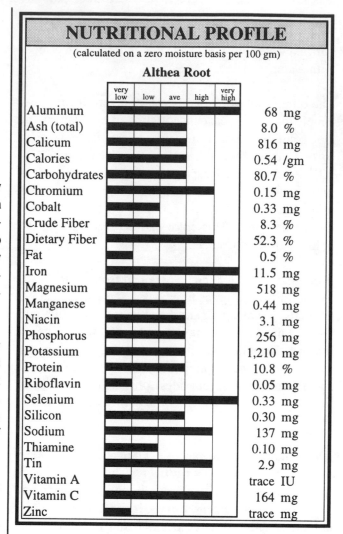

NUTRITIONAL PROFILE
(calculated on a zero moisture basis per 100 gm)

Althea Root

	very low	low	ave	high	very high		
Aluminum						68	mg
Ash (total)						8.0	%
Calcium						816	mg
Calories						0.54	/gm
Carbohydrates						80.7	%
Chromium						0.15	mg
Cobalt						0.33	mg
Crude Fiber						8.3	%
Dietary Fiber						52.3	%
Fat						0.5	%
Iron						11.5	mg
Magnesium						518	mg
Manganese						0.44	mg
Niacin						3.1	mg
Phosphorus						256	mg
Potassium						1,210	mg
Protein						10.8	%
Riboflavin						0.05	mg
Selenium						0.33	mg
Silicon						0.30	mg
Sodium						137	mg
Thiamine						0.10	mg
Tin						2.9	mg
Vitamin A						trace	IU
Vitamin C						164	mg
Zinc						trace	mg

mucilage content varies seasonally and is highest in fall and winter. Marshmallow also has substantial quantities of calcium and magnesium. These metals precipitate (harden) polysaccharides and further study would probably show an abundance of these minerals concentrated in the older structural cells of the root.

Marshmallow's ability to **bind** and **eliminate toxins** allows the body to cleanse itself. For this reason, it is added to **arthritis, laxative, infection, female tonic, vermifuge** and other **cleansing formulas**. It is also a major constituent of poultices. Marshmallow is well known for treating **kidney** and **bladder infections**.

In diuretic formulas, marshmallow is traditionally thought to **soothe the urinary tract**. However, the polysaccharides are not absorbed from the digestive tract. The active principles for diuretic action are volatile acids, oils and tannins which irritate the urinary tract and stimulate the production of urine and mucous.

Marshmallow is also popular as an **expectorant** for the respiratory system. It must be used topically as a decoction to **soothe the throat** since the mucilage is not absorbed by the digestive tract.

Medicinal Properties

Definite Action
    The benefits of viscous fiber
        Lowers bowel transit time
        Absorbs toxins form the bowel
        Regulates intestinal flora
        Acts as a demulcent to mucous membranes of the bowel
Probable Action
    Diuretic (volatile oil)
Possible Action
    Expectorant (?)

The plant contains 25-30% polysaccharides (mucilage) and 25-30% starch, which accounts for its demulcent effects on the digestive tract.

The non-absorbable polysaccharides coat the mucous membranes of the digestive tract and absorb toxins from the digestive tract. They can have no demulcent effect on the urinary or respiratory tract since they are not absorbed.

Tannins and volatile oils in the fresh root are responsible for the **diuretic effects** of marshmallow. Their presence irritates the mucous membranes of the urinary tract sufficiently that mucous is secreted to sequester the toxins. This results in other toxins being sequestered and subsequently purged from the urinary tract.

Typical Daily Usage

Fresh root: 1/8 to 1/3 cup
Dried root: 2-5 gm
Extract: 3.5 gm dried root, 17.5 ml alcohol, 17.5 ml water

Traditional Formulas

Gymnema combination
Pumpkin and Cascara combination
Plantain combination
Slippery Elm combination
Black Cohosh and Golden Seal combination
Raspberry and Dong Quai combination
Ginger and Dong Quai combination
Golden Seal and Juniper combination
Golden Seal and Bugleweed combination
Chamomile and Passionflower combination
Marshmallow and Fenugreek combination
Ephedra and Passionflower combination
Marshmallow and Plantain combination
Ginseng and Parsley combination

Chemical Constituents

Aromatic compounds
    Volatile oils (0.05 - 0.2%)
        not characterized
    Fixed oils and Resins
    Astringent compounds
Tannins
Bitter compounds
    Saponins
        Sterols
Mucilaginous compounds
    Polysaccharides: 25-35%
        Pectin: 11%

Nutrients of note

Water when fresh: 89.2%
Water when air dried: 10.3%
Starch: 37%
Sugars: 11% (rhamnose, galactose)

Asparagus root
Asparagus officinale (Liliaceae)

Properties: bitter, diuretic, laxative, blood purifier, antirheumatic

Systems affected: urinary, digestive, structural

Folk History and Use

Asparagus is a well-known culinary herb. It is a dioecious perennial plant with feathery, scale-like leaves and an erect stem that has many branches. The stem is cut when it is a four to six inch spear and used as a vegetable. The bitter root is used medicinally.

Asparagus is a **blood purifier** that has a **diuretic** and **laxative** effect. It is noted for the pungent odor it imparts to urine after one consumes it. It has been used to treat **rheumatism, neuritis, dysuria, parasites** and rarely in folk remedies fori.

Medicinal Properties

Probable action
Diuretic (?)
Laxative (?)
Antirheumatic (?)

Asparagus contains a variety of bitter principles. Flavonoids include rutin, quercetin, kaempferol and others. Saponins and their glycosides include a group of 18 known asparagosides. Two bitter compounds called officinalisins have also been identified in the root. The root is rich in acidic compounds as well but no tannins have been identified. These include asparagusic acid and other sulfer containing acids. These compounds likely contribute to the odor imparted to urine. No mechanisms have been proven to explain the medicinal properties of asparagus. Flavonoids are common in bitter herbs and often produce blood purifying effects. The other bitter compounds may contribute to these actions.

Typical Daily Usage

Fresh root: 1 tablespoon
Dried root: 1.5 gm
Extract: 1.5 gm dried root, 7 gm alcohol, 8 gm
water

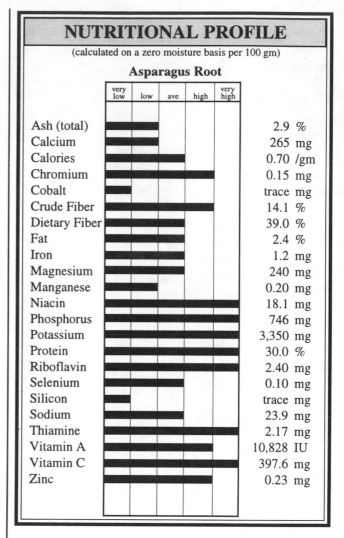

NUTRITIONAL PROFILE
(calculated on a zero moisture basis per 100 gm)

Asparagus Root

	very low	low	ave	high	very high	value
Ash (total)						2.9 %
Calcium						265 mg
Calories						0.70 /gm
Chromium						0.15 mg
Cobalt						trace mg
Crude Fiber						14.1 %
Dietary Fiber						39.0 %
Fat						2.4 %
Iron						1.2 mg
Magnesium						240 mg
Manganese						0.20 mg
Niacin						18.1 mg
Phosphorus						746 mg
Potassium						3,350 mg
Protein						30.0 %
Riboflavin						2.40 mg
Selenium						0.10 mg
Silicon						trace mg
Sodium						23.9 mg
Thiamine						2.17 mg
Vitamin A						10,828 IU
Vitamin C						397.6 mg
Zinc						0.23 mg

Traditional Formulas
Yellow Dock and Pau D'Arco combination

Chemical Constituents

Astringent compounds
Acidic compounds
Asparagusic acid and others
Bitter compounds
Saponins
Asparagosides A to I
Sitosterol, sarsapogenin and others
Flavonoids
Rutin, quercetin, kaempferol
Others

Officinalisins 1 and 2
Mucilaginous compounds
Polysaccharides
Gum: 11%

Nutrients of Note
Water when fresh: 90%
Water when air dried: 7.2%

Astragalus root
Astragalus membranaceus (Leguminosae)

Properties: bitter, immune stimulant, antiseptic,
diuretic, antispasmodic, carminative

Systems affected: immune, urinary, repiratory

Folk History and Use

Astragalus is the root of the membranous milk vetch, a perrenial lugume native to Northern China and Mongolia. It has fern-like fronds of leaves that grow about six inches long and a branched tap root about eight inches long. It bears one inch seed pods that resemble miniature soybeans.

Astragalus is important to Chinese folk medicine. It enhances the metal element of Chinese philosophy which has to do with the body's defenses. It has been used to treat **infections** of the mucous membranes of the body especially the urinary and respiratory tracts. It is commonly combined with ginseng as a prophylactic against **winter colds** and **viruses**. Some say it is used to **prevent cancers**. It is also said to **reguvenate the digestive organs** and **regulate blood sugar**.

It is especially famous in cases of **diabetes** for reducing the complications of poor circulation such as high blood pressure and failure to heal wounds.

Astragalus has been used to treat **infections, diabetes, edema, nephritis, ulcers,** and **prolapse of digestive organs**.

Medicinal Properties

Definite action
    Immune stimulant (bitter principles)
    Diuretic (bitter principles)
    Antiseptic (bitter principles)
    Antispasmodic (bitter principles)
    Carminitive (bitter principles)
Probable action
    Antitumor (?)
    Diaphoretic (?)

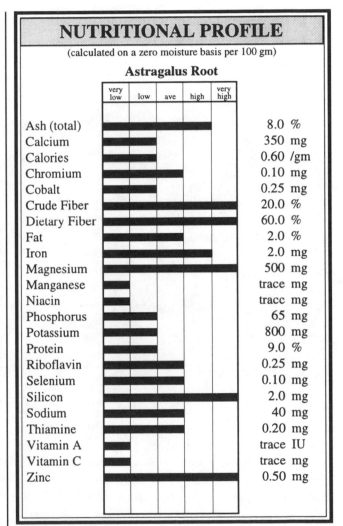

NUTRITIONAL PROFILE
(calculated on a zero moisture basis per 100 gm)

Astragalus Root

	very low	low	ave	high	very high		
Ash (total)						8.0	%
Calcium						350	mg
Calories						0.60	/gm
Chromium						0.10	mg
Cobalt						0.25	mg
Crude Fiber						20.0	%
Dietary Fiber						60.0	%
Fat						2.0	%
Iron						2.0	mg
Magnesium						500	mg
Manganese						trace	mg
Niacin						trace	mg
Phosphorus						65	mg
Potassium						800	mg
Protein						9.0	%
Riboflavin						0.25	mg
Selenium						0.10	mg
Silicon						2.0	mg
Sodium						40	mg
Thiamine						0.20	mg
Vitamin A						trace	IU
Vitamin C						trace	mg
Zinc						0.50	mg

Astragalus contains bitter principles that are thought to be responsible for its folk medical claims. These compounds have not been characterized, but crude extracts of the root have shown a variety of important properties.

The bitter extracts of astragalus are **diuretic, antiseptic** and **antispasmodic**. One study shows that these extracts stimulate the activity of white blood cells, an important component of the immune system.

Typical Daily Usage

Fresh root: 2-4 tablespoon
Dried root: 3-6 gm
Extract: 4.5 gm dried root, 22 ml alcohol, 23 ml water

Traditional Formulas

Biota and Zizyphus combination
Ginseng and Licorice combination
Dong Quai and Peony coimbination
Astragalus and Ganoderma combination
Ginseng and Phaffia combination
Anemarrhena and Astragalus combination
Eucommia and Achyranthes combination
Alisma and Hoelen combination

Chemical Constituents

Aromatic compounds
 Essential oil
 Bitter compounds
Saponins
 (not characterized)
 Flavonoids
 Rutin, Quercetin and others
Mucilaginous compounds
 Polysaccharides
  Gum: 10%

Nutrients of note
Water when fresh: 84%
Water when air dried: 6.7%

Barberry bark
Berberis vulgaris (Berberidaceae)

Properties: bitter, antidiarrheal, antipyretic, astringent, bitter tonic, antihemorrhagic, antifungal, antibiotic

Systems affected: digestive, circulatory

Common Names: pipperidge bush, berry

Folk History and Use

Barberry is a deciduous spiny bush that grows to be 10 to 15 feet tall. It is native to Europe and has been naturalized in the Eastern half of the United States. It has spiny, holly shaped leaves, yellow flowers and dark red to black berries. The bark of the trunk and root is bitter tasting and astringent. It contains alkaloids that provide a number of well established effects particularly in the digestive system. It contains the same type of alkaloids as goldenseal root and oregon grape root. Barberry is much less expensive than these other two plants and bark is much more renewable environmentally than are roots.

Barberry is noted in folk medicine as a cure for nearly every **gastrointestinal ailment, lymphatics, urinary tract** and **respiratory infection**. It has been used as a bitter tonic and **antypyretic**. Berberine, the primary

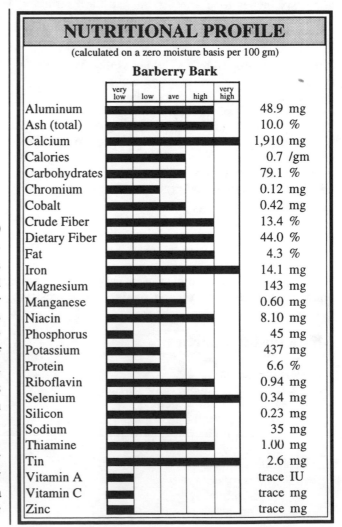

NUTRITIONAL PROFILE

(calculated on a zero moisture basis per 100 gm)

Barberry Bark

	very low	low	ave	high	very high	value
Aluminum						48.9 mg
Ash (total)						10.0 %
Calcium						1,910 mg
Calories						0.7 /gm
Carbohydrates						79.1 %
Chromium						0.12 mg
Cobalt						0.42 mg
Crude Fiber						13.4 %
Dietary Fiber						44.0 %
Fat						4.3 %
Iron						14.1 mg
Magnesium						143 mg
Manganese						0.60 mg
Niacin						8.10 mg
Phosphorus						45 mg
Potassium						437 mg
Protein						6.6 %
Riboflavin						0.94 mg
Selenium						0.34 mg
Silicon						0.23 mg
Sodium						35 mg
Thiamine						1.00 mg
Tin						2.6 mg
Vitamin A						trace IU
Vitamin C						trace mg
Zinc						trace mg

alkaloid, is a potent **antibiotic, astringent** and **antifungal**. When taken for infections, it controls the overgrowth of candida albacans as well as functioning as a bactericide. This is a real advantage over conventional antibiotics. Berberine is also used in eye washes both for its astringency to get the red out and to eliminate infection. It also controls infectious diarrhea and increases the production of digestive enzymes.

Barberry has traditionally been used to **treat infectious diarrhea, respiratory infections, poor appetite, fever, candidiasis** and **hemorrhages**.

Medicinal Properties

    Definite action
        Antibiotic (alkaloids)
        Antipyretic (alkaloids)
        Antihemorrhagic (alkaloids)
        Antifungal (alkaloids)
        Antidiarrheal (alkaloids)
        Bitter tonic (alkaloids)
    Probable action
        Sedative (alkaloids)
        Antispasmodic (alkaloids)

Barberry contains bitter alkaloids that are responsible for its action. Berberine and related akaloids impart a yellow color to the bark and root. These alkaloids have been shown to have bactericidal activity for which they are most noted. In addition, the alkaloids **reduce fever, calm the nerves, constrict capillary blood flow, reduce muscle spasms** and **lower blood pressure**.

The antimicrobial activity of barberry is most pronounced in the colon since its alkaloids are 2-4 times as bactericidal in alkaline pH as in neutral environments.

Berberine is more potent as a fever reducer than is aspirin. It also mobilizes the white blood cells of the immune system.

In summary, barberry can be used with success in treating most infectious conditions of the digestive, urinary and respiratory systems.

Typical Daily Usage

    Fresh bark: 1-2 tablespoon
    Dried bark: 1.5-3 gm
    Extract: 2 gm dried root, 10 ml alcohol, 10 ml water

Traditional Formulas
    Cascara combination
    Cascara and Dong Quai combination
    Gentain and Cascara combination
    Ginger and Barberry combination
    Dandelion and Barberry combination

Chemical Constituents

    Astringent compounds
        Tannin
    Bitter compounds
        Alkaloids: 3%
            Berberine and others

Nutrients of Note
    Water when fresh: %
    Water when air dried: %
    Starch: 9%

Bayberry bark
Myrica cerifera (Myricaceae)

Properties: astringent, stimulant

Systems Affected: digestive, circulatory, structural

Common Names: American bayberries, candle berry, wax berry, wax myrtle, tallow shrub, American vegetable wax

Folk History and Use

Bayberry is perhaps the most popular astringent herb because of its combination of stimulant effects and astringency. The most renowned use of bayberry bark is as a prime ingredient in Samuel Thompson's Composition tea, which combines stimulant herbs like capsicum, with bayberry to cleanse the body of toxins. There are several variations of composition tea, but they all combine astringents with stimulant herbs to produce **diaphoretic, diuretic** and **laxative effects that eliminate toxins**.

Bayberry is native to the evergreen forests of the Eastern United States and has been naturalized in all of Europe. It prefers coastal low lands and open fields near streams and pine barrens.

The bayberry bush is covered by a bluish wax that is boiled off the leaves and berries and used in candle making and medicated soaps. It contains aromatic, antibacterial agents. Burning a bayberry wax candle on Christmas day until it burns itself out is a Christian tradition that is supposed to bring good luck.

The generic name for bayberry, myrica, is derived from the Greek "tamarisk" and cerifera comes from the Latin "cera" meaning wax and "fero" meaning to bear.

The astringent properties of bayberry are readily apparent in its traditional uses. The Swedish and Welsh used bayberry bark to tan calfskin and made a strong extract that was spread on baseboards each spring to kill insects and vermin.

Early American settlers used the powdered bark in place of toothpaste as an abrasive and to cure gingivitis. A tea was also gargled to treat throat inflammations.

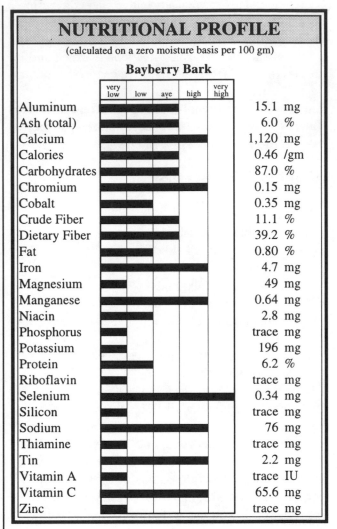

NUTRITIONAL PROFILE
(calculated on a zero moisture basis per 100 gm)

Bayberry Bark

	very low	low	ave	high	very high	
Aluminum						15.1 mg
Ash (total)						6.0 %
Calcium						1,120 mg
Calories						0.46 /gm
Carbohydrates						87.0 %
Chromium						0.15 mg
Cobalt						0.35 mg
Crude Fiber						11.1 %
Dietary Fiber						39.2 %
Fat						0.80 %
Iron						4.7 mg
Magnesium						49 mg
Manganese						0.64 mg
Niacin						2.8 mg
Phosphorus						trace mg
Potassium						196 mg
Protein						6.2 %
Riboflavin						trace mg
Selenium						0.34 mg
Silicon						trace mg
Sodium						76 mg
Thiamine						trace mg
Tin						2.2 mg
Vitamin A						trace IU
Vitamin C						65.6 mg
Zinc						trace mg

In India, a variation of composition tea using ginger and bayberry was used to produce diaphoretic effects to combat cholera. In large doses, this formula is used as an emetic.

The native Americans used bayberry to combat **dysentery, diarrhea, fevers** and **uterine hemorrhaging**.

Modern herbalists use bayberry to treat **polyps**.

In an early Journal of Materia Medica, Dr. Charles A. Lee summed up the use of bayberry bark as follows:

> Bayberry bark possesses tonico-astringent properties which entitle it to a very respectable rank among our indigenous astringents. Reduced to a powder, it is acrid and styptic to

the taste, and in doses of one drachm causes a sensation of heat in the stomach, followed by vomiting and purging, and sometimes diuresis. A decoction has been long used in diarrhoea, dysentery, uterine hemorrhage, dropsies succeeding fevers, and as a gargle in affections of the throat.

When chewed, it acts as a sialagogue, useful in toothache and to stimulate tender, spongy or bleeding gums. Bayberry bark is also used as a poultice and for jaundice, especially the form termed black jaundice. In the early 1800's, bayberry bark and lobelia constituted almost a complete materia medica for herbalists such as Thompson.

Medicinal Properties

Definite Actions
    Astringent
        Internally to digestive tract
        Externally to skin
    Antibacterial (flavonoids and tannins)
Probable Actions
    Increases circulation (?)

The actions of bayberry are due to two major groups of phenolic compounds, the tannins and flavonoids.

The tannins are responsible for the astringent or tissue tightening properties of the herb and make it useful in **scrofulous skin conditions** and **inflamed areas of the mouth and digestive tract**.

The flavonoids impart an antibacterial property to the plant that make it useful for treating various **infections** internally and externally.

The triterpene sapogenins of bayberry may impart a purge stimulus to the digestive tract and provide the stimulant properties assigned to it by folk remedies.

Typical Daily Usage

Fresh bark: 1-3 tablespoon
Dried bark: 1.5-3 gm
Extract: 2 gm dried bark, 10 ml alcohol, 10 ml
    water

Traditional Formulas

Ginseng combination
Eyebright combination
Bayberry and Ginger combination

Chemical Constituents

Aromatic compounds
    Volatile Oils: 0.2-0.4%
    Fixed Oils and Resins
        Resin - acrid, astringent
        Saturated Fatty acids
            palmitic
            stearic
            myristic
            lauric
Astringent compounds
    Tannins
        tannic acid
        gallic acid
    Flavonoids
        myricitrin and others
Bitter compounds
    Saponins
        Triterpene sapogenins
            myricadiol
            taraxerol
            taraxerone
            urocadiol

Nutrients of Note

Water when fresh: 78.2%
Water when air dried: 13.8%
Starch: 6%
Sugars: 9% (glucose)

Bilberry fruit

Vaccinium myrtillus (Ericaceae)

Properties: bitter, anti-inflammatory, antithrombotic, antispasmodic, decreases capillary permeability

Systems affected: structural, circulatory

Common Names: huckleberry, whortleberry, hurtleberry

Folk History and Use

Bilberry is a shrubby perennial plant that grows in most temperate climates of the world. It is one of a group of 200 berry producing plants that produce edible fruits. Most of the Ericaceae family is native to the forests of Europe but most grow well and have been naturalized in the United States. Most of the family including blueberries, grapes and black currents contain the purple colored flavonoids called anthocyanidins. These bitter compounds are responsible for the medicinal properties of the fruits. Much discussion continues about which species and varieties are the most effective. Indeed, the country and even locale where a particular plant is grown is considered important in determining the effectivness of the fruit.

The anthocyanidins of bilberry have considerable pharmacologic activity. They are especially used as anti-aging substances. These bitter compounds inhibit collagen destruction, scavenger free radicals, reduce capillary permeability, increase blood circulation to peripheral blood vessels and the brain, reduce inflammation and pain and relieve muscle spasms. It is one of the most popular over-the-counter drugs in Europe.

It is so effective that a single dose is said to improve one's night vision within hours.

It has traditionally been used to treat **poor night vision, bruising, capillary fragility, varicose veins, poor circulation, raynaud's disease, circulation complications due to diabetes, rheumatoid arthritis, gout** and **peridontal disease**.

Medicinal Properties

Definite action
  Prevents collagen destruction (flavonoids)
  Antioxidant (flavonoids)
  Anti-inflammatory (flavonoids)
  Decrease capillary permeability (flavonoids)
  Antithrombotic (flavonoids)
  Antispasmodic (flavonoids)
Possible action
  Urinary antiseptic (?)
  Inhibits stone formation (?)

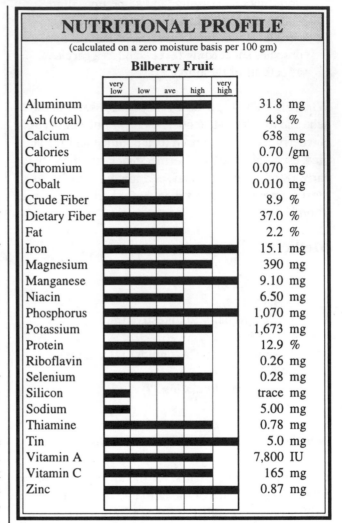

NUTRITIONAL PROFILE
(calculated on a zero moisture basis per 100 gm)

Bilberry Fruit

	very low	low	ave	high	very high		
Aluminum						31.8	mg
Ash (total)						4.8	%
Calcium						638	mg
Calories						0.70	/gm
Chromium						0.070	mg
Cobalt						0.010	mg
Crude Fiber						8.9	%
Dietary Fiber						37.0	%
Fat						2.2	%
Iron						15.1	mg
Magnesium						390	mg
Manganese						9.10	mg
Niacin						6.50	mg
Phosphorus						1,070	mg
Potassium						1,673	mg
Protein						12.9	%
Riboflavin						0.26	mg
Selenium						0.28	mg
Silicon						trace	mg
Sodium						5.00	mg
Thiamine						0.78	mg
Tin						5.0	mg
Vitamin A						7,800	IU
Vitamin C						165	mg
Zinc						0.87	mg

This herb is becoming more important to the aging populations of the world. This fruit and its extracts have marvelous anti-aging properties. Bilberry was first studied for its effects on poor night vision. Indeed, regular use of the fruit results in quicker adjustment to darkness and glare and improved visual acuity both at night and in bright light during the day. Bilberry may be useful in the prevention and treatment of **glaucoma** since it strengthens connective tissue and prevents free radical damage.

In the control of diabetes short term, one's blood sugar is lowered and long term, one's circulatory system is preserved. Connective tissue is not destroyed and capillaries function more normally.

In other chronic degenerative diseases, like rheumatoid arthritis, the inflammation and pain are reduced while damage to connective tissue is kept to a minimum.

This is an important fruit to add to one's daily diet. Blueberries and black currant fruit may also be as useful as bilberry but not yet as popular for their medicinal properties.

Typical Daily Usage

Fresh fruit: 1/2-1 cup
Dried fruit: 12-24 gm
Standardized extract: 1/2 gm (25% anthocyanidin)

Traditional Formulas

Eyebright combination

Chemical Constituents

Aromatic compounds
  Essential oil
  Resin
Astringent compounds
  Tannin
Bitter compounds
  Flavonoids
    Anthocyanidins
Mucilaginous compounds
  Polysaccharides
    Pectin: 5%

Nutrients of Note

Water when fresh: 92%
Water when air dried: 8%
Sugars: 15% (glucose, fructose, galactose, arabinose)

Black Cohosh Root
Cimifuga racemosa (Ranunculaceae)

Properties: bitter, astringent, antispasmodic, alterative, emmenagogue, diuretic estrogenic

Systems Affected: reproductive, nervous, respiratory, circulatory

Common Names: bugbane, rattleroot, squawroot, snakeroot, black snakeroot

Folk History and Use

Black cohosh is a tall, stately plant having perennial roots that is native to the eastern forests of the United States and Canada. Early American settlers found that black cohosh was widely used by American Indian tribes. They made a poultice of the bruised root and applied it to poisonous snake bites. The Winnebagos, Penobscots and Dakotas, in particular, used it internally as well as externally for snake bites. They also used a decoction of the root to treat **coughs, chest difficulties, diarrhea** and **irregular menstruation**.

The botanical name of black cohosh is derived from the Latin "cimex" meaning bedbug and "fugere" meaning to drive or fly away, in reference to its repellant action on bedbugs. The species name is from the Latin "racemosus" meaning full of flowers.

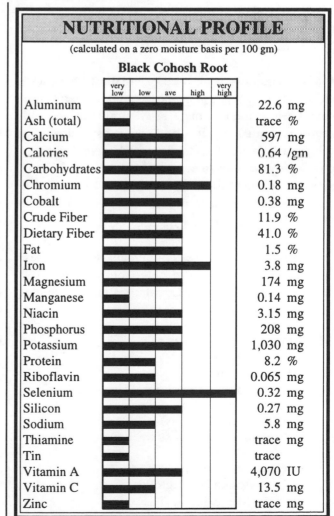

NUTRITIONAL PROFILE
(calculated on a zero moisture basis per 100 gm)

Black Cohosh Root

	very low	low	ave	high	very high		
Aluminum						22.6	mg
Ash (total)						trace	%
Calcium						597	mg
Calories						0.64	/gm
Carbohydrates						81.3	%
Chromium						0.18	mg
Cobalt						0.38	mg
Crude Fiber						11.9	%
Dietary Fiber						41.0	%
Fat						1.5	%
Iron						3.8	mg
Magnesium						174	mg
Manganese						0.14	mg
Niacin						3.15	mg
Phosphorus						208	mg
Potassium						1,030	mg
Protein						8.2	%
Riboflavin						0.065	mg
Selenium						0.32	mg
Silicon						0.27	mg
Sodium						5.8	mg
Thiamine						trace	mg
Tin						trace	
Vitamin A						4,070	IU
Vitamin C						13.5	mg
Zinc						trace	mg

Among the common names for this plant are black snakeroot, in reference to its use to treat snake bites, and black cohosh, cohosh being of unknown origin, but probably a Native American name.

Although reports vary, the use of black cohosh by American settlers dates back to between 1696 and 1850. During the 19th century, it was used in New York hospitals in the treatment of rheumatism, although the medical establishment later eliminated this practice. Its use in the treatment of rheumatism has been widespread and still continues in some areas. For example, in Georgia it is mixed with other herbs in whiskey. Historically, other uses have included treatment for **scarlet fever, measles, smallpox, asthma, scrofula, St. Vitus' dance, bronchitis, intercostal myalgia, sciatica, whooping cough, tinnitus, pericarditis, angina pectoris, gonorrhea in men, spermatorrhea, seminal emission, sexual weakness, dyspepsia, hysteria, menopause** and **general difficulties involving the female reproductive system**.

The herb is taken in small doses as it contains salicylic acid, a gastric irritant. Overdoses are easily identified by nausea and headache.

Black cohosh has been used externally to heal sores and puncture wounds. The most common internal uses have been in the treatment of **rheumatism** and **pulmonary conditions**. It is best known as a remedy for various ailments of the female reproductive system, including **dysmenorrhea, amenorrhea** and **difficult pregnancy** and **childbirth**. It was listed as official in the U.S. Pharmacopia from 1820 to 1936 and was listed in the National Formulary from 1935 to 1950.

Parallel to its use by Western herbalists, the Chinese have independently used species of cimicifuga, native to China, like C. foetida, C. dahurica and C. simplex for very similar purposes.

Medicinal Properties

> Definite Action
> > Binds to estrogen receptor sites (saponins)
> > Diuretic (tannins)
> > Diaphoretic (tannins)
> > Stimulates uterine contractions in childbirth
> Possible Action
> > Cardiostimulant
> > Increases gastric secretions

The actions of this herb have not been fully investigated. However, a significant pattern develops when one compares the known constituents with the traditional uses. First, black cohosh has been shown to have compounds which bind to estrogen receptors in the body. Second, the tannins, phenols and phenolic glycosides in black cohosh are all astringent and irritating to various systems of the body.

Such constituents as tannins, gallic acid and pseudotannins, including isoferulic acid and the salicylates, are irritants to the skin, lungs and kidneys, which result respectively in diaphoretic, expectorant and diuretic action. Salicylic acid is so irritating it is used to remove warts. The stimulation by irritation mechanism can be readily applied to the action of black cohosh as an emmenagogue, since irritation of the uterus would result in menstrual flow and uterine contractions. Increased gastric secretions can also be explained by this mechanism.

The drastic action of the irritant principles in black cohosh are not lethal, but overdoses are characterized by nausea and headache. Care, however, should be exercised by those using black cohosh with pregnant women, since the irritating principles that cause uterine contraction could potentially cause excessive hemorrhage.

Cimicifugin, the ranunculoside in black cohosh, exhibits antispasmodic and sedative properties in the fresh root. When the root is cut or bruised, an enzyme is released which reacts with cimicifugin to produce protoanemonine, which is unstable in water but, when dried, is readily oxidized to an anemonic acid which has no physiological activity. The process is much akin to the enzymatic action that takes place in garlic, the difference is that the active principle is destroyed in black cohosh and created in garlic when the herb is bruised.

This property of black cohosh was known as early as 1870, as the U.S. Dispensatory states:

> No doubt it [black cohosh] also contains when fresh, a volatile principle, with which its virtues may be in some degree associated; as we are confident that it is more efficacious in the recent state than when long kept.

The traditional virtues of this herb are best extracted by using hot water and preferably alcohol on the fresh root. Early settlers extracted whole roots with whiskey and drank it as a rheumatism cure.

The antispasmodic and sedative properties of black cohosh are only present in the whole, fresh root. The dried, powdered black cohosh in common use today contains only the irritating principles described above.

Much work remains to determine the complete action of black cohosh. It contains a saponin alkaloid and triterpene glycoside, which are not characterized and may or may not have physiological action.

Typical Daily Usage

Fresh root: 1-3 tablespoon
Dried root: 1.5-3 gm
Extract: 2 gm dried root, 10 ml alcohol, 10 ml water

Traditional Formulas

Black Cohosh combination
Black Cohosh and Blessed Thistle combination
Black Cohosh and Golden Seal combination
Black Cohosh and Raspberry combination
Alfalfa and Yucca combination
Dandelion and Parsley combination
Valerian and Black Cohosh combination
White Willow and Valerian combination

Chemical Constituents

Aromatic compounds
Volatile oils: 0.1-0.4%
Fixed oils and resins: 3-5%
  Cimicifugin
  Saturated fatty acid
    palmitic
  Unsaturated fatty acid
    oleic
Astringent compounds
Tannins - astringent principles
    Isoferulic acid - pseudotannin, astringent,
      possibly diuretic
  Salicylic acid - irritant, analgesic
  Gallic acid - astringent
Bitter compounds
Saponins - detected but not characterized
  Triterpene glycosides
    actein
    cimigoside
Mucilaginous compound
  Mucilaginous gum

Nutrients of note

Water when fresh: 79%
Water when air dried: 6.7%
Sugars: 10% (glucose, sucrose)
Starch: 8%

Black Walnut fruit rind

Juglans nigra (Juglanaceae)

Properties: astringent, vermifuge, iodine source

Systems affected: digestive, glandular

Folk History and Use

Black walnut is the name of a large deciduous tree that is native to Europe and has been naturalized into most temperate climates of the world for use as an ornamental or shade tree. It produces greenish-yellow fruits a little larger than a golf ball. The seed is edible but herbalists are more interested in the fruit rind than the seed. As the fruit of the black walnut tree ripens, the rind loosens and the seed is easily separated. The yellow rind has a black pulp that stains everything it touches. Its medicinal properties also come from these black colored tannins.

Its fruit rinds have been used to tan animal skins and to assist in wound healing. Black walnut tones and helps heal inflamed and damaged tissues. It is also said to be effective in enhancing the elimination of various microbes from the bowel. Herbalists also recognize it as a thyroid stimulant since it is relatively rich in the trace mineral iodine.

Black walnut has traditionally been used to treat **hemorrhoids, intestinal worms, wounds** and **bruises**.

Medicinal Properties

Definite action
  Astringent (tannin)
  Iodine supplement
Probable action
  Vermifuge (tannin)

Black walnut is typical of astringent plants. Its action is based on its tannin content. Tannins work topically to tone the body tissues they come in contact with. They function by precipitating free proteins which are generally present only in damaged and inflamed tissues. The term tannin comes from its use in tanning animal skins. This makes black walnut useful in treating inflammatory conditions of the bowel with special usefulness in treating hemorrhoids.

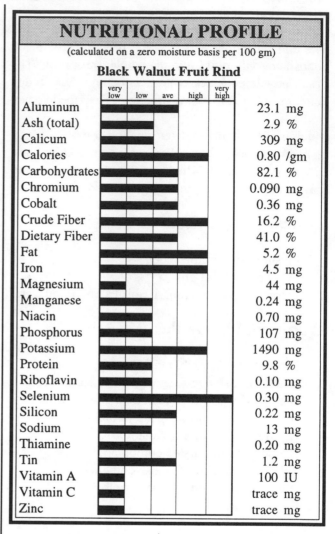

NUTRITIONAL PROFILE
(calculated on a zero moisture basis per 100 gm)

Black Walnut Fruit Rind

	very low	low	ave	high	very high		
Aluminum						23.1	mg
Ash (total)						2.9	%
Calicum						309	mg
Calories						0.80	/gm
Carbohydrates						82.1	%
Chromium						0.090	mg
Cobalt						0.36	mg
Crude Fiber						16.2	%
Dietary Fiber						41.0	%
Fat						5.2	%
Iron						4.5	mg
Magnesium						44	mg
Manganese						0.24	mg
Niacin						0.70	mg
Phosphorus						107	mg
Potassium						1490	mg
Protein						9.8	%
Riboflavin						0.10	mg
Selenium						0.30	mg
Silicon						0.22	mg
Sodium						13	mg
Thiamine						0.20	mg
Tin						1.2	mg
Vitamin A						100	IU
Vitamin C						trace	mg
Zinc						trace	mg

The tannins in black walnut are also thought to encourage the elimination of unwanted microbes in the colon. Herbalists believe that the acidic nature of tannins make life uncomfortable for the alkaline loving yeasts and microbes that can infect the bowel. Acid producing flora like lactobacillus acidophilous seem unaffected by the presence of tannins.

The content of iodine in black walnut is greater than most herbs. I have not been able to find any printed history of its use as an iodine supplement. Many herbalists report great success using black walnut to treat **thyroid deficiency conditions**.

Typical Daily Usage

Fresh fruit rind: 2-3 teaspoon

Dried fruit rind: 1-1.5 gm
Extract: 1 gm dried fruit rind, 5 ml alcohol, 5 ml water

Traditional Formulas

Chickweed and Cascara combination
Gentain and Cascara combination
Ginseng combination
Irish Moss and Kelp combination
Goldenseal and Bugleweed combination

Chemical Constituents

Aromatic compounds
   Resin

Astringent compounds
   Tannin: 28%
Bitter compounds
   Flavonoids
      Quercetin
Mucilaginous compounds
   Polysaccharides
      Gum: 8%

Nutrients of note
Water when fresh: 88%
Water when air dried: 6%
Sugars: 5% (fructose, glucose)
Iodine: 15 ppm

Blessed Thistle herb
Cnicus benedictus (Compositae)

Properties: bitter, galactagogue, emmenagogue, stimulant, diaphoretic, emetic

Systems affected: digestive, glandular, circulatory, urinary

Folk History and Use

Blessed thistle is native to Asia and the Mediterranean region. It has been cultivated in Europe and the United States as a medicinal herb.

Any farmer knows thistles for their ability to quickly inhabit cultivated ground. Summer hikers know them for their sting on bare legs, but when the spines are ground with the rest of the plant, the sting disappears and the plant becomes quite useful as a medicinal herb.

The term "blessed" was applied centuries ago to this plant from its reputation as a cure all, a remedy even for the Black Plague of the Middle Ages.

Its generic name "cnicus" is derived from the Greek "knekos" of safflower, a name that was formerly attached to thistles. It is also termed "carduus" by some taxonomists from the Latin word meaning spiny.

Benedictus is from the Latin meaning blessed, which was derived from the plant's curative properties, considered a gift from God.

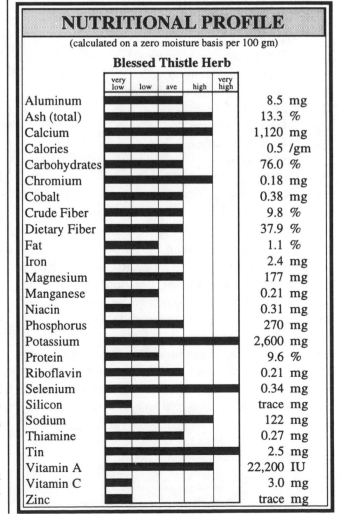

NUTRITIONAL PROFILE
(calculated on a zero moisture basis per 100 gm)
Blessed Thistle Herb

	very low	low	ave	high	very high		
Aluminum						8.5	mg
Ash (total)						13.3	%
Calcium						1,120	mg
Calories						0.5	/gm
Carbohydrates						76.0	%
Chromium						0.18	mg
Cobalt						0.38	mg
Crude Fiber						9.8	%
Dietary Fiber						37.9	%
Fat						1.1	%
Iron						2.4	mg
Magnesium						177	mg
Manganese						0.21	mg
Niacin						0.31	mg
Phosphorus						270	mg
Potassium						2,600	mg
Protein						9.6	%
Riboflavin						0.21	mg
Selenium						0.34	mg
Silicon						trace	mg
Sodium						122	mg
Thiamine						0.27	mg
Tin						2.5	mg
Vitamin A						22,200	IU
Vitamin C						3.0	mg
Zinc						trace	mg

The herb has a feeble, disagreeable odor and an intensely bitter taste. Extracts of the plant are nauseating and until recently herbalists had replaced blessed thistle with more pleasant tasting herbs like chamomile. Since the introduction of hard shell gelatin capsules, the popularity of this herb is on the rise.

Herbalists use it as a female tonic to **increase mothers' milk** and treat **painful menstruation**.

Large doses produce an **emetic** and **expectorant** effect. Its bitter glycosides are said to **stimulate appetite** and act as a **tonic to the digestive tract**. Large doses are also said to produce a **diaphoretic** and **general stimulant** action.

In the last century, blessed thistle has received a reputation for its action on the internal organs such as the liver and kidneys. Homeopaths have touted it most highly in this regard and use a tincture to treat jaundice, hepatitis and arthritis.

Medicinal Properties

Definite Actions
    Emetic (bitter glycosides)
    Astringent (tannins)
    Antibacterial(bitter glycosides)
Probable Actions
    Gastric aperitive (?)
    Diuretic(tannins)
Possible Actions
    Galactogogue (?)
    Emmenagogue (?)
    Liver purifier (?)

Chemically, little is known about the physiological actions of this herb. Cnicin, a bitter glycoside, has been identified only as the stinging principle present in the spines. It is, however, thought to be the emetic and gastric stimulant principle in blessed thistle.

Early man believed that ingesting bitter herbs gave strength that could be used to combat illness. Physiologically, bitter herbs stimulate various organs of the body into a reflex action that triggers the glands into action, producing various effects. In blessed thistle, the organs effected are thought to be the liver and female reproductive organs.

Typical Daily Usage

Fresh herb: 2-4 tablespoon
Dried herb: 3-6 gm
Extract: 4.5 gm dried herb, 22 ml alcohol, 23 ml water

Traditional Formulas

Black Cohosh and Blessed Thistle combination
Black Cohosh and Golden Seal combination
False Unicorn and Golden Seal combination
Raspberry and Dong Quai combination
Dandelion and Parsley combination
Yerba Santa combination

Chemical Constituents

Aromatic compounds
    Volatile Oils
    Fixed Oils and Resins
Astringent compounds
Sequiterpene lactone glycoside
    Cnicin
    Tannin
Mucilaginous compound
    Mucilage: 12-20%

Nutrients of note

Water when fresh: 86.7%
Water when air dried: 9.4%
Sugars: 12% (glucose, sucrose)
Starch: 8%

Blue Cohosh root
Caulophyllum thalictroides (Berberidaceae)

Properties: bitter, antispasmodic, anti-inflammatory, antifungal, antiseptic, estrogenic, laxative, vermifuge

Systems affected: glandular, digestive

Common Names: pappoose root, squawroot, blue ginseng, yellow ginseng

Folk History and Use

Blue cohosh is a perennial herb that grows in the deciduous forests of the eastern United States and Canada. Its name blue cohosh comes from its dark blue seeds. The demand for the plant is not great enough to warrant cultivation and the roots of blue cohosh look similar to others. It is differentiated by its characteristic irritation of the tongue when chewed.

Blue cohosh has been compared to goldenseal in its effects. Indeed, some have used it as an effective control for chronic yeast infections. Today its use is mostly limited to **regulating the menstual cycles of women** and **combatting painful menstruation**.

Most of its folk history comes from its use by Native Americans. It developed quite a reputation for reducing the pain and spasms of menstruation and to stimulate menstrual flow. Most importantly, it was used to **induce labor**. Indeed pregnant women should avoid the use of blue cohosh.

The bitter principles in blue cohosh constrict peripheral blood vessels in a manner similar to nicotine. They also cause uterine contractions and are antifungal.

Blue cohosh has traditionally been used to treat **spasmodic dysmenorrhea, amenorrhea, premenstrual syndrome, candidiasis, vaginitis, fiberous cystic disease, constipation** and as a **vermifuge**.

Medicinal Properties

Definite action
Increases blood pressure (alkaloids)
Peripheral vasoconstrictor (alkaloids)
Uterine stimulant (saponins)
Laxative (bitter principles)
Antifungal (bitter principles)
Antimicrobial (bitter principles)

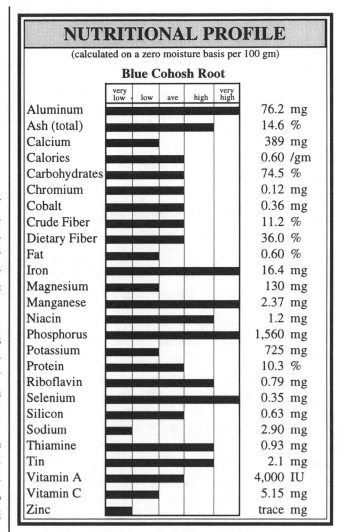

NUTRITIONAL PROFILE
(calculated on a zero moisture basis per 100 gm)

Blue Cohosh Root

	very low	low	ave	high	very high	
Aluminum						76.2 mg
Ash (total)						14.6 %
Calcium						389 mg
Calories						0.60 /gm
Carbohydrates						74.5 %
Chromium						0.12 mg
Cobalt						0.36 mg
Crude Fiber						11.2 %
Dietary Fiber						36.0 %
Fat						0.60 %
Iron						16.4 mg
Magnesium						130 mg
Manganese						2.37 mg
Niacin						1.2 mg
Phosphorus						1,560 mg
Potassium						725 mg
Protein						10.3 %
Riboflavin						0.79 mg
Selenium						0.35 mg
Silicon						0.63 mg
Sodium						2.90 mg
Thiamine						0.93 mg
Tin						2.1 mg
Vitamin A						4,000 IU
Vitamin C						5.15 mg
Zinc						trace mg

Blue cohosh contains bitter principles that are responsible for its action. The root is irritating and harsh. It raises one's blood pressure and constricts blood flow to the peripheral blood vessels and the heart. It can also relieve the pain and cramps associated with menstruation and induce labor.

Blue cohosh is a relatively complicated herb to use. It appears that the dose required for balancing the menstrual cycle changes throughout the cycle. If too much is taken intestinal cramping and headaches often occur. This probably explains why its use is now restricted nearly completely to **inducing labor during childbirth**.

If one could overcome the plant's harsh irritating side-effects it would be a good candidate in treating many infections and inflammatory conditions.

A final note of caution, blue cohosh causes uterine stimulation and should not be taken by pregnant women.

Typical Daily Usage

Fresh root: 1/2-1 teaspoon
Dried root: 0.25-0.5 gm
Extract: 0.5 gm dried root, 3 gm alcohol, 2 gm water

Traditional Formulas

False Unicorn and Goldenseal combination

Chemical Constituents

Bitter compounds
  Saponins
    Caulosaponin and others
  Alkaloids
    Caulophylline, baptifoline and others
  Flavonoids
    Leontin, hederagenin and others
Mucilaginous compounds
  Polysaccharides
    Gum: 16%

Nutrients of note

Water when fresh: 89%
Water when air dried: 7%
Starch: 14%

Boneset herb
Eupatorium perfolium (Compositae)

Properties: bitter, diaphoretic, antipyretic, laxative, stimulant, expectorant

Systems Affected: circulatory, structural, respiratory, urinary

Folk History and Use

Boneset is a common plant in the marshes of the eastern half of the United States and Canada. The plant grows to about three feet high and has a distinctive double leaf from which it derives its scientific name. Its double leaf looks like a single line that has been speared in the middle by the stem. Its species name "perfolia" means through the leaves.

Boneset is most famous for its use in reducing fevers. Native Americans also used it to treat aches and pains of the structural system and to assist in the **healing of broken bones**. Many of the early uses of boneset were topical plasters and poultices being its most common use. Infusions of the plant did not become popular until the snake oils of the mid 1900's.

Its common name, boneset, was derived from its ability to break fevers associated with influenza. The fevers in these cases were described as going to the bone or bone-fever.

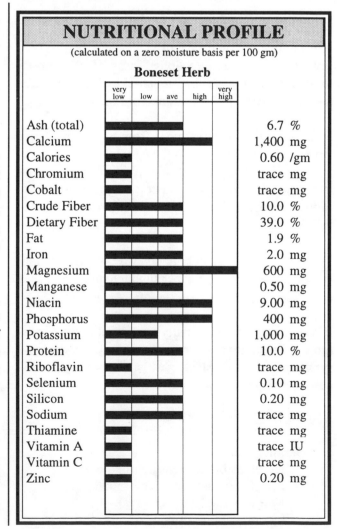

NUTRITIONAL PROFILE
(calculated on a zero moisture basis per 100 gm)

Boneset Herb

	very low	low	ave	high	very high		
Ash (total)						6.7	%
Calcium						1,400	mg
Calories						0.60	/gm
Chromium						trace	mg
Cobalt						trace	mg
Crude Fiber						10.0	%
Dietary Fiber						39.0	%
Fat						1.9	%
Iron						2.0	mg
Magnesium						600	mg
Manganese						0.50	mg
Niacin						9.00	mg
Phosphorus						400	mg
Potassium						1,000	mg
Protein						10.0	%
Riboflavin						trace	mg
Selenium						0.10	mg
Silicon						0.20	mg
Sodium						trace	mg
Thiamine						trace	mg
Vitamin A						trace	IU
Vitamin C						trace	mg
Zinc						0.20	mg

It has traditionally been used to treat **fever, influenza, respiratory allergies, chills, rheumatism, bruises, broken bones, urinary tract infection** and **jaundice**.

Medicinal Properties

Definite action
 Diaphoretic (flavonoids, essential oil)
 Laxative (flavonoids)
 Antipyretic (flavonoids)
Probable action
 Expectorant (essential oil)
 Circulatory stimulant (essential oil)

Boneset has been studied quite extensively. Reducing fevers and inducing sweating is quite a competitive market already filled with inexpensive drugs like aspirin, so conventional medicine has largely left this herb to traditional practitioners. Boneset contains one of the broadest array of chemicals in the herbalists' apothecary. All four of the major chemical types are present.

No one chemical is responsible for its action. The flavonoids and the sesquiterpene lactones in the essential oil appear to work together in an as yet undetermined fashion to produce the **antipyretic** and **diaphoretic** effect. The essential oil also irritates mucous membranes resulting in its **expectorant** effect. The irritation may also **stimulate peristalsis**.

Besides the bitter and aromatic components of the herb, it contains the mucilaginous polysaccharride inulin which could mitigate the harshness of the herb. Tannins are also present which tone inflamed tissue. One study also mentions the presence of pyrrolizidine alkaloids. These are apparently of the same chemical class as the hepatoxic alkaloids found in comfrey. As with comfrey, the early use of boneset was topically to **reduce fevers** and **reduce the swelling due to bruises** and **broken bones**. This may be the safest and best use of this herb.

I have found this herb to be one of the most versatile of medicinal plants. It may be employed nearly anywhere there is **inflammation, pain** or **infection**. Its flavonoids have even shown some **antitumor** properties.

Typical Daily Usage

Fresh herb: 2-4 teaspoon
Dried herb: 1-2 gm
Extract: 1.5 gm dried herb, 7 ml alcohol, 8 ml
 water

Traditional Formulas

Fenugreek combination

Chemical Constituents

Aromatic compounds
 Essential oil
  Terpenoids
   Sesquiterpene lactones
    Eupafolin and others
   Diterpenes
    Dendroidinic acid and others
   Triterpenes
    Alpha-amyrin and others
   Sesquiterpenes
    Chromenes
 Resin
Astringent compounds
 Tannin
Bitter compounds
 Saponins
  Sitosterol and others
 Alkaloids
 Flavonoids
  Eupatorin, quercetin, kaempferol,
   astragalin and others
Mucilaginous compounds
 Polysaccharides
  Inulin: 15%

Nutrients of note
Water when fresh: 91%
Water when air dried: 7%

Bupleurum root
Bupleurum chinense (Umbelliferae)

Properties: bitter, antipyretic, diaphoretic, sedative, anti-inflammatory, antidepressant

Systems affected: nervous, digestive, circulatory

Common names: hare's ear

Folk History and Use

Bupleurum is a perennial herb that is native to the northern provinces of China. It now grows wild in Northern Europe. Its common name is hare's ear which describes the shape of its leaves. The plant has a brown, carrot-like root and yellow flowers. The Doctrine of Signatures requires that this herb be useful in treating liver and gallbladder ailments because of the yellow color of its flowers.

Bupluerum has been an important herb in Chinese folk medicine for over 2000 years. It was first used to treat fevers including malaria and blackwater fever. In today's folk medicine it is used to treat stress conditions. These conditions are known in Chinese philosophy as excessive wood disorders. They often involve an overtaxed liver and gall bladder. They are often associated with lifestyle. These disorders include **premenstrual syndrome, spasmodic dysmenorrhea, fevers, depression, inflammatory skin conditions** and **tumors**.

Medicinal Properties

    Definite action
        CNS depressant (saponins)
        Anti-inflammatory (saponins)
        Diaphoretic (saponins)
        Antipyretic (saponins)
    Probable action
        Antidepressant (saponins)
        Analgesic (saponins)
        Antiseptic (saponins)

Bupleurum contains bitter saponins that show anti-inflammatory and CNS suppressing activity. Bupleurum was a relatively minor herb in Chinese folk medicine but modern society and its stresses have elevated it to prominence. The need to enhance liver function to combat the toxins of our time and the need to calm the nerves has become very important today. Bepleurum is said to relieve the side effects of steroid use. These effects include insomnia, high blood pressure, irritability and inflammatory skin conditions. These conditions could apply to nearly every teenager in industrialized society.

Typical Daily Usage

Fresh root: 1-2 teaspoon
Dried root: 0.5-1 gm
Extract: 1 gm dried root, 5 ml alcohol, 5 ml water

Traditional Formulas

Dong Quai and Peony combination
Bupleurum and Peony combination

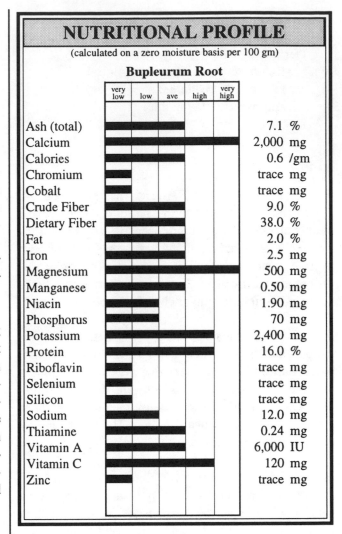

NUTRITIONAL PROFILE
(calculated on a zero moisture basis per 100 gm)

Bupleurum Root

	very low	low	ave	high	very high		
Ash (total)			■			7.1	%
Calcium					■	2,000	mg
Calories		■				0.6	/gm
Chromium	■					trace	mg
Cobalt	■					trace	mg
Crude Fiber			■			9.0	%
Dietary Fiber				■		38.0	%
Fat		■				2.0	%
Iron				■		2.5	mg
Magnesium					■	500	mg
Manganese			■			0.50	mg
Niacin		■				1.90	mg
Phosphorus	■					70	mg
Potassium				■		2,400	mg
Protein				■		16.0	%
Riboflavin		■				trace	mg
Selenium		■				trace	mg
Silicon		■				trace	mg
Sodium		■				12.0	mg
Thiamine			■			0.24	mg
Vitamin A		■				6,000	IU
Vitamin C		■				120	mg
Zinc	■					trace	mg

Dandelion and Purslane combination
Bupleurum and Cyperus combination
Pinellia and Citrus combination
Anemarrhena and Astragalus combination
Forsythia and Schizonepeta combination

Chemical Constituents

Aromatic compounds
   Resin
Bitter compounds
   Saponins

Saikogenin and others
Flavonoids
   Quercetin and others
Mucilaginous compounds
   Polysaccharides
     Gum: 12%

Nutrients of note

Water when fresh: 89%
Water when air dried: 6.9%
Sugars: 6% (glucose, fructose)

Burdock root
Arctium Lappa (Compositae)

Properties: mucilaginous, alterative, diuretic, diaphoretic (fresh), urinary tonic, demulcent

Systems affected: circulatory, urinary, digestive

Common Names: lappa, lappa minor, thorny burr, beggar's buttons, clothburr

Folk History and Use

Burdock is a common weed which grows in almost any uncultivated space. As its name suggests, it is a dock which bears seeds in big round bristly cones that stick to clothing and animal fur.

The plant is native to Europe and Asia, but has been introduced and naturalized in all temperate parts of the world. The hooked burrs of this large, handsome plant have been the play things of children for a very long time. The worldwide spread of the species must, in part, be attributed to childhood pranks. In "As You Like It" Shakespeare makes this observation:

ROSALIND: How full of briers is this working-day world!
CELIA: They are but burs, cousin, thrown upon thee in holiday foolery. If we walk not in the trodden paths, our very petticoats will catch them.

The Greek words "arktos" meaning bear and "lappa" meaning to seize are used as the scientific names of this plant and also describe its fruits. The English "bur" came from the French word for woolly "bourre." The word dock is from Old English referring to large leaves.

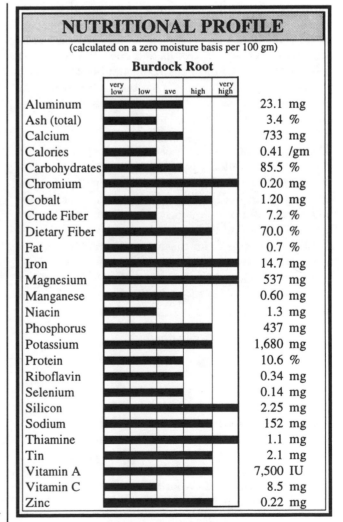

NUTRITIONAL PROFILE
(calculated on a zero moisture basis per 100 gm)
Burdock Root

	very low	low	ave	high	very high	
Aluminum						23.1 mg
Ash (total)						3.4 %
Calcium						733 mg
Calories						0.41 /gm
Carbohydrates						85.5 %
Chromium						0.20 mg
Cobalt						1.20 mg
Crude Fiber						7.2 %
Dietary Fiber						70.0 %
Fat						0.7 %
Iron						14.7 mg
Magnesium						537 mg
Manganese						0.60 mg
Niacin						1.3 mg
Phosphorus						437 mg
Potassium						1,680 mg
Protein						10.6 %
Riboflavin						0.34 mg
Selenium						0.14 mg
Silicon						2.25 mg
Sodium						152 mg
Thiamine						1.1 mg
Tin						2.1 mg
Vitamin A						7,500 IU
Vitamin C						8.5 mg
Zinc						0.22 mg

The stalks, cut before the flower is opened and stripped of their rind, form a delicate vegetable, similar in flavor to asparagus when boiled and a pleasant salad when eaten raw with vinegar.

On first examination, the root has a mild, sweet mucilaginous taste indicative of its **demulcent** properties. However, as one becomes more familiar with burdock root, he recognizes subtle astringent and bitter notes.

Though the carbohydrate content of this root predominates, it is more than a mucilaginous herb. Western herbalists have long used burdock for its **demulcent** action both externally and internally and for its **alterative effects on the blood** and **urinary system**. During the Middle Ages, remedies for kidney stones contained burdock in the belief that a stony character in a medicine would cure the stony ailment.

The Chinese, while recognizing burdock's demulcent properties, found it more valuable as a **healer of hot (yang) conditions**. Its **diaphoretic** and **diuretic** properties made it valuable for eliminating **excess nervous energy, sweating out toxins** and **cooling the heat of infections**. The Chinese also consider burdock to be a strengthening aphrodisiac. It has been cultivated in the Orient for food and is still considered a staple to the Japanese where it is known as Gobo.

The most popular western use of burdock root is as a primary herb in **blood purifier** formulas. These formulas are based on the traditional concept that diuretic and alkalizing herbs will neutralize acids and toxins and expel them more quickly. The actual mechanism is more likely due to its mucilage preventing the absorption of toxins from the digestive tract and its diuretic effect. By absorbing toxins from ingested food and those produced by intestinal flora, viscous fiber eliminates the source of many of the toxins. This allows the body to heal itself.

Medicinal Properties

    Definite Actions
        The benefits of viscous fiber
            Lowers bowel transit time
            Absorbs toxins from bowel
            Balances intestinal flora
            Demulcent action on digestive tract
        Astringent (tannin)
        Bacteriostatic (volatile oil)
        Fungistatic (volatile oil)
    Probable Actions
        Diaphoretic (volatile oil)
        Diuretic (volatile oil)

Carbohydrates predominate in burdock making up over 70% of the air-dried root. Inulin makes up 40-50% of the root with the remaining carbohydrates being mucilage, various monosaccharides and starch. The carbohydrates are responsible for the demulcent effects of burdock and add viscous fiber to the diet.

Tannins present in burdock are responsible for burdock's subtle astringent taste and contribute to the diuretic effect.

Volatile oils (many of which are acidic or phenolic in nature), especially in fresh roots, account for the diaphoretic and urinary tonic effects in burdock. Since the Japanese and Chinese use burdock as a staple food, they eat fresh roots. In the West, burdock is dried, ground and often stored before use. The volatile oils in dried burdock root are probably diminished sufficiently that no diaphoretic effect is present, but still strong enough to contribute to the diuretic effect. The difference in preparation of this herb must certainly account for the different usage patterns of this herb. Burdock also has a slight bacteriostatic effect due to a small quantity of polyolefins in the volatile oils.

The mineral profile of burdock is just the opposite of most mucilaginous herbs. However, burdock is not merely a mucilaginous herb. It is also a cleansing herb (alterative, diuretic) and it seems that nature gave burdock a strong, balanced mineral profile to replace the minerals that are inevitably purged during the cleansing processes.

Unlike potatoes which contain moderate quantities of vitamin C, our analysis of burdock showed very little. This is surprising since it is reported historically to be an antiscorbutic (meaning it was supposed to help cure scurvy, a vitamin C deficiency condition). The vitamin C value may be low only in the dried root and present in the fresh root as we only analyzed dried burdock root.

Typical Daily Usage

    Fresh root: 1/4-1/2 cup
    Dried root: 6-12 gm
    Extract: 9 gm dried root, 45 ml alcohol, 45 ml
        water

Traditional Formulas

    Alfalfa and Yucca combination
    Pau D' Arco and Yellow Dock combination
    Red Beet and Yellow Dock combination
    Ephedra and Senega combination
    Cedar Berry combination

Chemical Constituents

Aromatic compounds
    Volatile oils
        Acids
            acetic
            propionic
            butyric
            isovaleric (acrid odor)
        Polyacetylenes: 0.001-0.002% (Bacterio static)
            1,11- tridecadiene and others
            arctic acid
        Terpenes
    Fixed oils and Resins

        Saturated fatty acids
            lauric acid and others
Astringent compounds
    Tannins
    Pseudotannins
        chlorogenic acid
        caffeic acid
Mucilaginous compounds
    Mucilage: 5-12%
    Inulin: 40-50%

Nutrients of Note
Water when fresh: 76.5%
Water when air dried: 9.3%
Sugars: 15% (glucose)
Starch: 12%

Butcher's Broom root
Ruscus aculeatus (Liliaceae)

Properties: bitter, diuretic, antithrombotic, vasoconstrictor

Systems Affected: circulatory, urinary

Common Names: box holly, Jew's myrtle

Folk History and Use

Butcher's broom is a low, evergreen shrub native to the Mediterranean region, southern and western Europe and the southern United States. It belongs to the liliaceae or lily family. Common names for it are box holly and Jew's myrtle. Its name is derived from the stiff-jointed, leaf-like twigs which were formerly used by butchers to clean their cutting boards.

Its medicinal applications involve the use of the root (rhizome), which has been found by ancient peoples and modern medicine alike to be one of nature's most potent remedies for a wide spectrum of **circulatory ailments** ranging from **thrombosis** and **phlebitis** to **varicose veins** and **hemorrhoids**. The root has been used medicinally as a **diuretic,** an **anti-inflammatory, to prevent atherosclerosis** and **circulatory insufficiency**.

The ancient healers of the Mediterranean give butcher's broom a written history of more than 2000 years.

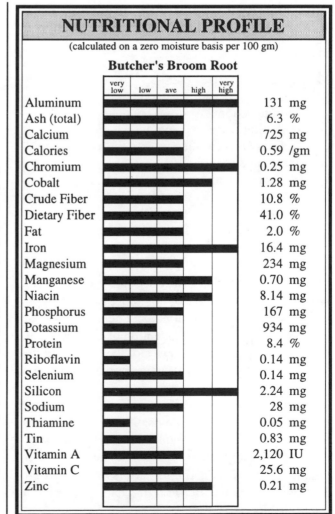

NUTRITIONAL PROFILE
(calculated on a zero moisture basis per 100 gm)

Butcher's Broom Root

	very low	low	ave	high	very high	
Aluminum						131 mg
Ash (total)						6.3 %
Calcium						725 mg
Calories						0.59 /gm
Chromium						0.25 mg
Cobalt						1.28 mg
Crude Fiber						10.8 %
Dietary Fiber						41.0 %
Fat						2.0 %
Iron						16.4 mg
Magnesium						234 mg
Manganese						0.70 mg
Niacin						8.14 mg
Phosphorus						167 mg
Potassium						934 mg
Protein						8.4 %
Riboflavin						0.14 mg
Selenium						0.14 mg
Silicon						2.24 mg
Sodium						28 mg
Thiamine						0.05 mg
Tin						0.83 mg
Vitamin A						2,120 IU
Vitamin C						25.6 mg
Zinc						0.21 mg

Theophrastus(c. 325 B.C.), the Greek naturalist and philosopher, praised the healing powers of Ruscus aculeatus. He reported seeing "lame people get up and walk" and "swelling become normal again after treatment" with what he called "the miracle herb."

Pliny (c. 60 A.D), the Roman scholar who wrote many treatises on the healing properties of herbs, described swellings (varicose veins) that "became flat again after patients took the powdered root of the whisk-broom plant."

Dioscorides recommended butcher's broom as an aperient (appetite stimulant) and diuretic.

During the Middle Ages, it was used as a food and gained a reputation for its power to relieve "a heavy feeling in the legs."

Recently, scientists and doctors have shown butcher's broom administered orally to be efficacious in treating **hemorrhoids** and **varicose veins**. It has also been shown to **prevent postoperative thrombosis** and **relieve phlebitis**. It also contains a known **diuretic** principle.

Medicinal Properties

> Definite action
>> Antithrombotic (saponins)
>> Decreases capillary permeability (flavonoids and saponins)
>> Diuretic (saponins)
> Anti-inflammatory (saponins)
> Possible actions
>> Hepatonic (?)

Butcher's broom contains steroidal saponins as the primary active principles. They act on the blood vessels by stimulating the release of norepinephrine. This produces a vasoconstricting effect and decreases the capillary permeability. The production of norepinephrine lengthens the time required to clot the blood and thus explains its use to prevent postoperative thrombosis.

The vasoconstricting effect makes it useful in reducing varicose veins and hemorrhoids. Its ability to decrease capillary permeability provides an anti-inflammatory effect. Heavy legs and swelling associated with menstruation, pregnancy and long-term standing can produce pools of lymphatic fluid that can be affected by butcher's broom.

The presence of flavonoids, like rutin, are known to generally strengthen blood vessels and reduce capillary fragility. This aids in the prevention of varicose veins.

The root also contains glycolic acid, which is a diuretic principle also found in parsley and juniper berries. Its mode of action is obscure, but probably irritates the kidney into a purge-cleanse cycle.

Many saponins are also diuretics, but the effect is not continuous and eventually stops after about a week as cholesterin in the body neutralizes the saponosides. Butcher's broom is thus not a good long-term diuretic.

The use of butcher's broom is recommended as a long-term preventative for the above mentioned circulatory conditions as the root shows little toxicity when ingested orally over long periods of time. It is not hemolytic and does not affect blood pressure.

Typical Daily Usage

1. Fresh root: 1-2 tablespoon
2. Dried root: 1.5-3 gm
3. Extract: 2 gm dried root, 10 ml alcohol, 10 ml water

Traditional Formulas

Black Cohosh combination

Chemical Constituents
> Volatile oils: 0.1-0.3%
>> glycolic acid
> Fixed oils and resins
>> euparone
>> chrysophanic acid
> Bitter compounds
>> Flavonoids
>>> Rutin: 0.03-0.04%
>> Saponins: 0.4-0.46%
>>> ruscogenin
>>> ruscin
>>> ruscoside
> Mucilaginous compounds
>> Mucilage: 10-15%

Nutrients of Note
Water when fresh: 69.8%
Water when air dried: 9.9%
Sugars: 8% (fructose, sucrose, glucose)
Starch: 12%

Capsicum fruit
Capsicum annum (Solanacea)

Properties: aromatic, stimulant, astringent, diaphoretic, antispasmodic, circulatory tonic, carminative, rubifacient

Systems Affected: circulatory, digestive

Common Names: cayenne, red pepper, bird pepper, African pepper

Folk History and Use

Since the dawn of civilization in South America, mankind has been fascinated by the seemingly innocuous plant with bright colored fruits that bite back when bitten. The earliest evidence of chile peppers in the human diet is from Mexico where excavations at Tamaulipas and Tehuacan contain chile seeds.

History books credit Christopher Columbus with discovering the chile pepper in the West Indies. Thinking it was another variety of black pepper, he misnamed the plant and brought seeds back to Europe after his first voyage. Explorers who followed soon learned that the pungent pod was an integral part of the Indian's culinary medical and religious lives.

From Europe, capsicum was introduced to Africa and India. It was introduced to England from India in 1548, and by 1650, capsicum was cultivated throughout northern Europe. Such were the trade routes of the day.

The most common use of capsicum by the South Americans was as a condiment, since their vegetable diet made them develop flatulence that capsicum helped correct.

The plant is a perennial, small shrub that grows in warm climates, but in most places it is cultivated as an annual. Several species have been described, but all are probably varieties of a single species.

Capsicum is a popular condiment. Many cultivated varieties have been developed. Some of the more mild forms are called paprika. Hungarian paprika is of particular note because of its delicate aroma. Green bell peppers with thick, fleshy skins are popular in North America. In Central and South America the thin skinned, pungent red and yellow peppers are used as main diet items, much as North Americans use toma-

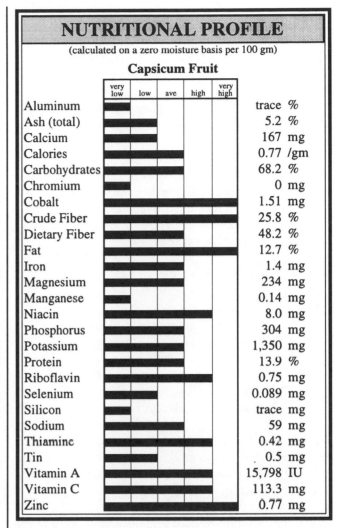

NUTRITIONAL PROFILE
(calculated on a zero moisture basis per 100 gm)

Capsicum Fruit

	very low	low	ave	high	very high		
Aluminum						trace	%
Ash (total)						5.2	%
Calcium						167	mg
Calories						0.77	/gm
Carbohydrates						68.2	%
Chromium						0	mg
Cobalt						1.51	mg
Crude Fiber						25.8	%
Dietary Fiber						48.2	%
Fat						12.7	%
Iron						1.4	mg
Magnesium						234	mg
Manganese						0.14	mg
Niacin						8.0	mg
Phosphorus						304	mg
Potassium						1,350	mg
Protein						13.9	%
Riboflavin						0.75	mg
Selenium						0.089	mg
Silicon						trace	mg
Sodium						59	mg
Thiamine						0.42	mg
Tin						0.5	mg
Vitamin A						15,798	IU
Vitamin C						113.3	mg
Zinc						0.77	mg

toes. The most pungent pepper is C. frutescence from which Tabasco sauce is made.

The most striking medicinal use of capsicum is as a catalyst herb in nearly every herbal combination conceivable. As a rule of thumb, capsicum is added to nearly all formulas except nervines. Its stimulant effects speed the circulation causing it to enhance digestion and absorption and thus the effectiveness of nearly any herbal formula.

Capsicum is used in this manner in formulas for **pain relief arthritis, female complaints, athletics, infection, heart, laxatives, diuretics, ulcers, thyroid balance, male tonic, cleansing** and **respiratory ailments**.

Samuel Thompson incorporated capsicum into his system of medicine. According to Thompson, illness is the result of loss of heat. Treatment of an illness required ridding the body of toxins and restoring the life heat. Capsicum was often his herb of choice because of its pungency.

Capsicum has also been used in poultices as an irritant and counter-irritant. Exposure to the pungent principle causes pain. Prolonged exposure deadens the nerves to any pain. Prolonged exposure to mucosa will make the mucosa insensitive to industrial pollution. As a condiment, capsicum stimulates the stomach to produce mucous which tends to sooth some intestinal ailments.

During the herbal resurgence in the early 1970's, capsicum played the major role in establishing encapsulated dry herb powders as a convenient safe dosage form for herbal remedies. Have you ever tried to swallow a teaspoon of capsicum before?

Medicinal Properties

Definite Action
Antibacterial (volatile oils, alkaloids)
Counter irritant (irritation) on mucous
membranes (alkaloids, volatile oil)
Rubifacient and vessicant on skin (alkaloids)
Diaphoretic (alkaloids)
Antispasmodic (alkaloids)

The alkaloids of capsicum, of which capsaicin is the principle active compound, are bitter, acrid and pungent. It is also a phenolic chemical, which makes it an antibacterial agent.

The volatile alkaloids capsicine provides many of the stimulant properties in capsicum, but have no narcotic (central nervous system) effects.

The volatile oil is also very pungent and provides a stimulant effect (irritation) to a variety of mucous membranes in the body.

The nutritional profile shows some interesting aspects. First, the calcium and magnesium content are below average so as not to interfere with the stimulant effects of the active principles.

Second, the trace mineral profile is generally below average as well. Since fruits store high concentrations of energy (fats) in a small space, they don't have much room for mineral storage.

Third, the high amount of vitamin A (beta-carotene) which adds to the fruit's physical color is responsible for healing properties related to the epithelial cells of mucous membranes (ulcers).

Typical Daily Usage

Fresh fruit: 1/4-1/2 teaspoon
Dried fruit: 100-300 mg
Extract: 200 mg dried fruit, 1 ml alcohol, 1 ml
water

Traditional Formulas

Capsicum and Garlic combination
Hawthorn combination
Capsicum and Myrrh combination
Cascara combination
Cascara and Dong Quai combination
Ginger combination
Black Cohosh combination
Black Cohosh and Golden Seal combination
False Unicorn and Golden Seal combination
Ginseng combination
Ginsing and Saw Palmetto combination
Golden Seal and Juniper combination
Kelp combination
Alfalfa and Yucca combination
Parthenium and Golden Seal combination
Parthenium and Myrrh combination
Ginseng and Gota Kola combination
Pollen and Ginseng combination
Valerian and Black Cohosh combination
Chamomile and Rose Hips combination
Bayberry and Ginger combination
Ephedra and Senega combination
White Willow combination
White Willow and Valerian combination
Ginseng and Parsley combination

Chemical Constituents

Aromatic compounds
Volatile oil: 0.5%
Fixed oils and Resins: 8%
carotenoids and others
Bitter compounds
Alkaloids: 0.3%
capsaicin and others

Nutrients of Note

Water when fresh: 74.2%
Water when air dried: 9.8%
Sugars: 7% (glucose, fructose)

Cascara Sagrada bark
Rhamnus purshiana (Rhamnaceae)

Properties: bitter, laxative, hepatic tonic, antispasmodic

Systems Affected: digestive, glandular

Folk History and Use

The bark of cascara sagrada is probably the most popular cathartic on earth. Traditionally used as a laxative by the North American Indians, its use became popular among the pioneers of the Pacific Northwest in the early 1800's.

Early settlers in the West made a cold infusion by soaking a piece of bark overnight and taking it as a tonic. They prepared a **laxative** potion by boiling fresh bark for several hours or by pouring boiling water over a small amount of pulverized dried bark and letting it cool. Rhamnus purshiana was described in 1805 and the bark was adopted into medical use in 1877.

Today, over-the-counter and prescription remedies, such as Pericolace by Mead-Johnson, are used by medical doctors and herbalists alike as moderate laxatives in cases of chronic constipation.

Early Spanish settlers called it sacred bark. Its common name "cascara" means bark and "sagrada" means sacred, denoting its use as a laxative and tonic.

Taxonomists named it Rhamnus from the Greek "Rhamnos" or buckthorn and "purshiana" after Fredrick Pursh, a German botanist.

This herb is a popular treatment for **chronic constipation** because it does not seem to be habit forming. It is said to increase the secretion of bile and seems to be **good for liver complaints**, especially in cases of an **enlarged liver**. Another reported use for this herb is in cases of **gas in the stomach (dyspepsia)** and in the treatment of **piles**, since it produces large, soft and painless evacuations.

The fresh bark tends to cause griping and nausea. Chemical changes in storage render it far more acceptable to the digestive system. However, large doses of the aged bark may still cause inflammation. Meanwhile, habitual use may induce chronic diarrhea with

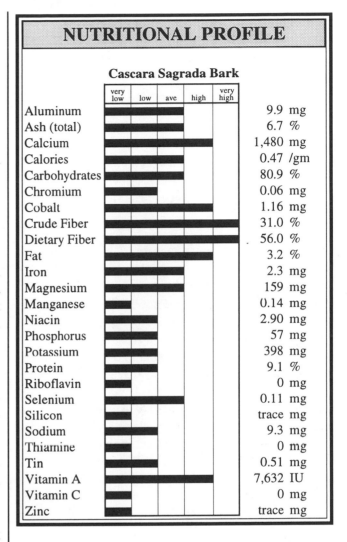

NUTRITIONAL PROFILE

Cascara Sagrada Bark

	very low	low	ave	high	very high	
Aluminum						9.9 mg
Ash (total)						6.7 %
Calcium						1,480 mg
Calories						0.47 /gm
Carbohydrates						80.9 %
Chromium						0.06 mg
Cobalt						1.16 mg
Crude Fiber						31.0 %
Dietary Fiber						56.0 %
Fat						3.2 %
Iron						2.3 mg
Magnesium						159 mg
Manganese						0.14 mg
Niacin						2.90 mg
Phosphorus						57 mg
Potassium						398 mg
Protein						9.1 %
Riboflavin						0 mg
Selenium						0.11 mg
Silicon						trace mg
Sodium						9.3 mg
Thiamine						0 mg
Tin						0.51 mg
Vitamin A						7,632 IU
Vitamin C						0 mg
Zinc						trace mg

weakness from excessive loss of potassium and over a long period, melanin will pigmentize the mucous membranes of the colon.

In the food and beverage industry, bitter cascara extract has been used in liqueurs. The debittered extract serves as a flavoring in soft drinks, ice cream and some baked goods.

The fruits of the tree are eaten raw or cooked but are said to give a transient reddish cast to the skin if consumed in excess.

Honey produced from the flowers of this plant is very dark, non-granulating and has a mildly laxative effect.

Medicinal Properties

Definite Action
    Stimulates peristaltic action in the colon
        (anthraquinone glycosides)
Probable Action
    Digestive aid (?)
Possible Action
    Anti-leukemic (?)
    Lithotriptic (?)
    Hepatic tonic (?)

The primary active principles are anthraquinone compounds, 10 to 20% being O-glycosides based on emodin, 80 to 90% being C-glycosides (aloin-like) including barbaloin.

These constituents have a **cathartic** effect through stimulating peristalsis of the large intestine and bring about their action in 6 to 8 hours. They are absorbed from the small intestine and act on the nerves of the large intestine. This stimulates motor propulsion in the colon. Because the anthraquinones are absorbed, the laxative effect can be transmitted to infants of nursing mothers taking cascara.

The fresh bark of cascara sagrada causes griping and nausea. Severe cramping may also occur. Weakness due to loss of potassium, pigmentation of the mucous membranes of the colon by melanin, discoloration of the urine and hypokalemia may also result from excessive intake. The USP standards for cascara bark require that it be aged at least one year before use.

Typical Daily Usage

Fresh bark: do not eat
Dried bark: 1-3 gm dried bark
Extract: 2 gm dried bark, 10 ml alcohol, 10 ml
    water

Traditional Formulas

Cascara combination
Cascara and Dong Quai combination
Chickweed and Cascara combination
Gentain and Cascara combination
Pumpkin and Cascara combination
Pau D' Arco and Yellow Dock combination

Chemical Constituents

Astringent compounds
    Tannin
Bitter compounds
    Anthraquinone glycosides: 6-10%
    Cascarosides A, B, C, D
    Frangulin
    Anthraquinones
    Barbaloin, chrysaloin and others

Nutrients of Note

Water when fresh: 72.3%
Water when air dried: 9.0%
Sugars: 5% (rhamnose, glucose)

Catnip herb
Nepeta cataria (Labiatae)

Properties: aromatic, sedative, antispasmodic, carminative, emmenogogue

Systems affected: nervous, digestive

CommonNames: nep, catmint, cat's wort

Folk History and Use

Catnip is the common name for a bushy herb that has dark green leaves and grows to about three feet high. It is native to Europe but is now established in most of the northeast United States and Canada. Both its Latin name and its scientific name are derived from the inability of cats to resist the aroma of the plant. Indeed it is used as a bait to trap wild cats and is supposed to ward off rats and insects.

It is supposed to produce euphoric feelings when smoked. The headache that follows provides a substantial deterrent to its abuse.

The plant and its extracts are available commercially in pet and health food stores. The essential oil of catnip produces the catnip response that stimulates most cats in unique ways that range from merely being frisky to euphoria and sexual stimulation. Its effects in humans appear to be just the opposite as in cats. It possesses an essential oil that contains sesquiterpene lactones that are chemically similar to those found in valerian root. Catnip is a sedative in humans and has traditionally been used to treat **insomnia, indigestion, nervousness, amenorrhea, flatulence, coughs, colds,** and **fevers.**

Medicinal Properties

    Definite action
        Sedative (nepetalactone)
        Antispasmodic (nepetalactone)

Catnip is an aromatic herb whose essential oil contains about 1% nepetalactone and related compounds. Nepetalactone is closely related in chemical structure to the valepotriates found in valerian root. Most of the scientific studies on catnip have been performed on cats.

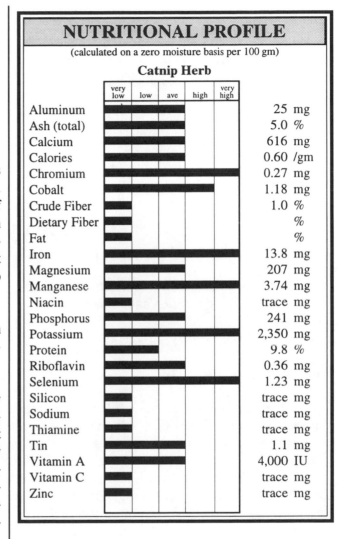

NUTRITIONAL PROFILE
(calculated on a zero moisture basis per 100 gm)

Catnip Herb

	very low	low	ave	high	very high		
Aluminum						25	mg
Ash (total)						5.0	%
Calcium						616	mg
Calories						0.60	/gm
Chromium						0.27	mg
Cobalt						1.18	mg
Crude Fiber						1.0	%
Dietary Fiber							%
Fat							%
Iron						13.8	mg
Magnesium						207	mg
Manganese						3.74	mg
Niacin						trace	mg
Phosphorus						241	mg
Potassium						2,350	mg
Protein						9.8	%
Riboflavin						0.36	mg
Selenium						1.23	mg
Silicon						trace	mg
Sodium						trace	mg
Thiamine						trace	mg
Tin						1.1	mg
Vitamin A						4,000	IU
Vitamin C						trace	mg
Zinc						trace	mg

There does not appear to be a direct correlation in humans. Indeed the effects seem to be nearly opposite in nature.

Catnip extracts, especially when used in conjunction with fennel oil, provide a safe and effective means for eliminating the effects of **colic** in young children. Catnip is one of the most popular herbs in stress formulas where it is included for its **sedative** effect. Perhaps the most popular use of catnip is as an herbal tea consumed just before bedtime. It has a very long list of folk uses which is understandable since it is often difficult to get a good night's sleep in today's fast paced world.

Typical Daily Usage

Fresh herb: 1-2 teaspoon
Dried herb: 0.5-1 gm
Extract: 1 gm dried herb in a cup of boiling
water

Traditional Formulas

Gentain and Cascara combination
Senna combination
Ginger and Barberry combination
Papaya and Peppermint combination
Alfalfa and Yucca combination
Ephedra and Passionflower combination

Chemical Constituents

Aromatic compounds
Volatile oil
Sesquiterpene lactones: 1%
Nepetalactone and others
Resin
Astringent compounds
Tannin

Nutrients of Note

Water when fresh: 88%
Water when air dried: 6.4%

Celery Seed
Apium graveolens (Umbelliferae)

Properties: aromatic, antirheumatic, urinary antiseptic, blood purifier, antioxidant, sedative

Systems affected: urinary, structural

Folk History and Use

Celery is a common garden vegetable that has been
cultivated in countless varieties. It is an erect biennial
plant grown for its stalks, leaves and seeds. Celery
seed and its oil is used as a food condiment. Its flavor
is familiar in many soups, sauces and in sausage. Its
seed oil is also used in the fragrance and pharmaceutical industries. Seed oil is most often obtained from
France where it meets market demand for the perfume,
as well as the food industry where it is used in soaps,
detergents and skin care preparations.

Celery seed appeared in popular snake oils of the 1900's
as a cure for **depression, rheumatism** and **arthritis**.
Herbalists consider the seed to have **tonic, sedative**
and **blood purifying properties**. It has also been used
to treat **urinary tract infections**. It is most noted for
its use in treating the **pain** and **depression associated
with rheumatic disorders**.

Medicinal Properties

Definite action
Antirheumatic (essential oil)
Sedative (essential oil)
Urinary antiseptic (essential oil)

NUTRITIONAL PROFILE
(calculated on a zero moisture basis per 100 gm)

Celery Seed

	very low	low	ave	high	very high		
Ash (total)						3.2	%
Calcium						800	mg
Calories						0.8	/gm
Chromium						trace	mg
Cobalt						0.2	mg
Crude Fiber						17.1	%
Dietary Fiber						32.0	%
Fat						6.6	%
Iron						12.0	mg
Magnesium						73	mg
Manganese						0.63	mg
Niacin						1.20	mg
Phosphorus						466	mg
Potassium						576	mg
Protein						16.9	%
Riboflavin						0.06	mg
Selenium						0.02	mg
Silicon						0.45	mg
Sodium						212	mg
Thiamine						0.12	mg
Vitamin A						6,000	IU
Vitamin C						170	mg
Zinc						0.12	mg

Celery seed possesses an essential oil thought to be responsible for its action. The oil is antiseptic, antioxidant and antirheumatic. Herbs used to combat rheumatism and rheumatic conditions are commonly called blood purifiers. Celery seed is no exception. It purifies the blood by increasing urinary output and relieving inflammation and muscle spasms as a byproduct of its antiseptic property.

Typical Daily Usage

Dried seed: 1-2 gm
Extract: 2 gm dried seed, 10 ml alcohol, 10 ml water

Traditional Formulas

Alfalfa and Yucca combination

Chemical Constituents

Aromatic compounds
    Essential oil: 20%
        Apiol and others
    Resin
Bitter compounds
    Flavonoids
        quercetin and others

Nutrients of Note

Water when fresh: 79%
Water when air dried: 8%
Sugars: 7%(glucose, maltose)

Chamomile flowers (German)
Anthemis noblis (Compositae)

Properties: aromatic, carminative, anti-inflammatory, antiseptic, antibacterial, stimulant, antifungal, nervine

Systems Affected: urinary, nervous, digestive, circulatory

Common Names: German chamomile, garden chamomile, ground apples, pin heads

Folk History and Use

Perhaps no plant was better known to the common folk of the Middle Ages than chamomile. Old herbals dismiss a discussion on the uses of chamomile as "lost time and labor," since knowledge of this herb was so widespread.

The plant is native to Eurasia and its first reported use was by early Egyptians who dedicated chamomile to their gods because of the people's belief in the plant's curative powers. It has since been cultivated in North and South America and is presently cultivated in Belgium, France and England.

Besides its medicinal virtues, chamomile finds widespread use as a flavoring agent. It is used in most major food categories including alcoholic beverages such as vermouth and a variety of bitter tonics, non-alcoholic beverages (teas), desserts, candies, etc.

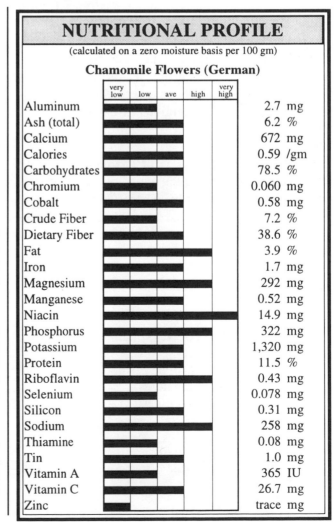

NUTRITIONAL PROFILE
(calculated on a zero moisture basis per 100 gm)

Chamomile Flowers (German)

	very low	low	ave	high	very high		
Aluminum						2.7	mg
Ash (total)						6.2	%
Calcium						672	mg
Calories						0.59	/gm
Carbohydrates						78.5	%
Chromium						0.060	mg
Cobalt						0.58	mg
Crude Fiber						7.2	%
Dietary Fiber						38.6	%
Fat						3.9	%
Iron						1.7	mg
Magnesium						292	mg
Manganese						0.52	mg
Niacin						14.9	mg
Phosphorus						322	mg
Potassium						1,320	mg
Protein						11.5	%
Riboflavin						0.43	mg
Selenium						0.078	mg
Silicon						0.31	mg
Sodium						258	mg
Thiamine						0.08	mg
Tin						1.0	mg
Vitamin A						365	IU
Vitamin C						26.7	mg
Zinc						trace	mg

Chamomile is the most popular herbal tea flavor in the world. It not only provides a stimulating, carminative and hypnotic action, but also a pleasant, apple-like flavor to teas.

The Greeks named it "ground apple" because of its scent and morphology. The name chamomile is derived from "kamai" (on the ground) and "melon" (an apple). The Spaniards call it "Manzanilla" or "a little apple," which is also the name of an alcoholic beverage flavored with chamomile.

Chamomile is also used to add a golden tint to hair and to scent chamomile shampoo formulas. It has also been used as an enema or douche and as a pomade for bathing. The Arabians used it in massage oils.

Both Chamaemelum nobile L. All. (Roman chamomile) and Matricaria recutita L. (German chamomile) have been used for centuries for medicinal purposes. Both produce essential oils containing azulenes such as chamazulene, but vary in appearance. German chamomile oil is characteristically more blue than Roman chamomile oil.

As medicinal agents, the two have been used for similar complaints. The amount of research conducted with German chamomile indicates that there is more interest in this plant. The production of Roman chamomile has been dropping.

One note of caution to users of chamomile flowers: they contain pollen and often are adulterated with minor quantities of other herbs. These can cause allergic reactions in some people. Therefore, those who are sensitive to these substances should take proper precautions.

Medicinal Properties

Definite Actions
    Antimicrobial effects (volatile oils)
    Anti-inflammatory (volatile oils)
    Antispasmodic action on smooth muscles
    (volatile oils, flavonoids)
    Antithrombotic (coumarins)

Probable Actions
    Analgesic (volatile oils)
    Antipyretic (volatile oils)

The major effects of chamomile are due to its volatile oils. Therefore, it is imperative that the freshest herb be used before the oils evaporate. Most tea bags are double sealed to insure freshness, but lose the seal when opened. Be sure to purchase high quality teas in boxes of 16 bags or less.

The actions of chamomile are strongest on the liver and kidneys where the volatile oils apparently stimulate the organs to purge themselves of toxins. To avoid a loss of volatile oils in the herb, an extract is conveniently described under preparations which can be added to teas to strengthen them. The extract may also be used alone.

Chamomile is a well studied herb and most of its folk uses have been verified chemically. The volatile oils are **bactericidal** and **fungicidal**, especially against gram positive bacteria (e.g. staphylococcus aureus) and candida albicans. The oil is also **analgesic, antispasmodic, anti-inflammatory, antipyretic** and **antianaphylatic (hypo allergenic)**.

The major constituents of the oils are: chamazulene (antimicrobial, antispasmodic, anti-inflammatory), farinesene, (-) bisabolol (anti-inflammatory) and en-yn-dicycloether (smooth muscle relaxant). Azulenes have been documented to be both hypo allergenic and anti-inflammatory.

Azulenes were shown to prevent **allergic seizures** in guinea pigs as long as 60 minutes after administration. The prevention of allergic seizures suggests that azulenes work by inhibiting the release of histamine.

(-)Bisabolol is one of the principle components of German chamomile. It is anti-inflammatory, antibacterial, antimycotic and ulcer protective with a low toxicity. (-)Bisabolol inhibited ulcer development induced by indomethacin, stress and ethanol in animals. The time was decreased by (-)bisabolol for the healing of ulcers from chemical stress (such as acetic acid) or heat coagulation.

The medicinal properties of German chamomile are most often attributed to chamazulene, -bisabolol and its oxides and cis-en-yn-dicycloether. However, the flavonoids and coumarins must also be considered active principles.

Many flavonoids exert the following beneficial effects on capillaries:

    a) chelation of metals, retarding vitamin C oxidation

    b) antithrombotic effects

    c) stimulation of the pituitary-adrenal axis

Many flavonoids have antiviral and antibacterial activity as well. Both flavonoids and the coumarins have an antispasmodic muscle relaxant effect.

Typical Daily Usage

Fresh flowers: 2-4 tablespoon

Dried flowers: 3-6 gm

Extract: 4.5 gm dried flowers, 22 ml alcohol, 23 ml water

Traditional Formulas

Plantain combination

Dandelion and Parsley combination

Chamomile and Passionflower combination

Chamomile and Rose Hips combination

Uva Ursi combination

Chemical Constituents

Aromatic compounds

    Volatile oil: 0.24-1.9%

        Azulenes and related compounds

    Fixed oils and resins: 3%

Astringent compounds

    Flavonoids - antispasmodic

        apigenin, rutin, luteolin, quercimeritin and others

    Coumarins - antispasmodic, antithrombotic

        umbelliferone

        herniarin

Mucilaginous compounds

    Polysaccharides

        mucilage of d-galactouronic acid

Nutrients of note

Water when fresh: 81.2%

Water when air dried: 10.6%

Sugars: 9% (glucose, fructose, galactose)

Starch: 4%

Chaparral herb
Larrea tridenta (Zygophyllaceae)

Properties: bitter, antiseptic, antibiotic, parasiticide, alterative, expectorant, diuretic

Systems Affected: digestive, respiratory, circulatory

Common Names: greasewood, creosote bush

Folk History and Use

Chaparral is a strongly scented, olive green shrub native to the Sonoran, Mojave and Chihuahuan deserts of the southwestern United States and northern Mexico.

Chaparral is an Indian name referring broadly to any dense thicket of shrubs growing in alkali soils. Today it is better known as the greasewood or creosote bush. This is in reference to the characteristic odor it pervades, especially after a rainstorm.

The Maricopa and Pima Indians of the United States boiled the branches to extract the gum. The decoction was used for stomach and digestive difficulties.

Spanish colonizers of the southwest deserts found the Native Americans using an aqueous extract of the leaves and twigs as a tea to treat a wide variety of ailments, including **arthritis, cancer, venereal disease, tuberculosis, bowel cramps, rheumatism** and **colds**. One unusual folk use is as a hair tonic where it is said to grow hair on balding scalps. A recent remedy attributed to chaparral is taking the residue of LSD out of the system to prevent recurrences of hallucinations. Chaparral is also in common use as a **blood purifier**.

Medicinal Properties

Definite Action
    Antimicrobial (volatile oil)
    Antioxidant (NDGA)
Probable Action
    Expectorant (volatile oil)
    Diuretic (volatile oil)
    Antispasmodic (flavonoids)
Possible Action
    Antitumor (NDGA)

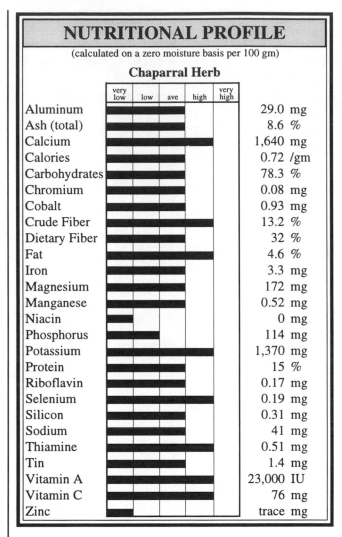

NUTRITIONAL PROFILE
(calculated on a zero moisture basis per 100 gm)
Chaparral Herb

Nutrient	Amount
Aluminum	29.0 mg
Ash (total)	8.6 %
Calcium	1,640 mg
Calories	0.72 /gm
Carbohydrates	78.3 %
Chromium	0.08 mg
Cobalt	0.93 mg
Crude Fiber	13.2 %
Dietary Fiber	32 %
Fat	4.6 %
Iron	3.3 mg
Magnesium	172 mg
Manganese	0.52 mg
Niacin	0 mg
Phosphorus	114 mg
Potassium	1,370 mg
Protein	15 %
Riboflavin	0.17 mg
Selenium	0.19 mg
Silicon	0.31 mg
Sodium	41 mg
Thiamine	0.51 mg
Tin	1.4 mg
Vitamin A	23,000 IU
Vitamin C	76 mg
Zinc	trace mg

As might be expected, most of the attention focused on chaparral tea in recent years is concerned with the use of the herb and its principal ingredient, nordihydroguaiaretic acid (NDGA), as an anticancer agent. NDGA is a potent antioxidant, especially for fats and oils. As such, it was once thought to be potentially useful in the treatment of cancer. Early studies in rats did indicate that NDGA exerted an inhibitory effect on some tumor cells, but follow-up studies with the tea in human beings have not confirmed the rat studies.

Further study on the antitumor potential of chaparral seems in order since other antioxidants such as beta-carotene and vitamins C and E have found a place in both **cancer prevention** and **cancer therapy**.

Other properties of chaparral are more straight forward. One known active agent is the resin which makes up 15 to 20% of the herb. This phenolic resin provides **antimicrobial, antioxidant** and **antispasmodic** effects associated with the herb. NDGA has been widely studied and has proven to be antibacterial, antifungal and antiparasitical. It is especially effective against skin bacteria.

The antispasmodic effects are probably provided by the flavonoids which include ternatin, herbacetin and gossypetin. The volatile oils, as well as the phenolic resin, account for its irritating properties that provide the stimulus for the **expectorant** and **diuretic** effects of the herb.

The traditional uses of chaparral in rheumatism and cold formulas are based on this irritation stimulus that rid the body of toxins. This herb also has antibiotic principles that affect the intestinal flora as well.

Typical Daily Usage

Fresh herb: 2-4 tablespoon
Dried herb: 3-6 gm
Extract: 4.5 gm dried herb, 22 ml alcohol, 23 ml water

Traditional Formulas

Alfalfa and Yucca combination
Pau D' Arco and Yellow Dock combination
Ephedra and Senega combination
Cedar Berry combination

Chemical Constituents

Aromatic compounds
 Volatile oils: 0.1-0.25%
 Terpenes
  pinenes, limonene, camphor, calamenene and others
 Vinyl ketones - provide characteristic odor of the plant
  l-hexen-3-one
  l-hepten-3-one
 Other ketones
  2-heptanone
  2-undecanone
 Fixed oil and Resin: 3.1-5%
Astringent compounds
Resin: 15-20%
 Flavonoids
  ternatin, gossypetin, and herbacetin
 Lignanes
  Nordihydroguariaretic acid (NDGA) and others
Mucilaginous compounds
 Polysaccharides
  Gum: 12%

Nutrients of Note

Water when fresh: 67.1%
Water when air dried: 6.2%
Sugars: 8% (sucrose)

Chickweed herb
Stellaria media (Caryophyllaceae)

Properties: bitter, diuretic, demulcent, antipyretic

Systems affected: circulatory, respiratory, urinary, digestive

Common Names: stitchwort, scarwort, satin flower, adder's mouth, starweed

Folk History and Use

Chickweed is one of the most common weeds in the world, native to all temperate regions of the world.

Chickweed is so common because it blooms as early as March and continues blooming throughout the summer. Its seeds are also easily scattered by the wind. Chickweed pollen is a common cause of allergies in the spring, yet the air dried herb very seldom provokes an allergic reaction.

The common name for chickweed comes from the old custom of using the seeds as birdfeed.

It is a mild herb that is very nutritious, providing large amounts of protein and minerals. The fresh tops are delicious boiled or as greens in a salad.

Chickweed is largely ignored by early herbalists because of its mild action and availability. Its most popular use is as a **poultice on external abscesses** and **rashes**, where it **removes the heat of infection and draws poisons** and **weakens infections**.

Internally it has been used as a **diuretic, eyewash** and as an **expectorant** in throat lozenges.

The most famous folk use of chickweed is an old wives' remedy for obesity. This is probably due to the diuretic action of chickweed.

Medicinal Properties

    Probable Actions
        Digestive aid (saponins)
        Diuretic (saponins)
        Regulation of intestinal flora (saponins)
        Vulnerary (topically) (saponins)
        The benefits of viscous fiber
            Lowers bowel transit time
            Absorbs toxins from bowel
            Regulates colonic bacteria and yeast
    Possible Actions
        Weight loss aid (?)
        Expectorant action (?)

NUTRITIONAL PROFILE
(calculated on a zero moisture basis per 100 gm)

Chickweed Herb

Nutrient	very low	low	ave	high	very high	Amount
Aluminum					■	196 mg
Ash (total)				■		15.7 %
Calcium				■		1,210 mg
Calories				■		0.43 /gm
Carbohydrates		■				60.2 %
Chromium		■				0.11 mg
Cobalt				■		1.21 mg
Crude Fiber		■				10.8 %
Dietary Fiber				■		32.9 %
Fat		■				4.8 %
Iron					■	25.3 mg
Magnesium					■	529 mg
Manganese				■		0.53 mg
Niacin			■			4.7 mg
Phosphorus		■				448 mg
Potassium		■				840 mg
Protein		■				21.7 %
Riboflavin	■					0.13 mg
Selenium	■					0.043 mg
Silicon					■	0.57 mg
Sodium		■				147 mg
Thiamine			■			0.21 mg
Tin	■					trace
Vitamin A				■		7,229 IU
Vitamin C		■				6.9 mg
Zinc		■				0.52 mg

The only known potentially active constituents of chickweed are yet to be characterized --the steroidal saponins. Saponins are emulsifying agents that cause water solutions containing them to foam. They have the ability to increase the permeability of many membranes of the body by partially dissolving them.

The saponins in chickweed are poorly absorbed through the intestinal walls, but apparently increase the permeability of the mucous membranes sufficiently to produce expectorant effects on the throat and increase the absorption of nutrients, especially minerals, from the digestive tract.

Chickweed is also a **mild diuretic**, but the effect is only temporary as the body produces cholesterin to neutralize this effect after about a week.

Externally the saponins of chickweed help **solubilize toxins in abscesses and rashes** and help **increase the effectiveness of bactericides** by increasing the permeability of bacterial cell walls.

Typical Daily Usage

Fresh herb: 1/4-1/2 cup
Dried herb: 6-12 gm
Extract: 9 gm dried herb, 45 ml alcohol, 45 ml water

Traditional Formulas

Chickweed and Cascara combination
Gentain and Cascara combination
Ginseng and Saw Palmetto combination
Red Beet and Yellow Dock combination

Chemical Constituents

Aromatic compounds
  Volatile Oil: 0.1-0.2%
  Fixed oils and Resins
    Saturated fatty acids
      palmitic and stearic
    Unsaturated fatty acids
      linoleic and oleic
Bitter compounds
  Saponins
    Steroidal saponins
Mucilaginous compounds
  Polysaccharides
    Mucilage: 20%

Nutrients of Note

Water when fresh: 91.7%
Water when air dried: 7.1%
Starch: 12%

Comfrey leaf
Symphytum officinale (Boraginaceae)

Properties: mucilaginous, demulcent, alterative, vulnerary, astringent

Systems Affected: digestive, liver

Common Names: gum plant, healing herb, knit bone, nipbone, knit back, boneset

Folk History and Use

Comfrey leaf formerly was highly esteemed as a vulnerary, but has come under fire in recent years because it contains a group of alkaloids (pyrollizidine) which are believed to be hepatoxic. As a result, comfrey has been banned from sale in many countries including Canada, Australia and Japan.

The virtues of comfrey are chiefly those of a mucilaginous herb with supporting astringent properties much like slippery elm bark.

Comfrey is native to Europe and Asia and has been cultivated in all temperate regions of the world.

Its name is derived from the Greek word "symphytos," or united, in reference to its corolla which is grown together.

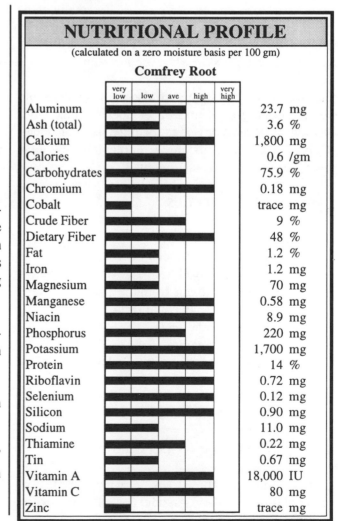

NUTRITIONAL PROFILE
(calculated on a zero moisture basis per 100 gm)

Comfrey Root

	very low	low	ave	high	very high	
Aluminum						23.7 mg
Ash (total)						3.6 %
Calcium						1,800 mg
Calories						0.6 /gm
Carbohydrates						75.9 %
Chromium						0.18 mg
Cobalt						trace mg
Crude Fiber						9 %
Dietary Fiber						48 %
Fat						1.2 %
Iron						1.2 mg
Magnesium						70 mg
Manganese						0.58 mg
Niacin						8.9 mg
Phosphorus						220 mg
Potassium						1,700 mg
Protein						14 %
Riboflavin						0.72 mg
Selenium						0.12 mg
Silicon						0.90 mg
Sodium						11.0 mg
Thiamine						0.22 mg
Tin						0.67 mg
Vitamin A						18,000 IU
Vitamin C						80 mg
Zinc						trace mg

Comfrey was strictly used externally until the early 1800's when Western herbalists began using it internally. In the 1800's, it was used solely as a **poultice for bone knitting, fractures,** or as a **pomade in the treatment of cuts, burns, skin ulcers, varicose veins, bronchitis** and **rheumatism.**

Comfrey has been credited with powerful healing qualities and a number of magical attributes as well. Culpepper claimed that comfrey leaf "is said to be so powerful to consolidate and knit together, that if they (comfrey leaves) be boiled with dismembered pieces of flesh in a pot it will join them together."

It is also reputed to possess the ability to **knit bones** together as well. This reputation has undoubtedly accounted for many of the common names (boneset, nipbone, knitbone, knitback, healing herb) by which this herb is known.

The leaf has been utilized in a decoction which is gargled or used as a mouthwash to relieve throat infections, hoarseness and bleeding gums. Externally, comfrey has been used in poultice form to treat wounds, bruises, sores and insect bites. The mucilage is believed to soften the skin when used in baths.

Comfrey leaves and shoots are also used as a vegetable and are often ground up in a blender or some other type of mechanical device to form the basis of "green drinks" which have become increasingly popular among health conscious individuals.

Medicinal Properties

    Definite Actions
        The benefits of viscous fiber
            Lowers bowel transit time
            Absorbs toxins from the bowel
            Regulates intestinal flora
            Demulcent effects
        Astringent (tannins)
            Cell proliferant action (allantoin)
    Probable Actions
        Hepatoxic (pyrollizidine alkaloids)
        Expectorant (tannins)
    Possible Actions
        Anti-inflammatory (alkaloids)

Comfrey is primarily used by Western herbalists to treat **internal (duodenal and gastric)** and **external ulcers.**

In addition, it functions as an **astringent, demulcent, emollient, hemostat, expectorant and cell proliferant** (wound healing).

Comfrey is used in the treatment of **colitis, varicose veins, assorted pulmonary complaints (pleurisy, bronchitis, bronchopneumonia), rheumatism, metritis, diarrhea** and **periostitis.** It is utilized as a **diuretic** and **bulk laxative** and is credited with **scar healing and sedative properties.** A decoction of the rhizome is still used in Europe as a **gargle for pharyngitis and tonsillitis.**

Allantoin is probably responsible for comfrey's healing properties, while the high percentage of mucilage explains the utilization of comfrey as a demulcent and bulk laxative. Its tannins are responsible for the astringent properties of the herb.

Recently, the safety of consuming comfrey has been questioned by several leading researchers. Comfrey contains up to eight (8) pyrollizidine alkaloids. Rats fed diets consisting of 0.5% comfrey leaves produced hemagioendothelial sarcoma (malignant tumors) of the liver and bladder. Hemagioendothelial sarcoma was also induced in rats fed diets consisting of 0.5% raw comfrey root.

Pyrollizidine alkaloids are also toxic in humans. An outbreak of acute intoxication (caused by ingesting wheat contaminated by Heliotropium) resulted in obstruction of the trunk or large branches of the hepatic vein. Veno-occlusive disease among a north Afghanistan community was caused by the ingestion of approximately 2 mg of toxic alkaloids a day over a period of two years.

Further research needs to be completed to determine the toxicity of comfrey. Until then, it seems wise to use this herb as the ancients did, for external use only.

Typical Daily Usage

    Fresh leaf: 1/4-1/2 cup
    Dried leaf: 6-12 gm
    Extract: 9 gm dried leaf, 45 ml alcohol, 45 ml water

Traditional Formulas

    Gentain and Cascara combination
    Comfrey combination

Chemical Constituents

Aromatic compounds
  Volatile oils: trace
Astringent compounds
  Tannins - pyrocatechol type
Bitter compounds
  Saponins
  Sitosterol and others
  Alkaloids - Pyrollizidine type
   Symphytine, echimidine, lycopsamine and

others
Flavonoids
  Isobauerenol and others
Allantoin: 1-2%
Mucilaginous compounds
  Mucopolysaccharides: 25-30%

Nutrients of Note

Water when fresh: 89%
Water when air dried: 7.5%
Sugars: 9% (glucose, fructose)

Cranberry fruit
Vaccinium macrocarpon (Ericaceae)

Properties:　　bitter, urinary acidifier, diuretic

Systems affected:　urinary

Folk History and Use

Cranberry fruit grows on evergreen shrubs in most damp places in the northeast quarter of the United States. The cranberry is of the same botanical family and genus as bilberry. Its tradition of use in folk medicine began when German physicians in the mid 1800's noticed that the urinary excretion of hippuric acid increased after drinking cranberry juice. Conflicting data from scientific studies have not determined how it works, but the consensus among regular drinkers of the juice point to its effectiveness in **preventing chronic urinary tract infections** and **in deodorizing the urine. Kidney** aliments are commonly treated with cranberry fruit.

Cranberry growers have withdrawn support of further studies of the plant because they cannot grow enough to meet the current demand. In an increasingly health conscious and aging society, cranberry is positioned as a good tasting, natural juice with at least perceived, if not proven, health benefits.

Medicinal Properties

Probable action
  Urinary acidifier (?)
  Bacteriostatic(?)
  Diuretic (?)

The reason for the scientific interest in cranberry is for its ability to lower the pH of urine. Acidifying the urine has two major benefits. First, urine becomes bacteriostatic at a pH of about five. At this pH, most chronic

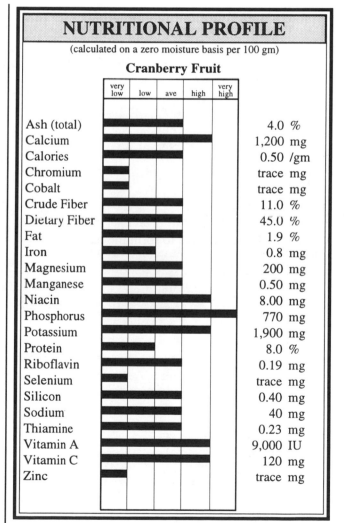

NUTRITIONAL PROFILE
(calculated on a zero moisture basis per 100 gm)
Cranberry Fruit

	very low	low	ave	high	very high	
Ash (total)						4.0 %
Calcium						1,200 mg
Calories						0.50 /gm
Chromium						trace mg
Cobalt						trace mg
Crude Fiber						11.0 %
Dietary Fiber						45.0 %
Fat						1.9 %
Iron						0.8 mg
Magnesium						200 mg
Manganese						0.50 mg
Niacin						8.00 mg
Phosphorus						770 mg
Potassium						1,900 mg
Protein						8.0 %
Riboflavin						0.19 mg
Selenium						trace mg
Silicon						0.40 mg
Sodium						40 mg
Thiamine						0.23 mg
Vitamin A						9,000 IU
Vitamin C						120 mg
Zinc						trace mg

urinary tract infections are prevented. Second, those who suffer from incontinence often develop the characteristic ammonia odor as E. coli bacteria proliferate in excreted urine. Acid urine would act as a deodorant of sorts to inhibit their growth and the resulting odor.

No one has yet found a mechanism or a particular chemical in cranberry fruit that can be called its active constituent. Reports on daily consumption of the juice accompanied by positive responses to kidney stones, chronic urinary tract infections and nephritis continue to make cranberry fruit an interesting folk medicine.

Typical Daily Usage

Fresh fruit: 1/2 cup
Dried fruit: 1 tablespoon
Extract: 15 gm dried fruit, 20 ml alcohol, 130 ml water

Chemical Constituents

Astringent compounds
  Fruit acids
    Citric, malic, quinic, benzoic and others
Bitter compounds
  Anthocyanins (color)
Mucilaginous compounds
  Polysaccharides
    Gum: 5%
    Pectin: 4%

Nutrients of Note

Water when fresh: 88%
Water when air dried: 9%
Sugars: 12 % (fructose, glucose)

Damiana leaf
Turnera diffusa (Turneraceae)

Properties: aromatic, diuretic, laxative, blood purifier, expectorant, aphrodisiac

Systems affected: circulatory, digestive

Folk History and Use

Damiana is an aromatic shrub native to the northwest desert region of Mexico. It is also found in the desert southwest of the United States and in many parts of South America. Its leaves are less than an inch long, yellowish brown and with a distinct aroma. Aztec legend states that damiana was a powerful aphrodisiac. This single evidence, it appears, has led to its use in liquor, and in most herbal energy and longevity formulas sold as health food.

More likely, damiana is a blood purifier with many of the same properties as parsley. Its essential oil is irritating to mucous membranes and may account for its success as a **diuretic, laxative, blood purifier** and **expectorant**. There is little evidence that sexual performance is enhanced with the use of damiana.

Damiana has traditionally been used to treat **coughs, colds, enuresis, nephritis, headaches** and **dysmenorrhea.**

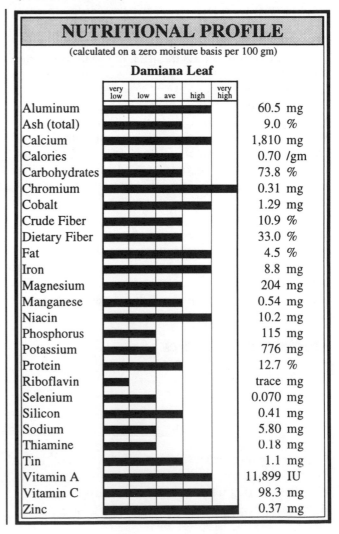

NUTRITIONAL PROFILE
(calculated on a zero moisture basis per 100 gm)

Damiana Leaf

Nutrient	very low	low	ave	high	very high	Value
Aluminum						60.5 mg
Ash (total)						9.0 %
Calcium						1,810 mg
Calories						0.70 /gm
Carbohydrates						73.8 %
Chromium						0.31 mg
Cobalt						1.29 mg
Crude Fiber						10.9 %
Dietary Fiber						33.0 %
Fat						4.5 %
Iron						8.8 mg
Magnesium						204 mg
Manganese						0.54 mg
Niacin						10.2 mg
Phosphorus						115 mg
Potassium						776 mg
Protein						12.7 %
Riboflavin						trace mg
Selenium						0.070 mg
Silicon						0.41 mg
Sodium						5.80 mg
Thiamine						0.18 mg
Tin						1.1 mg
Vitamin A						11,899 IU
Vitamin C						98.3 mg
Zinc						0.37 mg

Medicinal Properties

Definite action
    Expectorant (volatile oil)
    Laxative (volatile oil)
    Diuretic (volatile oil)
Possible action
    Aphrodisiac (?)

Damiana has been widely reported to be an **aphrodisiac**. This claim has not been supported by scientific study. It is more aptly described as a **blood purifier**. It contains an aromatic oil consisting promarily of terpenes. These are of the same chemical class of compounds as those found in juniper and parsley. These oils irritate mucous membranes and increase the production while decreasing the thickness of fluids produced by these membranes. In the case of damiana, the effect is most pronounced in the reproductive and urinary systems.

Typical Daily Usage

Fresh leaf: 1 teaspoon
Dried leaf: 0.5 gm
Extract: 0.5 gm dried leaf, 3 gm alcohol, 2 ml water

Traditional Formulas

Ginseng and Saw Palmetto combination

Chemical Constituents

Aromatic compounds
    Volatile oil: 1%
        Terpenes
            Cineole, pinene, thymol and others
    Resin: 6.5%
Astringent compounds
    Tannin: 4%
Bitter compounds
    Alkaloids
        (uncharacterized)
    Flavonoids
        Arbutin
Mucilaginous compounds
    Polysaccharides
        Gum: 15%

Nutrients of Note

Water when fresh: 79%
Water when air dried:6.8%
Sugars: 4% (sucrose, glucose)
Chlorophyllins: 7.5 %
Starch: 5%

Dandelion root
Taraxacum officinale (Compositae)

Properties: bitter, hepatonic, diuretic, stomachic, lithotriptic, astringent, cholagogue, galactogogue

Systems Affected: digestive, glandular, circulatory

Common Names: blow ball, cankerwort, lion's tooth, wild endive

Folk History and Use

Anyone who is responsible for the upkeep of lawns, yards or gardens can describe in detail the dandelion. It persists as bilious yellow disks despite painstaking efforts to eradicate it. Dandelions are short members of the sunflower (compositae) family. Western Europe and the Mediterranean both claim dandelion as a native plant, but its origin becomes moot as the wind-blown seeds now inhabit every temperate climate in the world.

Its widespread distribution may be a hint from Mother Nature that everyone has need of this plant.

Dandelion was first mentioned in the writings of Arabian physicians in the 10th and 11th centuries when they referred to it as Taraxacon. Later taxonomists changed this to Taraxacum, derived from the Greek "taraxos" meaning disorder and "akos" meaning remedy. The common name dandelion is from the French "dent de leon" meaning teeth of the lion in reference to the morphology of its leaves.

The root is used as a **laxative, tonic** and **diuretic** and also to treat **various liver** and **spleen ailments.** It is also used to treat **heartburn, rheumatism, gout** and **eczema.**

Dandelion is the principle herb of blood purifier formulas, kidney formulas and pancreas formulas.

Medicinal Properties

    Definite Action
        Diuretic (flavonoids)
        Laxative (essential oil)

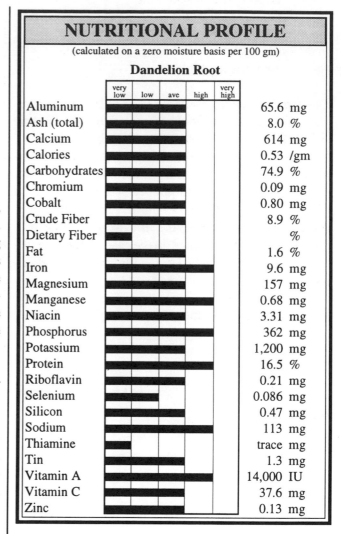

NUTRITIONAL PROFILE
(calculated on a zero moisture basis per 100 gm)
Dandelion Root

Nutrient	Value
Aluminum	65.6 mg
Ash (total)	8.0 %
Calcium	614 mg
Calories	0.53 /gm
Carbohydrates	74.9 %
Chromium	0.09 mg
Cobalt	0.80 mg
Crude Fiber	8.9 %
Dietary Fiber	%
Fat	1.6 %
Iron	9.6 mg
Magnesium	157 mg
Manganese	0.68 mg
Niacin	3.31 mg
Phosphorus	362 mg
Potassium	1,200 mg
Protein	16.5 %
Riboflavin	0.21 mg
Selenium	0.086 mg
Silicon	0.47 mg
Sodium	113 mg
Thiamine	trace mg
Tin	1.3 mg
Vitamin A	14,000 IU
Vitamin C	37.6 mg
Zinc	0.13 mg

    Antispasmodic (flavonoids)
    The benefits of viscous fiber
        Lowers bowel transit time
        Absorbs toxins from bowels
        Balances intestinal flora
        Demulcent action on digestive tract
    Bacteriostatic (essential oil)
    Fungistatic (essential oil)
    Diaphoretic (essential oil)

Dandelion contains bitter flavonoids that provide its diuretic properties. These compounds are very important to the actions of nearly all blood purifiers. Besides increasing the flow of urine, these compounds relieve muscle spasms and reduce inflammation.

Some of the medicinal virtues of dandelion can be explained by two concepts common to many mucilaginous herbs. Dandelion contains inulin and mucilage which sooth the digestive tract, absorb toxins from ingested food and regulate the colonies of intestinal bacteria which produce toxins intended to kill other bacteria as a self preservation instinct. That is, they help friendly flora thrive and inhibit unfriendly bacteria.

One way the mucilage does this is by absorbing bacteria produced bactericides meant to kill other bacteria. The mucilage thus allows the body to heal itself indirectly by removing a source of body pollution. Mucilaginous herbs often also contain volatile and bitter principles. These principles stimulate (by irritation) particular organs to produce mucous which sequesters toxins and helps eliminate them from the organ involved.

Dandelion contains oils and bitter resins that have a stimulating (irritating) effect on the liver and kidneys. Very few of the oils in dandelion are volatile and few properties are lost to drying and grinding this herb. The bitter resins are also responsible for the stomachic properties of this herb.

Perhaps the most important correlation of nutritional data to the effects of this herb is the abundance of minerals present in dandelion. Dandelion contains a very balanced mineral profile. Note the generous quantities of the electrolytes sodium and potassium. These help to balance the body's reaction to the diuretic effects produced by this herb.

Notice the high vitamin A content (beta-carotene). Since vitamin A is stored in the liver, the purging process stimulated by the bitter principles in dandelion would undoubtedly release some of the vitamin A stored in the liver and provide a ready supply of this essential nutrient to other body systems.

Typical Daily Usage

Fresh root: 1/4-1/2 cup
Dried root: 6-12 gm
Extract: 9 gm dried root, 45 ml alcohol, 45 ml water

Traditional Formulas

Chickweed and Cascara combination
Gentain and Cascara combination
Licorice combination
Golden Seal and Juniper combination
Alfalfa and Dandelion combination
Dandelion and Barberry combination
Dandelion and Parsley combination
Pau D' Arco and Yellow Dock combination
Dandelion and Purslane combination
Uva Ursi combination

Chemical Constituents

Aromatic compounds
  Essential oil: 0.5%
    Triterpenes
      taraxol, amyrin, taraxacin and others
    Fatty Acids
      Myristic, palmitic, stearic and lauric
    Carotenoids
Astringent compounds
  Pseudotannins
    caffeic acid and others
Bitter compounds
  Saponins
    Sitasterol and others
  Flavonoids
    Lutein, flavoxanthin, violaxanthin and
      others
Mucilaginous compounds
  Pectin: 12%
  Inulin: 30%

Nutrients of Note
Water when fresh: 85.7%
Water when air dried: 8.7%
Sugars: 10% (fructose, glucose, sucrose)

Devil's Claw root
Harpagophytum procumbens (Pedaliaceae)

Properties: bitter, antiarthritc, anti-inflammatory, analgesic

Systems Affected: immune, structural

Folk History and Use

Devil's claw is an African herb that takes its name from the clawlike shape of its root. It is native to the desert regions of southwest Africa. It is most commonly used to treat arthritis and other inflammatory conditions including allergies, headaches, nephritis and hepatitis.

Devil's claw is given to African women to relieve pain during pregnancy and delivery. It is especially popular in Europe where it is sold almost exclusively to treat the pain and inflammation of rheumatism and arthritis.

Herbalists consider this root to be one of the most useful blood purifiers in their materia medica.

Medicinal Properties

Definite action
Anti-inflammatory (harpagoside)
Analgesic (harpagoside)
Blood purifier (harpagoside)

Devil's claw has been studied with mixed results by scientists seeking a cure for a variety of chronic inflammatory conditions. German clinical studies do show it to **reduce the pain** and **inflammation of arthritis**. It has also been shown to **reduce serum cholesterol and uric acid levels**. No better description of a **blood purifier** has yet been given.

The plant owes its action and controversial performance in clinical studies to the bitter monoterpene glucoside called harpagoside and its related compounds. These bitter compounds apparently do not work like other antiarthritic drugs. No one quite knows how harpagoside works, so when it is compared to aspirin or indomethacin and the results don't always add up, the root is written off as another failed myth.

Devil's claw is too popular to be written off as a traditional legend. Its mode of action just hasn't been explained yet. Perhaps it is an immune modulator that works by some undiscovered mechanism?

Typical Daily Usage

Fresh root: 1-2 teaspoon
Dried root: 0.5-1 gm
Extract: 1 gm dried root, 5 ml alcohol, 5 ml water

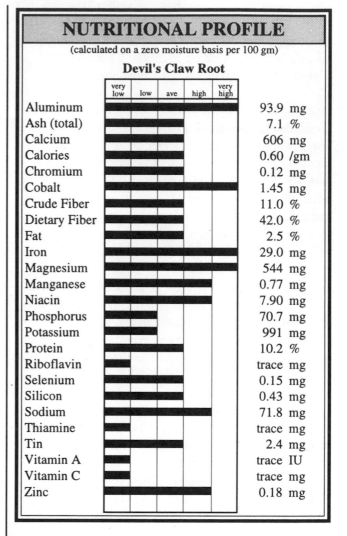

NUTRITIONAL PROFILE
(calculated on a zero moisture basis per 100 gm)

Devil's Claw Root

	very low	low	ave	high	very high		
Aluminum			■			93.9	mg
Ash (total)		■				7.1	%
Calcium			■			606	mg
Calories	■					0.60	/gm
Chromium		■				0.12	mg
Cobalt					■	1.45	mg
Crude Fiber			■			11.0	%
Dietary Fiber				■		42.0	%
Fat	■					2.5	%
Iron					■	29.0	mg
Magnesium				■		544	mg
Manganese		■				0.77	mg
Niacin				■		7.90	mg
Phosphorus		■				70.7	mg
Potassium	■					991	mg
Protein		■				10.2	%
Riboflavin	■					trace	mg
Selenium				■		0.15	mg
Silicon			■			0.43	mg
Sodium				■		71.8	mg
Thiamine		■				trace	mg
Tin		■				2.4	mg
Vitamin A	■					trace	IU
Vitamin C		■				trace	mg
Zinc				■		0.18	mg

Traditional Formulas

White Willow and Valerian combination

Chemical Constituents

Astringent compounds
Tannin
Bitter compounds
Harpagoside procumbide and others

Nutrients of Note

Water when fresh: 81%
Water when air dried: 5.3%
Sugars: 6% (fructose, glucose, stachyose, raffinose)

Dong Quai root
Angelica sinensis (Umbelliferae)

Properties: aromatic, uterine tonic, estrogenic, antispasmodic, alterative, liver tonic, hypotensive

Systems Affected: reproductive, structural, circulatory

Folk History and Use

Dong quai ranks next to licorice in frequency of use in Chinese herbal prescriptions. It comes principally from the three western Chinese provinces: Shansi, Shantung and Chili. It is a brown, fleshy root much like gentain root. The odor is very strong, resembling celery, and the taste is sweet, warm and aromatic.

The drug is much used by medical men in China in the **treatment of menstrual, chlorotic** and **purperal diseases of women**. It is used in **hemorrhages** of all kinds, **colds, fluxes, dyspeptic complaints, ague** and a large number of other difficulties. Its name is said to be derived from its asserted power to make the female revert to her husband, and much of its use is due to the wish of women to stimulate their reproductive organs in order to increase their opportunities of bearing children.

Women are highly regarded in Chinese culture. They are considered the spiritual teachers of the family. The well being and strength of women is an area of concern and specific research among the Chinese.

Dong quai is said by the Chinese to **increase blood flow to the reproductive organs of the female**. This makes it useful as a **menstrual balancer, aphrodisiac** and **postpartum healer**.

Dong quai was introduced into Western medicine in 1899 by the Merck company in the form of a liquid extract sold under the name of Eumenol and later in the form of Eumenol tablets. Eumenol was recommended for the treatment of menstrual disorders.

The Chinese believe tang kuei (the phonetic pronunciation of dong quai) is more compatible with vegetables than with fruit. It enjoys a harmonious medicinal relationship with ginger, lovage, marshmallow root, juniper berries, fennel seed and licorice root. It enhances the laxative aspects of rhubarb but doesn't go well with ginseng.

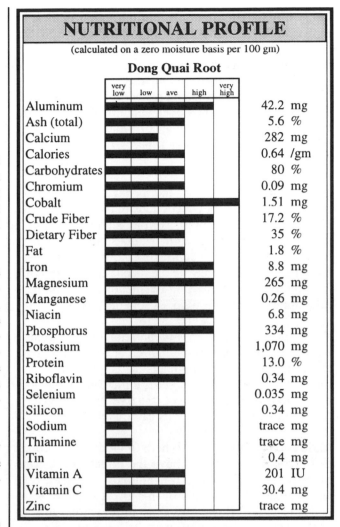

NUTRITIONAL PROFILE
(calculated on a zero moisture basis per 100 gm)

Dong Quai Root

	very low	low	ave	high	very high		
Aluminum						42.2	mg
Ash (total)						5.6	%
Calcium						282	mg
Calories						0.64	/gm
Carbohydrates						80	%
Chromium						0.09	mg
Cobalt						1.51	mg
Crude Fiber						17.2	%
Dietary Fiber						35	%
Fat						1.8	%
Iron						8.8	mg
Magnesium						265	mg
Manganese						0.26	mg
Niacin						6.8	mg
Phosphorus						334	mg
Potassium						1,070	mg
Protein						13.0	%
Riboflavin						0.34	mg
Selenium						0.035	mg
Silicon						0.34	mg
Sodium						trace	mg
Thiamine						trace	mg
Tin						0.4	mg
Vitamin A						201	IU
Vitamin C						30.4	mg
Zinc						trace	mg

The oral use of dong quai has been rejected by conventional medicine, but recent studies have shown its efficacy when injected. The Chinese base many of their claims for dong quai on an acupuncture therapy that involves injection of dong quai extract into the acupuncture point. Used this way, dong quai lowers blood pressure, is a diuretic and contracts (stimulates) smooth muscle, i.e. uterus, intestines and bladder.

Medicinal Properties

Definite Action
Diuretic Action (volatile oil)
Emmenagogue (volatile oil)
Uterine stimulant (volatile oil)
Estrogenic (volatile oil)

The active constituents of dong quai appear to be aromatic volatile oils that affect the uterus, liver, heart, blood pressure and nervous system. These compounds are called sequiterpene lactones and similar compounds are found in many medicinal plants.

Many of the benefits of the oral ingestion of the herb may also be due to its nutritional profile. It contains generous quantities of vitamin E, cobalt and iron. Many reports insist that dong quai contains vitamin B-12, that it is useful for treating **pernicious anemia**, but only lower plants like blue green algae produce vitamin B-12. Dong quai does, however, contain very high quantities of cobalt, a constituent of vitamin B-12. Dong quai, like many emmenagogue herbs, ranks high in iron content.

Dong quai's effects on the uterus have not been documented in humans, but decoctions of the herb do cause contractions on dog uteri. In one study using direct measurement of the myometrium, administration of dong quai enabled the contractions of the uterus to be more orderly. This may be the mechanism underlying its effectiveness in treating dysmenorrhea. The herb does appear to have a weak estrogenic effect.

When mice were fed a 5% preparation of dong quai, it increased the oxygen consumption of the liver without affecting the amount of nucleic acids present. This is thought to be a result of a general increase in metabolism. Dong quai also protects the liver from the effects of harmful chemicals such as carbon tetrachloride.

Various preparations of this herb (including decoctions and alcohol extractions) have the effect of lowering blood pressure in anesthetized animals. When the dosage is small, the duration of this effect is rather short and is usually followed by a rise in pressure. In controlled experiments on rats with artificial atherosclerosis, plaque formation was reduced. Dong quai also shows antibiotic and sedative properties.

Perhaps of most importance to the herbalist is the opposing continuum that exists between dong quai and black cohosh. Most women are benefitted by either one or the other. These two herbs seem to counterbalance each other when used in concert. Conventional science has not discovered how each of these individual herbs work and they cannot fathom how these herbs work when used in tandem.

Suffice it to say, dong quai usually works better with a little black cohosh, and black cohosh works better with a little dong quai. When dong quai predominates in the formula, cramping is relieved and menstrual flow is increased. When black cohosh predominates in the formula, menstrual flow is decreased and swelling is reduced.

Typical Daily Usage

Fresh root: 1-3 tablespoon
Dried root: 2-4 gm
Extract: 3 gm dried root, 15 ml alcohol, 15 ml water

Traditional Formulas

Biota and Zizyphus combination
Cascara and Dong Quai combination
Ginseng and Licorice combination
Papaya and Peppermint combination
Slippery Elm combination
Black Cohosh combination
Black Cohosh and Golden Seal combination
Black Cohosh and Raspberry combination
Raspberry and Dong Quai combination
Dong Quai and Peony combination
Ginger and Dong Quai combination
Bupleurum and Peony combination
Astragalus and Ganoderma combination
Bupleurum and Cyperus combination
Anemarrhena and Astralagus combination
Forsythia and Schizonepeta combination
Eucommia and Achyranthes combination

Chemical Constituents

Aromatic compounds
    Volatile oils: 0.4-0.7%
        Terpenes
            safrol, cadinene and others
        Sequiterpene lactones
            uncharacterized
    Fixed oils and Resin
        Saturated fatty acids
            palmitic, stearic and others
        Unsaturated fatty acids
            linoleic and oleic
Astringent compounds
    Phthalides
    Pseudotannin
    Liguistilide
Bitter compounds
    Saponin
        Sitosterol

Nutrients of Note

Water when fresh: 78.0%
Water when air dried: 9.0%
Sugars: 11 (sucrose, glucose)
Starch: 15%

Echinacea root

Echinacea purpurea (Compositae)

Properties: bitter, immune stimulant, alterative, antimicrobial, vasodilator sialagogue, analgesic

Systems Affected: immune, respiratory, digestive

Common Names: purple coneflower, black sampson

Folk History and Use

Echinacea is an annual herb that grows two or three feet high and native to the central and southwest United States. It has a purple flower and long hairy leaves. It is distinguished from other species of echinacea by the color of its flower and the size and shape of its root.

As early American settlers moved west in the early 1800's, they discovered Native Americans like the Kiowa tribe, who chewed on the root, swallowing the juice for relief of respiratory complaints. The Native Americans also considered it an aphrodisiac and analgesic of sorts that would give one more courage, stamina, tolerance to pain, etc. Echinacea was used as part of bravery rituals to help one better endure pain or hardship. The Native Americans valued echinacea not unlike the Chinese valued ginseng. The use of echinacea was quickly picked up by American settlers who gave it a prominent place in various alcoholic-based tonics.

The term "snakeroot" is a common synonym for echinacea, spun off from "snake oil" salesman who advertised it as a cure for snake bites. The origin of the "snakeroot" is often indicated in the echinacea of commerce as "Kansas snake root" or "Missouri snakeroot," etc., but all native snakeroots are one of two or three species of echinacea that are difficult to distinguish medicinally.

Another member of the compositae family, parthenium integrifolia, is also difficult to distinguish from the echinacea species and has often been substituted as the herb of commerce. This substitution has occurred for over a century since the e chinacea species were over harvested and exported to European markets in the late 19th century. The resulting derth of echinacea was filled by mixing parthenium with echinacea.

These two plants are distinguished by the color of their flowers. Echinacea has a purple flower while parthenium has a white flower.

Is it unclear at this time whether the medicinal value of echinacea exceeds that of parthenium, since the herb

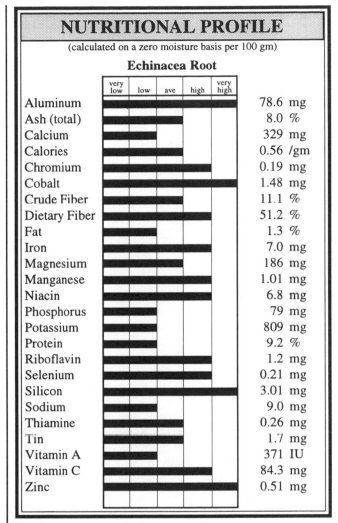

NUTRITIONAL PROFILE
(calculated on a zero moisture basis per 100 gm)

Echinacea Root

	very low	low	ave	high	very high	
Aluminum					■	78.6 mg
Ash (total)		■				8.0 %
Calcium		■				329 mg
Calories			■			0.56 /gm
Chromium		■				0.19 mg
Cobalt					■	1.48 mg
Crude Fiber			■			11.1 %
Dietary Fiber					■	51.2 %
Fat		■				1.3 %
Iron			■			7.0 mg
Magnesium				■		186 mg
Manganese			■			1.01 mg
Niacin				■		6.8 mg
Phosphorus		■				79 mg
Potassium			■			809 mg
Protein		■				9.2 %
Riboflavin				■		1.2 mg
Selenium			■			0.21 mg
Silicon					■	3.01 mg
Sodium		■				9.0 mg
Thiamine			■			0.26 mg
Tin		■				1.7 mg
Vitamin A			■			371 IU
Vitamin C			■			84.3 mg
Zinc		■				0.51 mg

sold as echinacea for the past fifty years has been almost entirely parthenium integrifolia.

The circumstances and confusion surrounding parthenium and echinacea is akin to the differences between panax and eleuterococcus ginsengs. They are different plants with similar folk uses. Parthenium is discussed fully elsewhere in this work. The name echinacea is derived from the Greek "echinos" or hedgehog in reference to its spine-like fruiting conehead.

Echinacea was listed in the National Formulary until 1950 and is still listed in the Homeopathic Pharmacopia. It is used primarily to treat disorders of the blood, such as **poisonous bites of insects and snakes, gangrene, carbuncles** and **abscesses**.

Recent studies show echinacea to have **immuno stimulant, antiviral, antiexudative, anti-inflammatory,** bacteriostatic and fungistatic properties. In practical use today, echinacea is used primarily to build resistance to infections of the respiratory and digestive tracts.

Medicinal Properties

Definite Action
  Immune stimulant (echinacin)
  Antimicrobial (echinacin)
  Sialagogue (echinacin)
  Expectorant (echinacin)
The benefits of viscous fiber (inulin)
    Lowers bowel transit time
    Absorbs toxins in the bowel
    Regulates colonic bacteria
Probable Action
  Anti-inflammatory (?)
Possible Action
  Antitumor (?)
  Digestive aid (?)

The proven actions of echinacea are due to water-soluble polysaccharides. They act by sequestering the attacks of various microbes and allow the body to heal itself. Upon reaching an infected area, the polysaccharides have an immunostimulant effect, which results in the production of leucocytes (white blood cells). The resulting phagocytic action of the leucocytes effectively eradicates a number of infectious organisms.

In addition, the polysaccharides exert a more specific effect on bacteria that secrete hyaluronidase such as streptococcus. The polysaccharide is able to form a complex with hyaluronidase in the same manner that viscous fiber absorbs toxins from the bowel. This prevents the bacteria from dissolving the intracellular glue and disrupting the cells. It is important to note that the polysaccharides are probably not absorbed into the bloodstream and are only effective when they physically come in contact with an infected area. This is why echinacea is most effective when used as the Native Americans did (i.e. as a poultice externally on infected areas and chewing slowly, swallowing the juice allowing the polysaccharides to coat the affected area of the throat or digestive tract).

Modern dosage forms such as lozenges, ointments and debittered extracts would facilitate convenience and palatability, but would produce no greater results than the Native Americans achieved.

The polysaccharides have also been shown to have antiviral activity, but the mode of action is obscure. The 1907 Merck Index lists echinacea as an aphrodisiac and analgesic. An extract was applied to the penis to alleviate impotence and sexual disfunction. This claim is probably due to the above-mentioned antimicrobial action acting upon venereal and other infections resulting from poor hygiene. As the infections cleared, one would have less pain in urination, etc. and thus more sexual pleasure.

Other actions of echinacea are less confirmed scientifically, but are worth mentioning:

1. The volatile oils contain polyacetylenes that show antibacterial and antifungal activity, but are probably lost in the drying and grinding processes. Their effects would only be available when using fresh roots.

2. A diene olefin has shown antitumor activity in vivo in mice, but no human testing has been performed.

3. Flavonoids present in echinacea may produce an antispasmodic effect on the respiratory and digestive tracts.

4. If the polysaccharides were absorbed systematically, many other infectious diseases would be affected by the use of echinacea. However, no evidence for this exists.

Typical Daily Usage

Fresh root: 1-2 tablespoon
Dried root: 3 gm
Extract: 3 gm dried root, 15 ml alcohol, 15 ml water

Traditional Formulas

Goldenseal and Bugleweed combination
Goldenseal and Echinacea combination

Chemical Constituents

Aromatic compounds
  Essential oil: 0.25%
    Polyacetylenes
    Echinacein
  Resin: 2%
    Betaine
    Echinacoside
Bitter compounds
  Flavonoids
Mucilaginous compounds
  Polysaccharrides
    Echinacin
    Gum: 8%
    Inulin:17%

Nutrients of Note

Water when fresh: 74.9%
Water when dried: 4.6%
Starch:12%

Elecampane root
Inula helenium (Compositae)

Properties: aromatic, anthelmintic, bactericidal, fungicidal, expectorant, sedative

Systems Affected: digestive, respiratory

Common Names: elf dock, scabwort, velvet dock, aunee

Folk History and Use

Elecampane is a perennial herb native to Europe and Asia that has been naturalized and grows throughout most of the temperate climates of North America. The herb is covered with soft hairs and grows up to five feet high. It possesses a starchy root made up primarily of the complex carbohydrate inulin from which its genus name is derived.

3% of elecampane root is an essential oil containing sesquiterpene lactones which account for most of its physiologic activity.

It has traditionally been used as an **expectorant** to treat **respiratory disorders** including **asthma and bronchitis,** and as a **vermifuge, bactericide** and **fungicide**.

Medicinal Properties

> Definite action
> Expectorant (inulin)
> The benefits of viscous fiber (inulin)
> Lowers bowel transit time
> Soothes inflamed tissue
> Regulates colonic flora
> Vermifuge (essential oil)
> Bactericide (essential oil)
> Fungicide (essential oil)

Elecampane contains an essential oil that consists primarily of sequiterpene lactones that have been successfully used as **anthelmintics** and for their **bactericidal** and **fungicidal** properties. This makes the herb useful for treating **diarrhea, dysentary** and **yeast infections of the bowel**.

The root also contains the complex carbohydrate inulin. This starchy material swells and forms a slippery suspension when mixed with digestive fluids. Marshmallow and burdock roots also contain a large proportion of inulin.

It is not surprising to find elecampane used for many of the same disorders as the other mucilaginous roots.

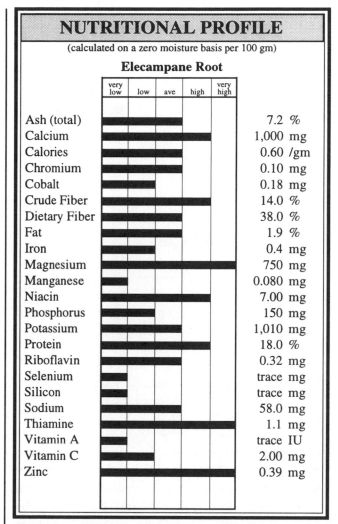

NUTRITIONAL PROFILE
(calculated on a zero moisture basis per 100 gm)

Elecampane Root

	very low	low	ave	high	very high		
Ash (total)						7.2	%
Calcium						1,000	mg
Calories						0.60	/gm
Chromium						0.10	mg
Cobalt						0.18	mg
Crude Fiber						14.0	%
Dietary Fiber						38.0	%
Fat						1.9	%
Iron						0.4	mg
Magnesium						750	mg
Manganese						0.080	mg
Niacin						7.00	mg
Phosphorus						150	mg
Potassium						1,010	mg
Protein						18.0	%
Riboflavin						0.32	mg
Selenium						trace	mg
Silicon						trace	mg
Sodium						58.0	mg
Thiamine						1.1	mg
Vitamin A						trace	IU
Vitamin C						2.00	mg
Zinc						0.39	mg

The inulin **sooths the lining of the digestive tract** and provides the benefits of viscous fiber. It also apparently elicits a **sympathetic expectorant response** to mucous membranes of the respiratory system.

Typical Daily Usage

Fresh root: 1-2 tablespoon
Dried root: 2-3 gm
Extract: 3 gm dried root, 20 ml alcohol, 10 ml water

Traditional Formulas

Elecampane combination

Chemical Constituents

Aromatic compounds
Essential oil
Sesquiterpene lactones

alantolactone and others
Bitter compounds
   Saponins
     Stigmasterol, sitosterol and others
Mucilaginous compounds
   Polysaccharides
     Inulin: 45%

Nutrients of Note

Water when fresh: 78%
Water when air dried: 6.1%

Ephedra herb
Ephedra sinica (Ephedraceae)

Properties: bitter, stimulant, diaphoretic, expectorant, astringent

Systems Affected: circulatory, respiratory, glandular

Folk History and Use

Ma haung, the common Chinese name for ephedra, is one of the most powerful medicinal plants. It is highly regarded in Chinese herbology, where it has been used for over 5,000 years to treat colds, coughs, fevers (including malaria), headaches and skin eruptions.

Its genus name, ephedra, comes from the Greek words "epi" upon and "edra" seat, since the plant climbs and grows upon rocks.

In Chinese characters, "ma" means astringent and "haung" means yellow, probably in reference to its taste and color. Ephedra is very easy to classify in both the Western and Chinese systems. Under the Chinese philosophy, ma haung is "yang" and provides a warming effect to the surface systems of the body (i.e. limbs, skin).

To the Western herbalist, ephedra is a classic bitter herb, since its bitter taste is provided by the active principle (alkaloids).

The habitat of ephedra is not confined to southern China, where it is found near the seacoast, but physiologically active species are also found in northwestern India, Tibet and Pakistan. Formerly, China supplied most of the American market until the 1950's when Pakistan became the sole exporter of ephedra for pharmaceutical use. Since the early 1980's, China has re-entered the international herb market and made ephedra more readily available and considerably less expensive.

NUTRITIONAL PROFILE
(calculated on a zero moisture basis per 100 gm)

Ephedra Herb

Nutrient	Value	Unit
Aluminum	6.3	mg
Ash (total)	5.6	%
Calcium	439	mg
Calories	0.62	/gm
Carbohydrates	81.7	%
Chromium	trace	mg
Cobalt	0.40	mg
Crude Fiber	9.8	%
Dietary Fiber	31.9	%
Fat	1.9	%
Iron	2.1	mg
Magnesium	211	mg
Manganese	0.54	mg
Niacin	9.0	mg
Phosphorus	323	mg
Potassium	1,320	mg
Protein	10.8	%
Riboflavin	1.1	mg
Selenium	0.12	mg
Silicon	0.31	mg
Sodium	43.0	mg
Thiamine	4.7	mg
Tin	1.1	mg
Vitamin A	6,211	IU
Vitamin C	72.1	mg
Zinc	0.21	mg

Today, Chinese ephedra is used in most decongestant formulas and to promote thermogenesis. Thermogenesis is the body's way of maintaining its body temperature. It does this by burning brown fat. Brown fat is located around your kidneys and near your sternum. This is survival fat and accounts for 15% of your caloric usage daily. This is 50% more than the caloric usage due to exercise. By promoting thermogenesis, more calories are burned and little physical effort is required. Chinese ephedra can raise your body temperature about one degree. This act will burn 45 pounds of calories in a year. Chinese ephedra is potentized by xanthines, meaning caffeine and cocao. This property is the basis of many weight loss programs.

Medicinal Properties

Definite Action
Vasoconstrictor, heart stimulant(alkaloids)
Bronchodilator (alkaloids)
Diuretic (alkaloids)
Contracts the uterus (ephedrine)
Mydriatic -- contracts the pupil (ephedrine)
Increases thermogenesis (ephedrine)

Few plants in the past century have attracted so much attention in Western medicine and herbology as ephedra. Ephedra and its active constituent, ephedrine, were popularized at the University of Peking in 1924 and promoted as a **decongestant** and **anti-asthmatic** agent. Scientists also showed that ephedrine was a **cardiac stimulant** and a **central nervous system stimulant**. In keeping with the philosophy of allopothy, chemical methods were employed to synthesize ephedrine, which resulted in the discovery of an entire new class of drugs, amphetamines.

Amphetamine-containing inhalers were very popular in the mid-1900's for the relief of nasal congestion and depression associated with influenza. Today, however, such inhalers are strictly controlled.

Ephedrine hydrochloride and pseudoephedrine both work when taken orally and, unlike amphetamines, are available without a prescription. Pseudoephedrine tablets (Sudafed, Contac, Primatene, and Bronkaid) are presently over-the-counter remedies for the relief of nasal congestion.

Ephedrine is a **vasoconstrictor** (vasopressor) and at the same time has a stimulant effect on the heart muscle, **increasing circulation and blood pressure**. This **forces more blood to the peripheral blood vessels** (i.e. brain and limbs), and provides a **stimulant action on the brain and nerve centers**, thus **reducing fatigue and weariness**. This effect also makes ephedra popular as a dieter's herb. As blood flow is diverted from the digestive tract to the limbs, **hunger instincts are lessened**. This property is most effective when ephedra is taken on an empty stomach, otherwise digestion in progress is merely slowed and indigestion can occur.

Ephedrine is also a **bronchodilator**, used in cases of **asthma, hay fever** and **emphysema** and as an aid to **relieve swollen mucous and sinus membranes**.

Ephedrine is known also for its **diuretic** action, its ability to **contract the uterus** and as a **mydriatic** (dilates the pupil) in the form of an eyewash.

Psuedoephedrine is similar to ephedrine, but it exhibits a more potent **diuretic** effect and no ability to contract the uterus. The alkaloids are quickly absorbed from the gastrointestinal tract and are unchanged when passed through the liver.

The alkaloids of ephedra do exhibit toxic properties with a minimum lethal dose of 500 mg per kilogram body weight (ephedrine) in adults. The Chinese prepare the herb by first removing the stem nodes, which are considered toxic for reasons other than their alkaloid content. Care should be exercised in the use of this plant when treating anyone, especially those with yin conditions (weak internal organs) or those with hypertension or heart conditions.

Typical Daily Usage

Fresh herb: 2-4 tablespoon
Dried herb: 3-6 gm
Extract: 4.5 gm dried herb, 22 ml alcohol, 23 ml water

Traditional Formulas

Pinellia and Citrus combination
Ephedra and Passionflower combination
Ephedra and Senega combination

Chemical Constituents

Astringent compounds
Tannins
Bitter compounds
Alkaloids: 0.8-2.5%
Ephedrine: 30-90% of total alkaloids
Pseudoephedrine: 5-20% of total alkaloids
Six other enantiomers and isomers of ephedrine

Nutrients of Note

Water when fresh: 79%
Water when air dried: 7.2%

Eyebright
Euphrasia officinalis (Scrophulariaceae)

Properties: astringent, alterative, hepatonic

Systems Affected: digestive, circulatory, eyes

Folk History and Use

No historical writings refer to eyebright until the 1400's, even though the herb was available to early Greek and Arab physicians like Dioscorides and Galen.

Eyebright is a native European annual herb. Its genus name, Euphrasia, is derived from the Greek "euphrosyne" meaning gladness in reference to its use in cleansing the eyes. It was popularized by medieval medical practitioners who probably assigned its use as an eye medicine from the Doctrine of Signatures:

> The purple and yellow spots and stripes which are upon the flowers of the eyebright doth very much resemble the diseases of the eye, as bloodshot, etc., by which signature it hath been found out that this herb is effectual for the curing of the same.

Few scientific studies have been performed on eyebright to determine its activity. Yet it remains in high esteem among Western herbalists for its use as an eyewash. Recently, the internal consumption of the herb has been popularized by the notion that eyebright has a stimulant, cleansing effect on the liver that is somehow indirectly beneficial to the eye. Some claim that this cleansing action on the liver releases stores of vitamin A in the blood, which in turn finds its way to the eye. It is highly unlikely the eye could be strengthened in this manner. Its function as an eyewash is due to its **antimicrobial**, volatile oil content and **astringent** tannins.

Medicinal Properties

    Definite Actions
        Antibacterial (volatile oils)
        Astringent (tannins)
    Possible Actions
        Hepatonic (?)

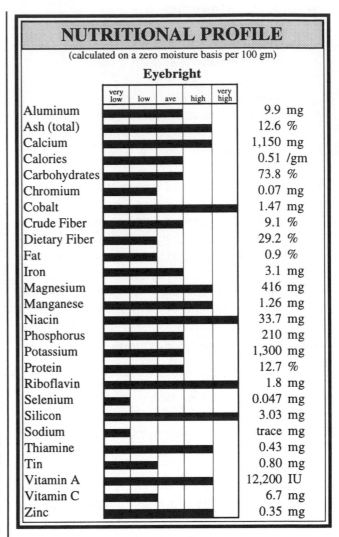

NUTRITIONAL PROFILE
(calculated on a zero moisture basis per 100 gm)
Eyebright

	very low	low	ave	high	very high	
Aluminum						9.9 mg
Ash (total)						12.6 %
Calcium						1,150 mg
Calories						0.51 /gm
Carbohydrates						73.8 %
Chromium						0.07 mg
Cobalt						1.47 mg
Crude Fiber						9.1 %
Dietary Fiber						29.2 %
Fat						0.9 %
Iron						3.1 mg
Magnesium						416 mg
Manganese						1.26 mg
Niacin						33.7 mg
Phosphorus						210 mg
Potassium						1,300 mg
Protein						12.7 %
Riboflavin						1.8 mg
Selenium						0.047 mg
Silicon						3.03 mg
Sodium						trace mg
Thiamine						0.43 mg
Tin						0.80 mg
Vitamin A						12,200 IU
Vitamin C						6.7 mg
Zinc						0.35 mg

Eyebright is a **blood purifier** that **enhances liver function**. Chinese philosophy gives every part of the universe an opposite. The liver is the internal organ that matches the eye as an external organ of the body. Therefore, any herb that strengthens the liver must also strengthen the eye.

Eyebright is similar, but much weaker in action, to golden seal when it comes to its use as an eyewash. It contains **astringent** and **antibiotic** principles that are useful for cleansing the eye. Systemic effects such as stimulation of the liver to release vitamin A are unfounded scientifically.

Typical Daily Usage

Fresh herb: 1/4-1/2 cup
Dried herb: 6-12 gm
Extract: 9 gm dried herb, 45 ml alcohol, 45 ml
water

Traditional Formulas

Eyebright combination

Chemical Constituents

Astringent compounds
Tannin
Pseudotannin
Resin (aucubin)
Bitter compounds
Flavonoids
Quercetin

Nutrients of Note

Water when fresh: 84.6%
Water when air dried: 7.8%

Fennel seed

Foeniculum vulagare (Umbelliferae)

Properties: aromatic, antispasmodic, carminative, diuretic, expectorant, stimulant, anti-inflammatory, antimicrobial

Systems Affected: digestive, urinary, respiratory

Folk History and Use

The Latin name for hay, "foenum," gave rise to both the scientific name and English name of this member of the carrot family. This plant is very pretty, with delicate, highly divided leaves and bright yellow flowers produced in large, flat, terminal umbells. The foliage, depending on the variety, can be bright green, red or purple. It is a native of Italy and is one of the most ancient cultivated plants.

Its use spread with civilization, especially from the Roman colonizing efforts centered in Italy. Pliny had twenty-two uses for fennel, but the most popular was as a flavoring for saltwater fish. Its culinary properties are to whiten, tenderize and deodorize the fish and stimulate the secretion of digestive fluids in one's stomach.

The odor of fennel seed is fragrant, the taste is warm, sweet and agreeable. The seed of commerce are frequently graded as longs and shorts. The longs are premium. Commercial fennel varies in quality, partly because of the care taken during harvest, but also because the product is very often adulterated. Care must be taken to ensure the seed has not been exhausted (the

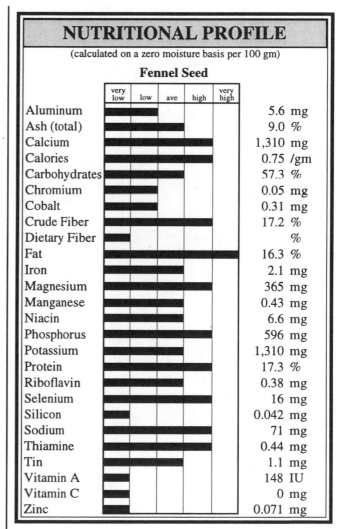

NUTRITIONAL PROFILE
(calculated on a zero moisture basis per 100 gm)
Fennel Seed

	very low	low	ave	high	very high		
Aluminum						5.6	mg
Ash (total)						9.0	%
Calcium						1,310	mg
Calories						0.75	/gm
Carbohydrates						57.3	%
Chromium						0.05	mg
Cobalt						0.31	mg
Crude Fiber						17.2	%
Dietary Fiber							%
Fat						16.3	%
Iron						2.1	mg
Magnesium						365	mg
Manganese						0.43	mg
Niacin						6.6	mg
Phosphorus						596	mg
Potassium						1,310	mg
Protein						17.3	%
Riboflavin						0.38	mg
Selenium						16	mg
Silicon						0.042	mg
Sodium						71	mg
Thiamine						0.44	mg
Tin						1.1	mg
Vitamin A						148	IU
Vitamin C						0	mg
Zinc						0.071	mg

oil removed), and that dirt, weed seed and other filth make the product unusable.

Fennel, in addition to being a kitchen herb and flavoring, is a **carminative** and acts to **depress the appetite**. In ancient times, it was believed that fennel had the power to restore sight. During medieval times, it was considered a magic herb and was hung over doors to repel witches and devils. Persisting to this day is the Western belief that it conveys **longevity, strength and courage**. The Chinese use fennel in a similar manner as in the West. It is also used as a **poultice for snake bites.**

Medicinal Properties

Definite Actions
Antimicrobial (volatile oils)
Antispasmodic (flavonoids)
Probable Actions
Carminative (volatile oils)
Increased gastric secretions (volatile oils)
Regulation of intestinal flora (volatile oils)
Diuretic (volatile oils)
Expectorant (volatile oils)

The volatile oils are responsible for most of the medicinal properties in fennel. The **carminative** action is primarily explained by **stimulation of the gastrointestinal mucous membrane**. This in turn **stimulates the pancreas to increase its secretions** and results in better and quicker **digestion** of food and less flatulence. The stimulated mucous membrane also results in the production of mucous which acts to isolate intestinal flora from oligosaccharides and other feed stock used by bacteria to produce gas.

The **expectorant, diuretic** and **general tonic** (stimulant) properties are also described as irritations which stimulate specific purging of organs. The mechanism of its **spasmolytic effect on smooth muscles** is probably due to its flavonoid content, and has been shown to be efficacious in studies with experimental animals. Many essential oils in fennel are **antimicrobial**. Alpha-pinene, for example, found in fennel is a major constituent of turpentine.

Typical Daily Usage

Fresh seed: 2-6 teaspoon
Dried seed: 1-3 gm
Extract: 2 gm dried seed, 10 ml alcohol, 10 ml alcohol

Traditional Formulas

Cascara and Dong Quai combination
Chickweed and Cascara combination
Senna combination
Ginger and Barberry combination
Papaya and Peppermint combination
Ginseng combination
Licorice and Red Beet combination
Dandelion and Barberry combination
Chamomile and Passionflower combination
Fenugreek combination

Chemical Constituents

Aromatic compounds
Volatile oil: 2-6%
Terpenes
anethole: 60-80%
fenchone: 10-15%
estragole, pinenes and others
Fixed oils and Resins: 9-28%
Unsaturated fatty acids
petroselenic, oleic, linoleic, vitamin E
and others
Bitter compounds
Saponins
Stigmasterol
Flavonoids (antispasmodic principles)
quercitin-3-glucuronide
rutin
isoquercitrin
quercitin-3-arabinoside
kaempferol-3-arabinoside
Coumarins (antithrombotic principles)
umbelliferone

Nutrients of Note

Water when fresh: 89.2%
Water when air dried: 8.8%

Fenugreek seed

Trigonella foenum-gracum (Leguminoseae)

Properties: mucilaginous, expectorant, tonic, astringent, demulcent, emollient

Systems Affected: digestive, respiratory, urinary

Folk History And Use

Fenugreek is an herb esteemed by the Greek, Roman and Egyptian societies for its culinary and medicinal virtues. Because fenugreek is native to southern Eurasia, its use spread with the expansion of Western civilization. Early Egyptians prepared a thick paste by soaking fenugreek seeds in water. This was used to prevent fevers, sooth stomach disorders and to treat diabetics. This practice is in common use to this day. In addition, the preparation is often used as an antibiotic or disinfectant.

In India , its culinary virtues make it an important ingredient in curry powders.

Fenugreek was first introduced to the Chinese in the Sung Dynasty (ca 1057 A.D.). The Chinese have since used fenugreek to treat kidney ailments, beri beri and male problems such as impotence.

Fenugreek extracts are used by farmers to flavor damaged hay, since the flavor is much enjoyed by cattle.

The species name, foenum gracum, is the Greek "hay from Greece," from which the common name fenugreek is derived. Its genus name, Trigonella, comes from the Greek "three sides" in reference to its flowers.

The most common uses of fenugreek today are culinary, such as providing a maple flavor for confectioneries. It is also used in commercially prepared spices.

In addition, some of its folk medicine properties have been studied and substantiated. One such study (Lloydia 39, #6) showed that an alcohol extract of the seeds could possibly be used as an **oral hypoglycemic** agent since it significantly **lowered blood glucose** levels in rats.

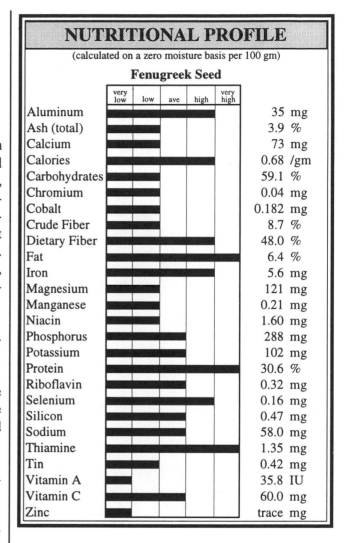

NUTRITIONAL PROFILE
(calculated on a zero moisture basis per 100 gm)

Fenugreek Seed

	very low	low	ave	high	very high	value	unit
Aluminum						35	mg
Ash (total)						3.9	%
Calcium						73	mg
Calories						0.68	/gm
Carbohydrates						59.1	%
Chromium						0.04	mg
Cobalt						0.182	mg
Crude Fiber						8.7	%
Dietary Fiber						48.0	%
Fat						6.4	%
Iron						5.6	mg
Magnesium						121	mg
Manganese						0.21	mg
Niacin						1.60	mg
Phosphorus						288	mg
Potassium						102	mg
Protein						30.6	%
Riboflavin						0.32	mg
Selenium						0.16	mg
Silicon						0.47	mg
Sodium						58.0	mg
Thiamine						1.35	mg
Tin						0.42	mg
Vitamin A						35.8	IU
Vitamin C						60.0	mg
Zinc						trace	mg

In folk medicine today, fenugreek is most commonly used for its **expectorant** properties. Like the other mucilaginous herbs, it causes the mucosa of the bowel to increase the production while decreasing the viscosity of protective fluid. This response in the digestive system triggers a **sympathetic response** in the other mucous membranes of the body. This is particularly noted in the **respiratory and urinary systems**.

It is usually a key component of **lung healing** and **expectorant** formulas. It seems particularly suited to relieving the symptoms of **allergies** such as **hay fever** and in resolving the **unproductive coughs** often found in humid climates.

Medicinal Properties

Definite Action
- The benefits of viscous fiber
  - Lowers bowel transit time
  - Absorbs toxins from digestive tract
  - Balances intestinal flora
  - Demulcent effect on digestive tract
- Hypoglycemic (alkaloids)
- Uterine stimulant (saponins)
- Antimicrobial (flavonoids)
- Antispasmodic (flavonoids)
- Expectorant (mucilage)

Fenugreek seeds are very nutritious and contain a wide variety of chemical constituents. The major effects of this seed are due to its mucilage content which causes it to swell in water and provides a source of viscous fiber. The seeds are rich in fixed oils which are often compared to cod liver oil preparations as it contains choline and vitamin A. These constituents (especially choline) oxidize to produce a distinct fishy odor.

Alkaloids consisting mainly of trigonelline, gentianine and corpine provide much of the flavor of roasted fenugreek. Trigonelline provides a **hypoglycemic** effect in rats but is converted to niacin and other pyridines and pyrroles when it is cooked.

Fenugreek also contains saponins and sapogenins consisting of diosgenin and yamogenin, which are starting materials for the synthesis of steroid hormones and related drugs. Agriculturists are looking at the potential of cultivating fenugreek for this purpose, since it is an annual herb and the time between planting and harvest is much shorter than for wild yam (dioscorea) species.

The saponin content of wild yam and fenugreek have been the source of much folklore since many have purported the idea that the saponins are somehow turned into steroids in the digestive tract and supply a natural anti-inflammatory agent. This, however, is not possible as the saponins are absorbed intact, provide a stimulation of the uterus and are oxytocic. The purpose of the human digestive tract is to break down molecules, not synthesize them.

The protein in fenugreek is high in lysine and tryptophan and low in sulfur-containing amino acids. Like most seeds, it contains energy concentrates of fats and phosphorus. It also contains generous quantities of iron.

Typical Daily Usage

Fresh seed: 1/4-1/2 cup
Dried seed: 6-12 gm
Extract: 9 gm dried seed, 45 ml alcohol, 45 ml water

Traditional Formulas

Gentain and Cascara combination
Fenugreek combination
Fenugreek and Thyme combination
Marshmallow and Fenugreek combination

Chemical Constituents

Aromatic compounds
- Fixed oils and Resins: 5%

Bitter compounds
- Saponins: 0.6-1.7%
  - Diosgenin, yamogenin, tigogenin, neotigogenin
- Alkaloids: 0.1-0.3%
  - Trigonelline, gentianine, carpaine

Flavonoids
- Vitexin, quercitin, luteolin

Mucilaginous compounds
- Polysaccharides: 15-28%
  - Galactomannan

Nutrients of Note

Water when fresh: 87%
Water when air dried: 8.4%
Sugars: 13% (glucose, arabinose, galactose)
Starch: 15%

Feverfew leaf

Chrysanthemum parthenium (Compositae)

Properties: bitter, anti-inflammatory, analgesic, tranquilizer, emmenogogue

Systems Affected: circulatory, nervous, structural

Common Names: feather few, febrifuge plant, featherfoil, pyrethrum

Folk History and Use

Feverfew is a flowering herb cultivated throughout the United States and Europe for its ornamental properties. Its common name feverfew is apparently a corruption of the word febrifuge in reference to its folk use as a fever reducer. During the Middle Ages, it was used to minimize the hang-over resulting from alcohol or opium use.

Early European settlers in America noticed that insects would not eat feverfew or even land on the plant. These astute observers subsequently planted it as a border and insecticide for their vegetable gardens.

Feverfew has been used to treat most of the same disorders treated by aspirin. It is most noted for its use in treating **migraine headaches, fever** and **arthritis**. Folk literature is so pointed about its effectiveness that it has caught the attention of scientists who have defined its chemistry and medicinal action to a great extent. Today, it is popularly used as a preventor of migraine headaches. It is also used to treat **menstrual pain, dysmenorrhea, asthma, inflammatory skin conditions** and **arthritis**.

Medicinal Properties

Definite action
    Anti-inflammatory (parthenolide)
    Prostaglandin antagonist (parthenolide)
    Antithrombotic (parthenolide)
    Serotonin inhibitor (parthenolide)

Feverfew leaf is rich in a group of chemicals called sesquiterpene lactones, parthenolide being the predominant one. These bitter compounds have a variety of physiologic effects that substantiate most of the folk uses of the leaf. They have been shown to **inhibit pros-**taglandin synthesis, decrease the rate at which blood clots, inhibit histamine and enzyme release from immune cells** and have a **mild sedative effect**. If you were to describe the action of common aspirin, you could use nearly the same language.

Prostaglandins are often associated with pain and inflammation. Platelet aggregation or blood clotting is thought to play a role in at least some migraine headaches. Histamine is associated with inflammation. Counteracting these conditions make the folk uses for feverfew reasonable.

Even though the physiologic results are similar, the parthenolides in feverfew do not work by the same method as salicylates and this has led investigators into

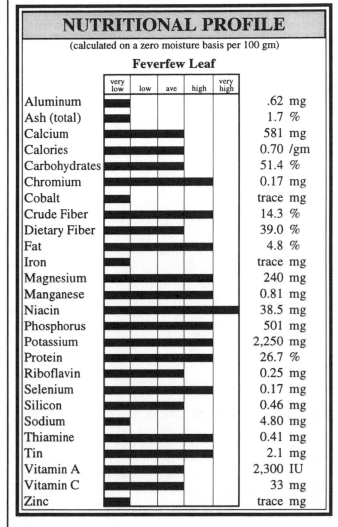

NUTRITIONAL PROFILE (calculated on a zero moisture basis per 100 gm) Feverfew Leaf	very low	low	ave	high	very high	
Aluminum	■					.62 mg
Ash (total)	■					1.7 %
Calcium	■	■				581 mg
Calories	■	■	■			0.70 /gm
Carbohydrates	■	■	■			51.4 %
Chromium	■	■	■	■		0.17 mg
Cobalt	■					trace mg
Crude Fiber	■	■	■	■		14.3 %
Dietary Fiber	■	■	■			39.0 %
Fat	■	■				4.8 %
Iron	■					trace mg
Magnesium	■	■	■			240 mg
Manganese	■	■				0.81 mg
Niacin	■	■	■	■	■	38.5 mg
Phosphorus	■	■	■	■		501 mg
Potassium	■	■	■	■		2,250 mg
Protein	■	■	■			26.7 %
Riboflavin	■	■				0.25 mg
Selenium	■	■	■	■		0.17 mg
Silicon	■	■	■	■		0.46 mg
Sodium	■					4.80 mg
Thiamine	■	■	■	■		0.41 mg
Tin	■	■	■	■		2.1 mg
Vitamin A	■	■	■			2,300 IU
Vitamin C	■	■				33 mg
Zinc	■					trace mg

an in depth study on its action to combat and prevent **migraine headaches**, an area in which aspirin is not always effective.

Finally, when one sees such a correlation between the action of this leaf and salicylates one must question the use of feverfew by pregnant women and very young children.

Typical Daily Usage

Fresh leaf: 1/4-1/2 teaspoon
Dried leaf: 0.2-0.4 gm
Extract: 0.3 gm dried leaf, 2 ml alcohol, 1 ml water

Traditional Formulas

Chamomile and Passionflower combination

Chemical Constituents

Aromatic compounds
  Essential oil
    Sesquiterpene lactones (bitter taste)
      Parthenolide and others
  Terpenes
    Camphor, l-borneol and others

Nutrients of Note

Water when fresh: 82%
Water when air dried: 5.8%

Garlic bulb
Allium sativum (Liliaceae)

Properties: aromatic, alterative, stimulant, diaphoretic, expectorant, antispasmodic, nervine, carminative, vulnerary

Systems Affected: circulatory, immune, respiratory, digestive

Folk History and Use

If the saying is true, "an apple a day keeps the doctor away," then garlic must be an apple. Garlic is a strongly scented perennial herb whose medicinal virtues are published worldwide in both folk and scientific literature.

"Allium" was the ancient Latin name for garlic. The English name is derived from "gar," a lance and "lac," a plant, in reference to the shape of the leaves. A close relative of the onion, garlic has an underground bud (bulb) which is divided into several distinct bulblets or cloves. This member of the lily family has a long written history of use in culinary, mystical and medicinal literature. The characteristic odor is the source of most of its notoriety.

A Moslem tradition says when Satan stepped out of the Garden of Eden after Adam's expulsion, garlic sprang up from under his left foot. The Egyptians took oaths in the name of garlic, the ancient Greeks gave offerings of garlic to their god, Hectare.

The odor of garlic has been responsible for many cultural and culinary restrictions. Horace, an ancient Greek writer, called it "more poisonous than hemlock." In ancient Greece, a person who smelled of garlic was

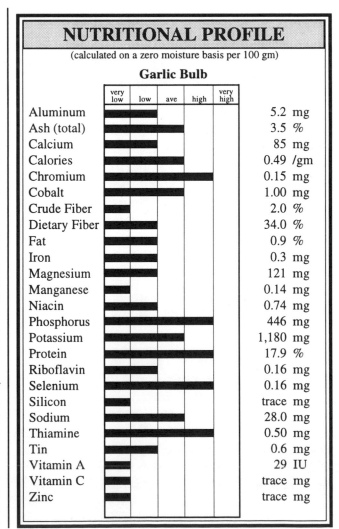

NUTRITIONAL PROFILE
(calculated on a zero moisture basis per 100 gm)

Garlic Bulb

	very low	low	ave	high	very high		
Aluminum		▓				5.2	mg
Ash (total)		▓				3.5	%
Calcium		▓				85	mg
Calories		▓				0.49	/gm
Chromium				▓		0.15	mg
Cobalt					▓	1.00	mg
Crude Fiber		▓				2.0	%
Dietary Fiber				▓		34.0	%
Fat		▓				0.9	%
Iron		▓				0.3	mg
Magnesium			▓			121	mg
Manganese	▓					0.14	mg
Niacin		▓				0.74	mg
Phosphorus				▓		446	mg
Potassium			▓			1,180	mg
Protein			▓			17.9	%
Riboflavin		▓				0.16	mg
Selenium		▓				0.16	mg
Silicon	▓					trace	mg
Sodium			▓			28.0	mg
Thiamine				▓		0.50	mg
Tin		▓				0.6	mg
Vitamin A	▓					29	IU
Vitamin C	▓					trace	mg
Zinc		▓				trace	mg

denied entrance into the temples of Cybele. The Romans attributed their success in conquering the world to garlic because "no invader would come into the country that smelled so strong." An old herbal, <u>Cole's Art of Simpling</u>, reports that if a garden is infested with moles, garlic will simply make them "leap out of the ground presently." Hungarian jockeys fasten cloves of garlic on the bridles of their horses with the belief that other horses, upon smelling the garlic, will fall behind.

The Neriades in ancient Greece, who worshipped a phallic-serpent god that seduced unprotected husbands, could be guarded against by displaying garlic. The Scandinavian mythical female, Huldra Talle-Maja, whose powers captured a woman's husband, was tricked into revealing the property of garlic she used to keep a bull from wandering off at night.

Hippocrates (460 B.C.), known as the father of medicine, used garlic for a variety of infections and intestinal disorders as well as for wounds, toothaches, leprosy, epilepsy and chest pains.

Aristotle (384 B.C.) said of garlic, "it is a cure for hydrophobia and tonic, is hot, laxative but bad for the eyes."

Disocorides, who lived in the first century A.D. and was a surgeon and physician in the Roman armies, described garlic with regard to the Doctrine of Signatures, in which the medicinal properties of the plant were revealed symbolically by its outward form. A plant such as garlic, with a long hollow stalk, would be good for all diseases of the windpipe. The following text is from <u>The Greek Herbal of Disocorides</u>, translated by J. Berendes:

> If eaten, garlic helps eliminate the tapeworm, it drives out the urine. It is good against snake bite with wine, or when crushed in wine. It is good against the bite of a rabid dog. It makes the voice clear, soothes continuous coughing, when eaten raw or boiled. Boiled with oregano it kills lice and bed bugs. <u>It clears the arteries.</u> Burnt and mixed with honey, it heals white skin spots, herpetic eruptions, liver spots, leprosy and scurvy. Boiled with pine wood and incense, it soothes toothache when solution is kept in the mouth...boiling the umbrel flower is good for a sitzbath to help the coming of menstruation and placenta. It is helpful for dropsy.

The Roman author and poet, Virgil (70-19 B.C.), knew that garlic was "essential to maintain the strength of harvesters" and garlic was valued as a tonic for the endurance of extreme temperatures while working in the fields.

Galen (131-200 A.D.), called garlic Poor Man's Treacle or Heal All. Pliny, the Roman naturalist, listed 61 diseases for which garlic was an effective treatment.

The Israelite slaves upon fleeing Egypt, disappointed in the diet of manna, wept saying, "We remember the fish which we were wont to eat in Egypt for nought; the cucumbers and the melons, and the leeks, onions and garlic" (Numbers 11:5).

The Talmud, the repository of Jewish civil and religious law, instructed the use of garlic and onion skin in the treatment of wounds and inflammation, and particularly for gynecological and menstrual disturbances. It is also mentioned in the "Ten Regulations of Ezra" as an aphrodisiac, "to eat garlic on Friday because of its salutary action."

In spite of its strong odor, garlic is used widely in food. The pungent, acrid volatile oils are generally driven off during cooking by various methods. The remaining fixed oils provide a distinct pleasant taste to many entrees, particularly in Mediterranean and mid-eastern cultures.

Garlic has been widely studied by chemists. Many **antibiotic, hypocholesterolemic, hypotension** and **antithrombotic** principles have been isolated from the bulb.

Unlike many herbs, there is a near consensus of opinion on the value of garlic in the diet from both culinary artists and medical practitioners.

In order to overcome the disagreeable odor of garlic, various methods have been proposed, tested and marketed to remove the odor without removing the virtues of the bulb.

The odorless garlic business focuses on removing or modifying allicin and related sulfur-containing compounds in garlic. One Japanese firm touts a patented anaerobic aging process by which alliinase is complexed so allicin cannot be produced. This process takes 18 months and results in an expensive product which is not truly odorless.

Most American manufacturers of odorless garlic products use various extraction and complexing processes to rid garlic of its unpleasant, bitter odor and taste, while leaving the pleasant odor behind. Most attempt to complex the allicin with ascorbic or citric acids. These products work by releasing allicin in the stomach so the odor is not concentrated on the breath. However, hard gelatin capsules or enteric coatings will give the same effect.

Despite the claims, proven or unproven, two facts remain. First, alliin, allicin and other sulfur-containing compounds have been shown to be active antimicrobial, hypotensive, antithrombotic, hypoglycemic and hypocholesterolemic agents. Second, they stink!

Medicinal Properties

Definite Action
Antimicrobial (allicin)
Antifungal (allicin)
Paraciticidal (allicin)
Antithrombotic (allicin)
Vasodilator (allicin)
Expectorant (allicin)
Digestive aid (allicin)
Hypoglycemic (allicin)
Hypocholesterolemic (allicin)
Hypolipidemic (allicin)
Immune stimulant (allicin)
Probable Action
Antitumor (?)
Circulatory stimulant(?)

Recently, scientific research has confirmed many of the traditional medicinal claims for garlic.

Garlic has been found to be effective in treating a myriad of conditions in the **circulatory, urinary, respiratory** and **digestive tracts** by a remarkably simple mechanism. Its vast arsenal of sulfur-containing volatile oils are readily absorbed and transported throughout the body (except through the brain blood barrier).

Unlike proteinaceous and polysaccharide drugs, garlic's oils can be effective against **infections** nearly anywhere in the body, which accounts for garlic's versatility. Thus, garlic is effective against conditions in the circulatory system by **lowering blood sugar, blood lipids, free cholesterol, low density lipoproteins** and **blood pressure** while at the same time **raising high density lipoproteins.**

In the circulatory system, it **eases bronchial secretions** making it useful in the treatment of **asthma**.

In the urinary system, volatile oils stimulate (by irritation) the cleanse by purge mechanism of the kidneys, which results in a **greater flow of urine.**

In the digestive system, garlic **stimulates the production of bile** and thus aids digestion.

The close chemical relationship of certain sulfur and selenium complexes has led researchers to look for anticancer links in the sulfur-containing molecules of garlic, using mechanisms already established for selenium as a starting point.

Ajoene, a trisulfide, has been shown to **increase the clotting time in blood** and thus **antithrombotic.**

Uncut garlic has much less odor than cut garlic because of the enzymatic process which occurs when it is cut. The enzyme, alliinase, which upon contact with alliin, forms the odorous allicin or garlic odor. In the live plant, the alliinase is separated from alliin. When the plant is disturbed (i.e. cut or bruised), the scent is produced. An instinct not unlike that of a skunk.

Recent reseach shows garlic to be an effective **immune stimulant**. When combined with anerobic exercise, garlic has shown to **increase the quantity, longevity and killing power of natural killer cells ten fold**.

On top of all these properties, garlic produces a **wide spectrum antimicrobial** effect on gram positive and gram negative bacteria fungus and certain worms.

A final word on the odor. Many employ chlorophyll to absorb the odor of garlic on the breath after a meal. Italians traditionally use chlorophyll rich parsley sprigs after an entree of garlic-rich food.

Typical Daily Usage

Fresh bulb: 1/4-1/2 cup
Dried bulb: 6-12 gm
Extract: 9 gm dried bulb, 45 ml alcohol, 45 ml water

Traditional Formulas

Capsicum and Garlic combination
Garlic combination
Hawthorn combination
Ginseng and Saw Palmetto combination
Golden Seal and Juniper combination

Chemical Constituents

Aromatic compounds
Volatile oil: 0.1-0.4%
Alliin (present in uncut garlic)
Allicin, Ajoene, and others
Terpenes
Citral, geraniol, and linalool
Fixed oil and resin:0.7-1.2%

Nutrients of Note

Water when fresh: 63.0%
Water when air dried: 5.4%
Sugars: 14% (glucose, maltose, fructose)
Starch: 8%

Gentain root

Gentiana lutea (Gentainaceae)

Properties: bitter, bitter tonic, anti-inflammatory, appetite stimulant

Systems Affected: digestive

Folk History and Use

Gentain root is the most famous bitter tonic in Western folk medicine. The plant is a perennial herb that produces a cluster of large yellow flowers. Folk legend holds that these yellow flowers are a sign that the plant will stimulate the production of bile. It is native to the alpine climates of the European Alps. Its roots range in color from light tan to dark brown. The darker roots are valued over the lighter roots and contain higher quantities of bitter constituents.

Gentain is most famous for its bitter taste. It is used as a flavoring in alcoholic bitters and vermouth. These drinks are customarily served before the evening meal to get the digestive juices flowing. A bitter tonic **stimulates the appetite, improves digesion by increasing the production of digestive enzymes and fluids and tones the tissues of the digestive tract**. Indeed, extracts of gentain have exhibited **strong anti-inflammatory action** in animal studies.

Gentain has traditionally been used to treat **chronic stomachache, gastritis, diarrhea, nausea, heartburn, anorexia, jaundice, throat inflammations** and **arthritis.**

Medicinal Properties

Definite action
Bitter tonic (bitter principles)
Anti-inflammatory (bitter principles)

Gentain has a characteristic bitter taste that is derived from a number of bitter glycosides. Care must be taken when harvesting the plant since its bitter principles degrade when dried too slowly. Its bitter principles include amarogentin and gentiopicrin. Amarogentin, when isolated in its pure form, is one of the most bitter substances known to man.

In addition, the root contains a group of alkaloids including gentisein, gentialutine and several xanthones.

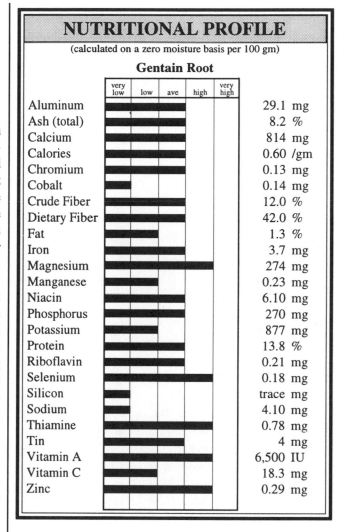

NUTRITIONAL PROFILE
(calculated on a zero moisture basis per 100 gm)

Gentain Root

	very low	low	ave	high	very high	
Aluminum						29.1 mg
Ash (total)						8.2 %
Calcium						814 mg
Calories						0.60 /gm
Chromium						0.13 mg
Cobalt						0.14 mg
Crude Fiber						12.0 %
Dietary Fiber						42.0 %
Fat						1.3 %
Iron						3.7 mg
Magnesium						274 mg
Manganese						0.23 mg
Niacin						6.10 mg
Phosphorus						270 mg
Potassium						877 mg
Protein						13.8 %
Riboflavin						0.21 mg
Selenium						0.18 mg
Silicon						trace mg
Sodium						4.10 mg
Thiamine						0.78 mg
Tin						4 mg
Vitamin A						6,500 IU
Vitamin C						18.3 mg
Zinc						0.29 mg

All these compounds contribute to the medicinal effects of the root. Studies confirm that consuming gentain extracts before eating **increases the production of digestive fluids and bile.**

Typical Daily Usage

Fresh root: 1/2-1 teaspoon
Dried root: 0.25-0.5 gm
Extract: 0.5 gm dried root, 3 ml alcohol, 2 ml water

Traditional Formulas
Gentain and Cascara combination
Ginseng combination
Dandelion and Parsley combination

Chemical Constituents

Aromatic compounds
    Volatile oil
Bitter compounds
    Bitter principles
        Amarogentin, gentiopicrin,
        gentiopicroside, swertiamarin
Alkaloids
    Gentianine, gentialutine and others
Flavonoids
    gentisein, gentisin and others

Nutrients of Note

Water when fresh: 78%
Water when air dried: 5.7%
Sugars: 10% (glucose)
Starch: 16%

Ginger root
Zingiber officinale (Zingiberaceae)

Properties: aromatic, diaphoretic, stimulant, carminative, anti-inflammatory, analgesic

Systems Affected: digestive, circulatory, structural

Common Names: Canada snake root, Indian ginger, Vermont snakeroot

Folk History and Use

Ginger is a reed-like plant that is native to the coastal region of India. It has been cultivated there since before written history began. The first mention being made in China about 400 B.C. The plant has since been naturalized and is cultivated in Jamaica, China, India, Africa and the West Indies. The Greeks and Romans used it as a spice.

Marco Polo reported seeing it in China between 1280 and 1290 A.D., and it was a particularly popular import item in Europe from the 11th to 13th centuries. Later, the Spaniards introduced the plant into the West Indies, and by 1547, it was so widely cultivated there that it was exported back to Spain. The British prize Jamaican ginger above all other, making unbleached Jamaican ginger their pharmacopeal standard.

Its generic name come from the Greek "zingiberis" and Arabic "zindschebil" or root of zindschi (India), which is interpreted "known already to the ancients." Its common name, ginger, is derived from the Sanskrit "gringa" or horn and "vera" meaning body, in reference to the shape of the root.

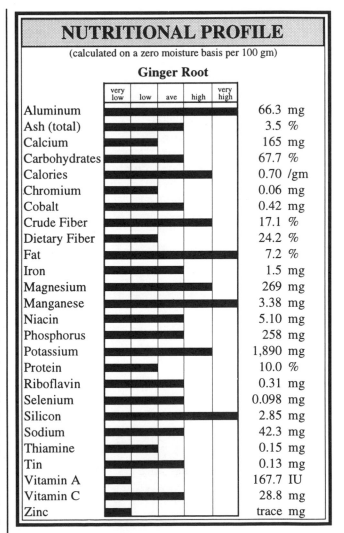

NUTRITIONAL PROFILE
(calculated on a zero moisture basis per 100 gm)

Ginger Root

	very low	low	ave	high	very high		
Aluminum						66.3	mg
Ash (total)						3.5	%
Calcium						165	mg
Carbohydrates						67.7	%
Calories						0.70	/gm
Chromium						0.06	mg
Cobalt						0.42	mg
Crude Fiber						17.1	%
Dietary Fiber						24.2	%
Fat						7.2	%
Iron						1.5	mg
Magnesium						269	mg
Manganese						3.38	mg
Niacin						5.10	mg
Phosphorus						258	mg
Potassium						1,890	mg
Protein						10.0	%
Riboflavin						0.31	mg
Selenium						0.098	mg
Silicon						2.85	mg
Sodium						42.3	mg
Thiamine						0.15	mg
Tin						0.13	mg
Vitamin A						167.7	IU
Vitamin C						28.8	mg
Zinc						trace	mg

The most popular use of ginger today is by the food industry where it is classed as a flavor and used in the manufacture of ginger ale and ginger beer, candies, pastries and cakes.

Folk medicine has used ginger to treat **indigestion, flatulence, diarrhea** and **loss of appetite**. It is considered **carminative, aphrodisiac, tonic, aperative** and **stomachic, especially for convalescents**. Teas have been made for **indigestion, stomach ache, malaria** and **fever**.

The Chinese value ginger as a **stimulating diaphoretic** and always add ginger to meat dishes to detoxify the meat. They use ginger externally to remove the heat of painful, inflamed and stiff joints. An oil extract of ginger is used in massage therapy for the treatment of **dandruff** and for **earaches**.

A study in The Lancet (March 2, 1982) showed ginger to be effective in treating **motion sickness**. Two gelatin capsules of ginger are more effective than 100 mg of dimenhydrinate (dramamine), an over-the-counter motion sickness remedy. To use ginger in this manner, take two capsules approximately 20-25 minutes before taking off in an airplane or boarding a ship and thereafter every 4 hours.

A favorite personal use of ginger is to place 2-3 tablespoonsful in a hot tub of water. This really relaxes my muscles and **relieves body pain**. It helps if you place the powdered ginger in a large tea bag so you don't have floaties in the bath with you.

Medicinal Properties

Definite Action
    Carminitive (essential oil)
    Hypocholesterolemic (essential oil)
    Diaphoretic (essential oil)
    Anti-inflammatory (essential oil)
    Analgesic (topically) (essential oil)
Probable Action
    Hypoglycemic (essential oil)
Possible Action
    Hallucinogen (?)

The volatile oils, oleo resins and proteolytic enzymes in ginger are **digestive stimulants** which trigger the production of digestive fluids. This helps combat the effects of **overeating, improper chewing or excessive motion** by helping to make the digestive process more efficient, **increasing gastric motility** and **neutralizing toxins and acids in the digestive tract**. This **carminative** action has been widely recognized for centuries and is the basis for most of its medicinal use.

The volatile oils are also stimulants that produce effects on the circulatory system, including **diaphoretic** action and **vasomotor stimulus**. The folk use of ginger in rheumatism remedies apparently has some basis as ginger is **hypocholesterolemic**, both to serum cholesterol and cholesterol stored in the liver. This makes ginger a **blood purifier** in folk terms. This may also help rid the body of other toxins that contribute to the inflammatory diseases.

The fresh juice of ginger has the ability to **reduce serum glucose levels** in test animals and may have use as a **hypoglycemic** agent, although its mode of action is obscure.

Finally, the phenolic oleo resins and volatile oils are also antimicrobial (antihelmintic and bactericidal).

Legends about hallucinogenic properties associated with ginger root are based on the consumption of ginger just before bedtime, but are as yet unsubstantial. Ginger has a longer shelf life than most aromatic herbs because of its protective root bark.

Typical Daily Usage

Fresh root: 2-4 tablespoon
Dried root: 3-6 gm
Extract: 4.5 gm dried root, 22 ml alcohol, 23 ml
    water

Traditional Formulas

Garlic combination
Agastache and Shengu combination
Cascara combination
Cascara and Dong Quai combination
Ginger combination
Senna combination
Ginger and Barberry combination
Ginseng and Licorice combination
Papaya and Peppermint combination
Slippery Elm combination
Black Cohosh combination
Black Cohosh and Golden Seal combination
False Unicorn and Golden Seal combination
Raspberry and Dong Quai combination
Ginger and Dong Quai combination
Bupleurum and Peony combination
Fushen and Dragon Bone combination
Bupleurum and Cyperus combination

Pinellia and Citrus combination
Bayberry and Ginger combination
White Willow and Valerian combination
Alisma and Hoelen combination
Ginseng and Parsley combination

Chemical Constituents

Aromatic compounds
  Essential oil: 1-3%
    Terpenes
      zingiberene, bisabolene, zingiberol,
      zingiberenol and others
  Fixed Oils and Resins:6-8%
    Lecithins and phosphatidic acid

Saturated fatty acids
  lauric, palmitic, stearic
Unsaturated fatty acids
  linoleic, oleic
Astringent compounds
  Oleo resin (phenolic pungent principles)
    gingerol, shogaols, zingerone

Nutrients of Note

Water when fresh: 93.0%
Water when air dried: 6.7%
Starch: 50-60%
Sugars: 8% (glucose, sucrose, fructose, raffinose)

Ginkgo leaf
Ginkgo biloba (Ginkgoaceae)

Properties: bitter, peripheral vasodilator, circulatory stimulant, antioxidant

Systems affected: circulatory, nervous

Common Names: maidenhair

Folk History and Use

Ginkgo is commonly called the maidenhair tree. It is commonly planted throughout the United States as an ornamental tree. During the Ice Age, it appears that the ginkgo tree was extincted in all but the central part of China. Fossils of the tree have been found from the Permian period of geologic time, making the species over 200 million years old. It has reached its popularity in ornamental horticulture because of its resistance to atmospheric and water pollution, insects and disease. It is also a long lived tree, reaching ages of 1,000 years. It grows to a height of over 100 feet and its leaves resemble a fan after which it developed its common maidenhair name. Its almond-like seed is used by oriental herbalists to **improve reproductive organ function** and to **treat respiratory ailments.**

Ginkgo leaf has a rich folk history for treating **poor circulation**. The shape of the leaf with its many fan segments were thought by early herbalists to represent the many vessels of the circulatory system poised for maximum circulation. The longevity of the tree itself

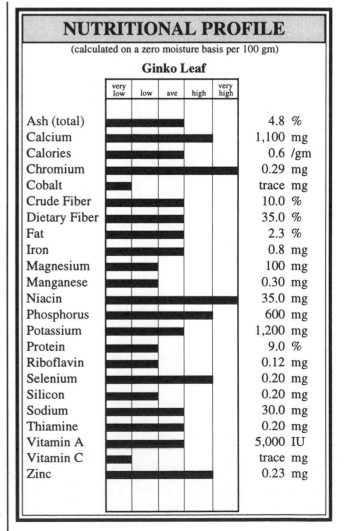

NUTRITIONAL PROFILE
(calculated on a zero moisture basis per 100 gm)

Ginko Leaf

	very low	low	ave	high	very high	Value	
Ash (total)						4.8	%
Calcium						1,100	mg
Calories						0.6	/gm
Chromium						0.29	mg
Cobalt						trace	mg
Crude Fiber						10.0	%
Dietary Fiber						35.0	%
Fat						2.3	%
Iron						0.8	mg
Magnesium						100	mg
Manganese						0.30	mg
Niacin						35.0	mg
Phosphorus						600	mg
Potassium						1,200	mg
Protein						9.0	%
Riboflavin						0.12	mg
Selenium						0.20	mg
Silicon						0.20	mg
Sodium						30.0	mg
Thiamine						0.20	mg
Vitamin A						5,000	IU
Vitamin C						trace	mg
Zinc						0.23	mg

and its ability to resist pollution and disease give it special place with folk practitioners. These observations alone point herbalists to its potential uses. Standardized concentrates of the bitter principles in ginkgo are sold all over the world but most especially in Europe and Japan. Studies have shown it to be effective in **increasing peripheral blood flow**. This makes it especially useful in treating **age related brain disorders, cerebral and vascular insufficiency, Raynaud's disease, chronic bronchitis, emphsyma** and to **prevent strokes**.

Medicinal Properties

Definite action
Peripheral vasodilator (bitter principles)
Inhibits platelet aggregation (bitter principles)
Antioxidant (bitter principles)

Ginkgo has demonstrated remarkable ability to **improve peripheral circulation**. All the anti-aging effects of better circulation go along with this ability: **increased energy, antioxidant effects, decreased blood clotting, better concentration, improved hearing** and others.

No one quite knows how it accomplishes its feats but its action is attributed to a group of bitter compounds that include flavonoids, hetersides and anthocyanidines. It is especially popular as a **longevity** drug in Japan and is gaining popularity in the United States as the population ages. Its active principles seem to wear off after six to eight hours so small doses are recommended three times a day for maximum effect. Ginkgo is currently being studied and shows promise in cases of dementis and Alzheimer's disease.

Typical Daily Usage

Fresh leaf: 1-2 tablespoon
Dried leaf: 2-3 gm
Extract: 2 gm dried leaf, 10 ml alcohol, 10 ml water

Traditional Formulas

Ginkgo and Hawthorne combination
Ginseng and Phaffia combination

Chemical Constituents

Aromatic compounds
Volatile oil
Terpenes
Astringent compounds
Tannin
Bitter compounds
Flavonoids
Ginkgo heterosides
pro-Anthocyanidines
Flavones: (sciaopitysin, ginkgetin, bilobetin, ginkgolic acid and others)

Nutrients of Note

Water when fresh: 76%
Water when air dried: 6.8%

Golden Seal root
Hydrastis canadensis (Ranunculaeae)

Properties: bitter, stimulant, antiseptic, alterative, diuretic, emmenagogue, astringent, hepatonic

Systems Affected: digestive, respiratory, glandular, circulatory

Common Names: yellow puccoon, ground raspberry, tumeric root, yellow root, orange root

Folk History and Use

Golden seal is an herb native to the eastern half of the North American continent. It grows in rich, shady woods, mainly in the mountains of North and South Carolina and the Appalachian highlands of Kentucky, Tennessee and West Virginia. Recently it is has been cultivated in the state of Washington. Golden seal is fast becoming rare in the wild and in most places must now be cultivated.

Its botanical name, hydrastis, is derived from the Greek "hydor" water and "aste" native, referring to its growing in moist places. The botanical name also could be derived from "hydor" water and "drao" to act, referring to the active principles of the drug.

Written history on golden seal begins in the 16th century when pioneers encountered Native Americans chewing it for mouth ulcers.

In Appalachia, a root tea is used as a tonic and to improve the appetite. A water infusion of the root was used by Indians and pioneers to treat watering eyes, which was probably hay fever. Powdered roots were applied over open cuts and wounds to encourage the formation of scabs. Appalachian Cherokees mixed this same powder with bear grease and rubbed it on the skin as an insect repellent. It was also used by the Cherokees as a cure for external cancers, although there is little modern evidence to support this practice. An infusion of leaves was also used to treat liver and stomach ailments.

The Native Americans used golden seal for many ailments and called it yellow root because of its bright

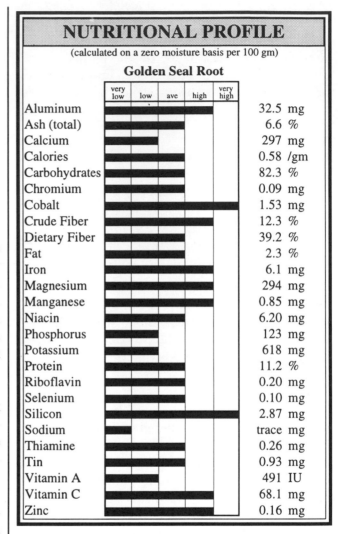

NUTRITIONAL PROFILE
(calculated on a zero moisture basis per 100 gm)

Golden Seal Root

	very low	low	ave	high	very high		
Aluminum						32.5	mg
Ash (total)						6.6	%
Calcium						297	mg
Calories						0.58	/gm
Carbohydrates						82.3	%
Chromium						0.09	mg
Cobalt						1.53	mg
Crude Fiber						12.3	%
Dietary Fiber						39.2	%
Fat						2.3	%
Iron						6.1	mg
Magnesium						294	mg
Manganese						0.85	mg
Niacin						6.20	mg
Phosphorus						123	mg
Potassium						618	mg
Protein						11.2	%
Riboflavin						0.20	mg
Selenium						0.10	mg
Silicon						2.87	mg
Sodium						trace	mg
Thiamine						0.26	mg
Tin						0.93	mg
Vitamin A						491	IU
Vitamin C						68.1	mg
Zinc						0.16	mg

yellow color. Golden seal was also used as a yellow dye for their clothes. In 1860, golden seal was declared an official drug in the U.S. Pharmacopoeia.

Medicinal Properties

Definite Action
   Vasoconstrictor (alkaloids)
   Increased bile production (alkaloids)
   Antibiotic (alkaloids)
   Astringent (alkaloids)
Probable Action
   Hypoglycemic (?)
   Hepatonic (?)
Possible Action
   Emmenagogue (?)

Golden seal's **vasoconstricting** effect makes it helpful as a bitter tonic to **tone mucous membranes**, especially for **gastric disturbances, cases of difficult or painful digestion** and in **nose bleeds** or other cases of **hemorrhages** and **bleeding**, such as from the pelvic tissues. It is excellent for **cleansing the eye** and in treating **conjunctivitis**.

Murine, a commercial eye preparation, formerly contained hydrastine hydrochloride and berberine chloride, the major alkaloids of golden seal. These salts are **hemostatic** and help constrict the eye reddening blood vessels that often result from irritated eyes. These alkaloids also act as **uterine stimulants**, although the mechanism of action is obscure.

While used mainly for its effect on the mucous membranes, this herb has favorable influences on all parts of the body. It is known to **improve the appetite** and **assist digestion** by **stimulating the production of bile**. It has been found valuable in cases of **stomach ulcers** and, in general, **aid to the nervous system**. The remainder of the therapeutic value of golden seal is due to its **antibiotic** effects. This has been shown to be effective against staphylococcus aureus and E. coli bacteria. Golden Seal is widely used to treat **infections of all kinds**.

In combination with bicarbonate of soda, this herb is excellent as a **mouthwash** and for **relief of sores in the mouth and the gums**. Used by itself, it is recommended for alleviating **pyorrhea**. Golden seal has also been used by doctors for **ulcers in the vagina and uterus**, as well as for **eczema** and **smallpox**.

Golden seal is one of the most rapidly effective of all herbal remedies. It is frequently recommended for the blisters of **herpes simplex**, especially in the genital area, as it seems to be able to **heal damaged or infected tissues**.

Herbalists have long claimed that golden seal exerts a **hypoglycemic** effect on the blood. This claim has not been investigated scientifically, but is deeply rooted in folk tradition. The tradition follows that golden seal is a male herb since many more women than men suffer from hypoglycemia.

Because of its long-term effect (2 months) on the intestinal flora, the use of golden seal should be alternated with bacteria supplements of friendly flora like lactobacillus acidophilus.

Typical Daily Usage

Fresh root: 1-2 tablespoon
Dried root: 1.5-3 gm
Extract: 2 gm dried root, 10 ml alcohol, 10 ml water

Traditional Formulas

Garlic combination
Capsicum and Myrrh combination
Cascara and Dong Quai combination
Gentain and Cascara combination
Ginger combination
Comfrey combination
Black Cohosh combination
Black Cohosh and Golden Seal combination
False Unicorn and Golden Seal combination
Golden Seal and Juniper combination
Eyebright combination
Golden Seal and Bugleweed combination
Parthenium and Golden Seal combination
Chamomile and Rose Hips combination
Ephedra and Senega combination
Cedar Berry combination
Ginseng and Parsley combination

Chemical Constituents

Astringent compounds
  Tannin - gallic acid
Bitter compounds
  Alkaloids: 5.5-7.0%
    Isoquinoline alkaloids
      berberine (0.5-6.0%), hydrastine
      (1.5-4%), canadine (0.25%) and others

Nutrients of Note

Water when fresh: 72.3%
Water when air dried: 7.9%
Sugars: 7% (fructose, galactose, glucose, sucrose, inositol)
Starch: 10-18%

Gotu Kola leaf
Centella asiatica (Umbelliferae)

Properties: bitter, alterative, antipyretic, brain tonic, nervine, diuretic

Systems Affected: nervous, urinary, circulatory

Folk History and Use

Gotu Kola is grown widely throughout the tropical areas of the world. It is commonly referred to as a creeping weed in most areas and is used as a ground cover in Java and Ceylon to retard soil erosion.

It is one of the most widely used herbs in ayurvedic (Indian) medicine, where it is used as a **nerve tonic** and for all ailments of the mind and nerves, including **epilepsy, schizophrenia** and **memory loss**.

The Chinese value gotu kola more as a plant that **increases longevity** and **brain capacity** than for any other purpose. An Indian proverb has been translated and reads: "A leaf or two a day will keep old age away."

Interest in gotu kola began with modern scientists investigating its use in longevity and brain capacity and found that gotu kola is of great value in **fever** and **inflammatory conditions**. It has been used for centuries to treat scrofulous skin diseases like **leprosy, syphlitic skin diseases** and **ulcers**. The Indians also value it for the treatment of **dysentery, ulcers, cholera, fever, headaches** and **stomach aches**.

Medicinal Properties

    Definite Action
        Antibacterial (saponins)
        Antifungal (saponins)
        Vulnerary (saponins)
        Antiulcer (flavonoids)
        Anti-inflammatory (flavonoids)
        Sedative (saponins)
    Probable Action
        Diuretic (volatile oil)
        Antispasmodic (flavonoids)
    Possible Actions
        Antifertility (?)
        Brain tonic (?)

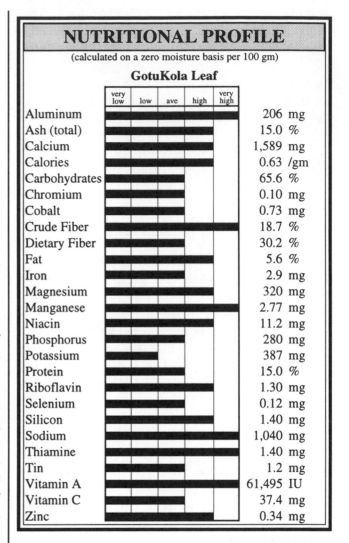

NUTRITIONAL PROFILE
(calculated on a zero moisture basis per 100 gm)
GotuKola Leaf

Nutrient	Value
Aluminum	206 mg
Ash (total)	15.0 %
Calcium	1,589 mg
Calories	0.63 /gm
Carbohydrates	65.6 %
Chromium	0.10 mg
Cobalt	0.73 mg
Crude Fiber	18.7 %
Dietary Fiber	30.2 %
Fat	5.6 %
Iron	2.9 mg
Magnesium	320 mg
Manganese	2.77 mg
Niacin	11.2 mg
Phosphorus	280 mg
Potassium	387 mg
Protein	15.0 %
Riboflavin	1.30 mg
Selenium	0.12 mg
Silicon	1.40 mg
Sodium	1,040 mg
Thiamine	1.40 mg
Tin	1.2 mg
Vitamin A	61,495 IU
Vitamin C	37.4 mg
Zinc	0.34 mg

The most active constituents of gotu kola are the triterpene saponins asiaticoside, Brahmoside and Brahminoside. Asiaticoside, in particular, exhibits the wide range of **antibiotic** activity of the herb. It has been found to be **bactericidal, fungicidal, ameobacidal, insecticidal** and **syphlitic skin diseases**.

As with all saponins, the mode of action is to weaken membranous tissues. By partially dissolving cell walls, various microbes become easier to kill. Therefore, it is used in scrofulous diseases like **leprosy**, where the saponins can, in this case, break down the waxy covering of the leprosy bacillis so they become susceptible to the body's immune system.

Asiaticoside is a **cell proliferant** and speeds wound healing by **stimulating mitosis** (cell division). It is thus useful in treating **gastric** and **duodenal ulcers**. Because it stimulates mitosis, asiaticoside has been classed as a possible carcinogen by some researchers.

The volatile oils produce a **diuretic** and **blood purifying** effect by producing a purge stimulus in the kidneys. The volatile oils also contain cholesteremic steroids like Beta-sitosterol that helps **lower serum cholesterol levels.**

Flavonoids present in the herb also produce **antispasmodic** effects on smooth muscles.

Gotu kola extracts are spermicidal to mice and this antifertility property is possible in humans, but not as yet demonstrated.

Because of the presence of the glycosides, Brahmoside and Brahminoside some sources indicate that massive doses of gotu kola can produce narcotic effects. The evidence for this effect is sketchy at best and is controversial. No toxic effects are listed in the British Herbal Pharmacopoeia, and gotu kola is considered to be quite safe by nearly all herbalists.

Typical Daily Usage

Fresh leaf: 1/4 cup
Dried leaf: 6 gm
Extract: 6 gm dried leaf, 30 ml alcohol, 30 ml water

Traditional Formulas

Chickweed and Cascara combination
Black Cohosh combination
Ginseng and Saw Palmetto combination
Ginseng and Phaffia combination
Ginseng and Gota Kola combination
Pollen and Ginseng combination

Chemical Constituents

Aromatic compounds
Volatile oil: 0.3-0.6%
Terpenes
beta-farnesene,germacrene,
beta-elemene, bicycloelemene and
others
Bitter compounds
Saponins: 0.25%
Asiaticoside, brahmoside, madecassoside
and others
Mucilaginous compounds
Pectin: 6%

Nutrients of Note

Water when fresh: 89.3%
Water when air dried: 7.8%
Sugars: 9% (glucose, rhamnose, inositol)

Gymnema leaf
Gymnema sylvestre (Asclepiadaceae)

Properties: bitter, hypoglycemic

Systems Affected: glandular, digestive

Folk History and Use

Gymnema is a tree native to Africa and India. It is now common throughout the world and is very popular in India and Japan. Its leaves have the unique ability to block out one's sense of sweetness when chewed. Granulated sucrose tastes like sand after chewing gymnema leaves. Sour, astringent and pungent tastes are not blocked by the herb, and the effect lasts 1-2 hours.

Its ability to block sweet tastes apparently led to the folk legend that gymnema could block the absorption of ingested carbohydrates (every dieter's dream). This claim has not been proven, but lunching after gymnema is quite disgusting to the palette. Gymnema is commonly used in **diet** formulas for these reasons.

Gymnema has been an important part of Ayurvedic medicine for some time and is one of the most popular herbal preparations sold in Japan today.

Its history and use is solely based on the management of blood sugar disorders like **diabetes**. Clinical studies show that it has proven ability to lower one's blood sugar.

Medicinal Properties

> Definite action
>   Hypoglycemic (gymnemin)
> Possible action
>   Appetite suppressant (?)

Gymnema owes its hypoglycemic properties to gymnemin and a group of related bitter compounds. Its mode of action has yet to be determined, but it probably works by increasing the efficiency with which insulin is released from stores in the body and by making individual cells in the body more sensitive to insulin. This last mechanism, if proven, would be very important to insulin dependent diabetics who build up an insulin tolerance over time.

Typical Daily Usage

> Fresh leaf: 1-2 tablespoon
> Dried leaf: 2-3 gm
> Extract: 2 gm dried leaf, 10 ml alcohol, 10 ml water

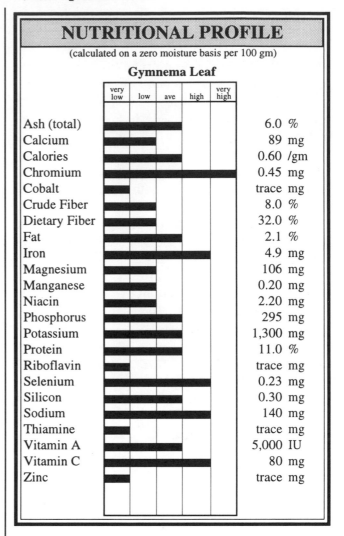

NUTRITIONAL PROFILE
(calculated on a zero moisture basis per 100 gm)

Gymnema Leaf

	very low	low	ave	high	very high		
Ash (total)						6.0	%
Calcium						89	mg
Calories						0.60	/gm
Chromium						0.45	mg
Cobalt						trace	mg
Crude Fiber						8.0	%
Dietary Fiber						32.0	%
Fat						2.1	%
Iron						4.9	mg
Magnesium						106	mg
Manganese						0.20	mg
Niacin						2.20	mg
Phosphorus						295	mg
Potassium						1,300	mg
Protein						11.0	%
Riboflavin						trace	mg
Selenium						0.23	mg
Silicon						0.30	mg
Sodium						140	mg
Thiamine						trace	mg
Vitamin A						5,000	IU
Vitamin C						80	mg
Zinc						trace	mg

Traditional Formulas

> Gymnema combination

Chemical Constituents

> Astringent compounds
>   Tannin
> Bitter compounds
>   Gymnemin and others

Nutrients of Note

> Water when fresh: 81%
> Water when air dried: 6%

Hawthorn berries
Crataegus oxycantha (Rosaceae)

Properties: bitter, cardiac tonic, diuretic, astringent, sedative

Systems Affected: circulatory, digestive

Folk History and Use

Hawthorn is a bushy, spiny shrub or small tree that produces brilliant red clusters of berries which are harvested in the fall. They are used in marmalades and jellies, and as an additive to flour in some parts of Africa and as a **heart tonic** by herbalists.

Hawthorn is native to the Mediterranean region including north Africa and all of Europe and central Asia. The tree was known to the ancient Greeks and mentioned by Dioscorides in his writings, but the berries were used only as a food by African tribesmen until the 19th century when it again became a folk medicine.

The tree was formerly regarded as sacred because of the Christian tradition that it furnished the crown of thorns prior to the crucifixion of Christ. In fact, a stand of the trees still inhabits a portion of the Mount of Olives outside Jerusalem.

Folk medicine holds hawthorn berries in high esteem for its effectiveness in treating both **high and low blood pressure, rapid pulse and arythmic heartbeat,** as a **prophylactic against angina pain** and in **atherosclerosis.**

The Native Americans used hawthorn to treat **rheumatism** and in Chinese medicine, another species of hawthorn is used as a **digestive aid.**

Medicinal Properties

> Definite Actions
>   Coronary vasodilator (flavonoids)
>   Hypotensive (flavonoids)
> Probable Actions
>   Antithrombotic (coumarins)
>   Digestive aid (saponins)
> Possible Actions
>   Anti-atherosclerotic (?)

During the past decade, some knowledge has been gained with respect to the action of hawthorn berries on the circulatory system. Claims of digitalis-like activity are apparently unfounded since hawthorn contains neither cardiotonic glycosides or cardiotonic alkaloids.

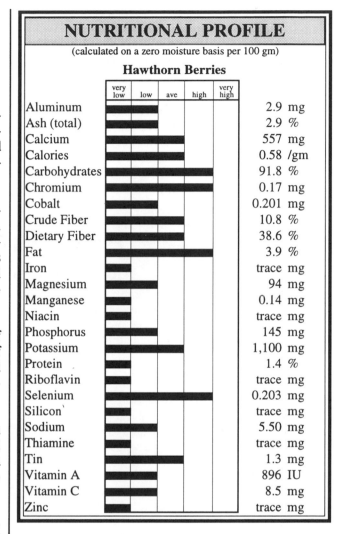

NUTRITIONAL PROFILE
(calculated on a zero moisture basis per 100 gm)

Hawthorn Berries

Nutrient	very low	low	ave	high	very high	Value
Aluminum		■				2.9 mg
Ash (total)		■				2.9 %
Calcium			■			557 mg
Calories		■				0.58 /gm
Carbohydrates				■		91.8 %
Chromium			■			0.17 mg
Cobalt		■				0.201 mg
Crude Fiber			■			10.8 %
Dietary Fiber			■			38.6 %
Fat				■		3.9 %
Iron	■					trace mg
Magnesium		■				94 mg
Manganese	■					0.14 mg
Niacin	■					trace mg
Phosphorus			■			145 mg
Potassium				■		1,100 mg
Protein	■					1.4 %
Riboflavin	■					trace mg
Selenium				■		0.203 mg
Silicon	■					trace mg
Sodium		■				5.50 mg
Thiamine	■					trace mg
Tin			■			1.3 mg
Vitamin A		■				896 IU
Vitamin C		■				8.5 mg
Zinc	■					trace mg

Instead, the active principles appear to be the flavonoids which slowly act on circulatory and cardiac problems by causing **dilation of the blood vessels**, especially the coronary arteries, and by causing some **reduction in blood pressure**. Hawthorn does not appear to be a cardio-toxic and seems to have no cumulative effects. Hawthorn should be taken with or immediately after a meal in order to avoid nausea. Toxicity has been noted only with very high doses.

Typical Daily Usage

> Fresh berry: 2-6 teaspoon
> Dried berry: 1-3 gm
> Extract: 2 gm dried berry, 10 ml alcohol, 10 ml water

Traditional Formulas

Ginkgo and Hawthorn combination
Hawthorn combination
Chickweed and Cascara combination
Licorice and Red Beet combination

Chemical Compounds

Aromatic compounds
    Volatile Oil: 0.1-0.25%
    Fixed Oils and Resins
        Saturated fatty acids
            lauric and palmitic
        Unsaturated fatty acids
            linoleic and linolenic
Astringent compounds
    Catechin
Bitter compounds
    Alkaloids
        Tyramine and others
    Flavonoids
        hyperoside, procyanidin, vitexin, quercitin
           and others
    Coumarins
        Aesculin

Nutrients of Note

Water when fresh: 72.1%
Water when air dried: 6.9%
Starch: 15-18%
Sugars: 12% (glucose, rhamnose)

Hibiscus flower
Hibiscus sabdariffa (Malvaceae)

Properties: astringent, antiseptic, diuretic, antispasmodic, digestive aid

Systems Affected: digestive, structural

Folk History and Use

Hibiscus is a flowering herb native to the tropics of Africa which is grown throughout most of the tropical climates of the world. It is an annual herb that reaches five feet or more and produces deep red flowers. Horticulturists and herbalists prize hibiscus flowers, while the textile industry turns the stems into burlap.

In its native land, hibiscus is used widely in food. It imparts a much desired flavor and color to jams, jellies, beverages and desserts. Egyptians use hibiscus flowers to **calm muscle spasms associated with heart and nerve disease**. The flowers are also included in **diuretic** and **laxative** herbal formulas.

Today it is used primarily by herbalists to impart a tart flavor and purplish color to herbal teas. It is often added to bulk **laxative** formulas as an **antispasmodic** and to improve their palatability.

Medicinal Properties

Definite action
    Astringent (fruit acids)
    Digestive aid (fruit acids)
Probable action
    Antispasmodic (?)
    Diuretic (?)
Possible action
    Antiseptic (?)

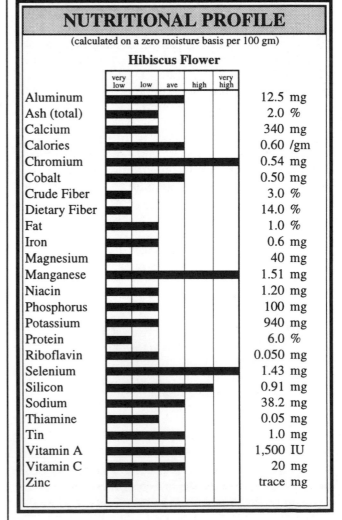

NUTRITIONAL PROFILE
(calculated on a zero moisture basis per 100 gm)

Hibiscus Flower

Nutrient	very low	low	ave	high	very high	Value
Aluminum						12.5 mg
Ash (total)						2.0 %
Calcium						340 mg
Calories						0.60 /gm
Chromium						0.54 mg
Cobalt						0.50 mg
Crude Fiber						3.0 %
Dietary Fiber						14.0 %
Fat						1.0 %
Iron						0.6 mg
Magnesium						40 mg
Manganese						1.51 mg
Niacin						1.20 mg
Phosphorus						100 mg
Potassium						940 mg
Protein						6.0 %
Riboflavin						0.050 mg
Selenium						1.43 mg
Silicon						0.91 mg
Sodium						38.2 mg
Thiamine						0.05 mg
Tin						1.0 mg
Vitamin A						1,500 IU
Vitamin C						20 mg
Zinc						trace mg

Hibiscus is an acidic herb that imparts an astringent note to herbal teas. In addition, it may help **calm muscle spasms** when combined with bulk laxatives like psyllium hulls. Its characteristic color is imparted by a group of anthocyanins. Anthocyanins are a class of chemicals that also give grapes and bilberries their color.

Typical Daily Usage

Fresh flowers: 1-2 teaspoon
Dried flowers: 0.5-1 gm
Extract: 1 gm dried flowers in a cup of boiling
water

Traditional Formulas

Psyllium combination

Chemical Constituents

Aromatic compounds
Volatile oil
Astringent compounds
Anthocyanins
ibiscin and others
Ibiscic acid: 25%
Bitter compounds
Saponins
sitosterol

Nutrients of Note

Water when fresh: 89%
Water when air dried: 7.9%
Sugars: 11% (fructose, glucose)
Fruit acids: 17% (citric, malic, tartaric)

Hops flowers

Humulus lupulus (Cannabaceae)

Properties: bitter, diuretic, nervine, antispasmodic,
bitter tonic, sedative

Systems Affected: digestive, urinary, respiratory

Folk History and Use

The most popular use of hops has been in the brewing of beer. Hops contributes the distinctive flavor and aroma of beer, as well as providing a natural preservative to the beverage, which is an effective **bacterioside**. The flowers are also eaten in place of asparagus, particularly in Belgium, while the oil is used in many perfumes.

Hops is native to Europe and North America where it is now widely cultivated. Its common name is derived from the old English "hoppan" to climb and its generic name humulus from the Latin "humus" or ground, i.e. the plant creeps on the ground unless supported. Its species name lupulus is from Pliny's lupus or little wolf because it strangles shrubbery when it climbs.

Hops has been used as a **calmative, nervine, stomachic, sedative** and **hypnotic**. It has been considered especially useful in alleviating **nervous stomach** conditions and in helping **produce sleep**. It is also a **diuretic** and **vermifuge**. One of the most popular folk uses is in a "hops filled pillow" which, when used to replace a standard pillow, is said to produce non-narcotic **sleep**.

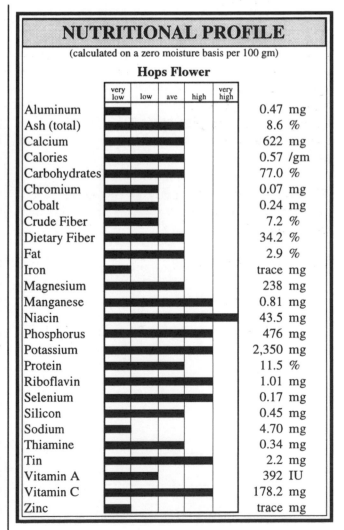

NUTRITIONAL PROFILE						
(calculated on a zero moisture basis per 100 gm)						
Hops Flower						
	very low	low	ave	high	very high	
Aluminum	■					0.47 mg
Ash (total)	■■■					8.6 %
Calcium	■■■■					622 mg
Calories	■■■					0.57 /gm
Carbohydrates	■■■■					77.0 %
Chromium	■					0.07 mg
Cobalt	■■					0.24 mg
Crude Fiber	■■					7.2 %
Dietary Fiber	■■■■					34.2 %
Fat	■					2.9 %
Iron	■					trace mg
Magnesium	■■■					238 mg
Manganese	■■■■■					0.81 mg
Niacin	■■■■■■				→	43.5 mg
Phosphorus	■■■■					476 mg
Potassium	■■■■					2,350 mg
Protein	■■■■					11.5 %
Riboflavin	■■■■					1.01 mg
Selenium	■					0.17 mg
Silicon	■■■					0.45 mg
Sodium	■					4.70 mg
Thiamine	■■■					0.34 mg
Tin	■■■■					2.2 mg
Vitamin A	■■					392 IU
Vitamin C	■■■					178.2 mg
Zinc	■					trace mg

Recorded cultivation of hops dates back to the middle of the 8th century. The use of hops in brewing dates back to the Middle Ages. It was introduced into England in 1524. Its use in brewing in England began in 1530 during the reign of Henry VIII. In 1787, it was first used in a pillow during an illness of King George III; the pillow was used in place of opiates to produce sleep. Several tribes of Indians in North America used it as a natural neutralizing agent for **hyperacidity** and **indigestion**.

Medicinal Properties

Definite Action
    Antibacterial (bitter principles)
    Antispasmodic (flavonoids)
Probable Action
    Diuretic (flavonoids)
    Appetite stimulant (bitter principles)
Possible Action
    Antitumor (?)

Hops has an overriding bitter taste due to the **antibiotic** bitter acids, humulone and lupulone. These irritating bitter acids, together with volatile oils, stimulate (primarily through irritation) the urinary tract and the lungs to purge themselves of toxins. This results in **diuretic** and **expectorant** effects. The oils also trigger the **production of digestive fluids**, aiding efficient **digestion**.

The **sedative** and **antispasmodic** properties of hops are apparently due to the various flavonoids present in the flowers of the plant.

Typical Daily Usage

Fresh flowers: 2-6 teaspoon
Dried Flowers: 1-3 gm
Extract: 2 gm dried flower, 10 ml alcohol, 10 ml
    water

Traditional Formulas

Kelp combination
Chamomile and Passionflower combination
Scullcap combination
Valerian and Black Cohosh combination
White Willow and Valerian combination

Chemical Constituents

Aromatic compounds
    Volatile oil: 0.3-1%
        Terpenes
            caryophyllenes, myrcene, farnesene
            and others
    Fixed oil and Resin: 3-12%
Astringent compounds
    Tannins
Bitter compounds
    Bitter acids
        umulone, lupulone
    Flavonoids
        Astragalin, quercitin, rutin, kaempferol and
        others

Nutrients of Note

Water when fresh: 81.4%
Water when air dried: 6.8%
Sugars: 12% (glucose)
Phosphlipids: choline

Horseradish root
Armoracia rusticana (Cruciferae)

Properties: bitter, expectorant, counterirritant

Systems Affected: respiratory, digestive

Folk History and Use

Horseradish root is a cruciferous vegetable of the same family as broccoli, cabbage and cauliflower. Like the other crucifers, it is a hardy plant that can be planted early in the year and harvested before the heat of the summer. It has been used as a spice for over 2,000 years. As with many spices, horseradish was first used to mask the taste and odor of spoiled meat. It is a pungent herb included as one of the five bitter herbs of Passover. Its association with meat dishes continues today where it is used as a condiment.

Its folk medical history is linked to its irritating effect on mucous membranes. In this regard, it is a **counterirritant** that elicits a sympathetic increase in the production of mucous by various membranes of the body. If you were eating spoiled meat on a regular basis, horseradish would irritate the mucous membranes of your digestive tract into producing a protective mucous coat that could prevent further irritation, inflammation, nausea and possibly absorb some of the putrified substances in the meat.

It has traditionally been used in respiratory formulas where an **expectorant** effect is desired. The sympathetic responses of mucous membranes throughout the body make it useful in treating **bronchitis**, as a **diuretic**, in **respiratory allergy formulas** and as a **vermifuge**. It is also an important **immune stimulant** included in many herbal formulas to increase the number of white blood cells circulating in the blood stream. Horseradish, a cruciferous vegetable, is a known **antioxidant**.

Medicinal Properties

    Definite action
        Expectorant (isothiscyanates)
        Counterirritant (isothiocyanates)
    Probable action
        Immune stimulant (?)

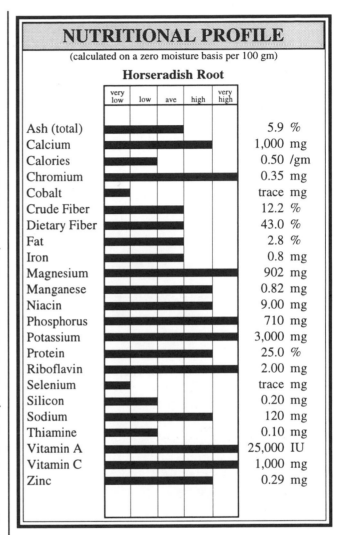

NUTRITIONAL PROFILE
(calculated on a zero moisture basis per 100 gm)

Horseradish Root

	very low	low	ave	high	very high		
Ash (total)						5.9	%
Calcium						1,000	mg
Calories						0.50	/gm
Chromium						0.35	mg
Cobalt						trace	mg
Crude Fiber						12.2	%
Dietary Fiber						43.0	%
Fat						2.8	%
Iron						0.8	mg
Magnesium						902	mg
Manganese						0.82	mg
Niacin						9.00	mg
Phosphorus						710	mg
Potassium						3,000	mg
Protein						25.0	%
Riboflavin						2.00	mg
Selenium						trace	mg
Silicon						0.20	mg
Sodium						120	mg
Thiamine						0.10	mg
Vitamin A						25,000	IU
Vitamin C						1,000	mg
Zinc						0.29	mg

Horseradish root increases the production while decreasing the production of fluids from mucous membranes it comes in contact with. This expectorant effect elicits a sympathetic response from mucous membranes in other parts of the body that it does not come directly in contact with. These effects seem to be most pronounced in the respiratory and urinary system. This accounts for the herbal use in folk remedies for **respiratory allergies** and **difficult urination.**

The action of horseradish is attributed to its pungent principles called isothiocyanates. The isothiocyanates in horseradish are only released by enzymatic cleavage when the root is crushed. It is similar to garlic in this respect.

Typical Daily Usage

Fresh root: 1-2 tablespoon
Dried root: 1.5-3 gm
Extract: 2 gm dried root, 10 ml alcohol, 10 gm
water

Traditional Formulas

Licorice combination
Dandelion and Barberry combination
Rosehips and Broccoli combination
Fenugreek combination

Chemical Constituents

Aromatic compounds
Volatile oil
Resin
Bitter compounds
Isothiocyanates
sinigrin
2-phenylethylglycosinolate

Nutrients of Note

Water when fresh: 82%
Water when air dried: 7%
Starch: 22%

Horsetail herb
Equisetum arvense (Equisetaceae)

Properties: bitter, diuretic, hemostatic, vulnerary, emmenagogue, carminative

Systems Affected: urinary, digestive

Common Names: shave grass, bottlebrush, pewterwort

Folk History and Use

Horsetail belongs to a family of flowerless plants that is distinguished by branched, jointed, hollow and striated stems with leaves that are reduced to scales.

The horsetails are primitive plants known in the fossil record as early as the carboniferous period. Anciently they are estimated to have reached 300 or more feet high, but today are only bushy ground cover around streams and wet places.

Various species of horsetail grow worldwide and are most famous as bottle brushes used in scouring, because of the silica-bearing striations they possess.

The name equisetum is derived from the Latin "equus" for horse and "seta" for tail, in reference to the copious branching of several species.

The Doctrine of Signatures assigned horsetail as a cure for **gout** and other **joint inflammations** because of the many unswollen joints it possesses.

NUTRITIONAL PROFILE
(calculated on a zero moisture basis per 100 gm)

Horsetail Herb

Nutrient	very low	low	ave	high	very high	Value	
Aluminum				■		37.8	mg
Ash (total)				■		10.6	%
Calcium				■		1,890	mg
Calories			■			0.53	/gm
Carbohydrates			■			73.7	%
Chromium					■	0.22	mg
Cobalt				■		0.53	mg
Crude Fiber				■		20.2	%
Dietary Fiber			■			31.2	%
Fat		■				2.7	%
Iron					■	12.3	mg
Magnesium				■		437	mg
Manganese		■				0.69	mg
Niacin				■		4.20	mg
Phosphorus		■				190	mg
Potassium					■	1,560	mg
Protein		■				11.4	%
Riboflavin		■				0.19	mg
Selenium			■			0.13	mg
Silicon					■	3.86	mg
Sodium			■			56.0	mg
Thiamine	■					0	mg
Tin		■				1.4	mg
Vitamin A				■		8,219	IU
Vitamin C			■			20.8	mg
Zinc	■					trace	mg

The Native Americans used horsetail to make mats and to polish woodwork. The Europeans used it during the Middle Ages to scour milk pails and as a finishing "rouge" on fine jewelry and cabinet work.

Horsetail is considered to be a **diuretic** and **astringent**. It induces **perspiration** during high fever and has primary effects in **correcting bladder problems**; it is used both as a **diuretic** and to help **control incontinence**, including **childhood enuresis**. Horsetail is also used as an **eye treatment**, especially for **conjunctivitis** and **inflammation of the lachrymal ducts**. It has been applied externally to treat both **hemorrhoids** and anal fissures. It has also been used to treat **menstrual clots.** Horsetail is commonly used to treat **tumors**.

Medicinal Properties

Definite Action
  Diuretic (tannins and flavonoids)
  Astringent (tannins)
  Antispasmodic (flavonoids)
  Antibacterial (flavonoids)
  Source of trace minerals, including organic
    silica

The major action of horsetail is as a **urinary tract astringent and diuretic**. These properties are produced by a combination of tannins and flavonoids present in the herb. Folk medicine refers to the ability of horsetail to **tone organs of the urinary tract and soothe the bladder**. This is best explained by the herb's ability to **tighten the inflamed epithelial tissues** with tannins and purge the urinary tract of toxins by **diuresis**. Concurrently, the flavonoids present in horsetail exert a **spasmolytic action on the smooth muscles** to **ease the painful spasms often associated with urinary tract infections**. Its flavonoids are also **antiseptic** and **help fight infections of the urinary tract**. Its **astringent** properties also make it useful topically as an **eyewash** and to **heal wounds**.

Many claims have been made regarding horsetail and its organic silicon content. Cabinetmakers use the herb as a final sandpaper, and homeopaths make tinctures of the herb as a silica supplement. Kervran, a French scientist, even proposed a theory for transmuting the organic silicon into calcium!

In spite of the unproven claims associated with the herb, horsetail is unique among the herbs because it does contain the highest amount of silicon of all the herbs and this silicon is in a bioavailable form. This property makes horsetail popular in **skeletal strengthening** formulas.

Typical Daily Usage

Fresh herb: 2-4 tablespoon
Dried herb: 3-6 gm
Extract: 4.5 gm dried herb, 22 ml alcohol, 23 ml
  water

Traditional Formulas

Ginseng and Saw Palmetto combination
Alfalfa and Yucca combination
Dandelion and Parsley combination
Horsetail and Gelatin combination
Marshmallow and Plantain combination

Chemical Constituents

Astringent compounds
  Tannin
Bitter compounds
  Saponins
    Sitosterol and others
      Equisetrin, equisetonin, articulatin
  Flavonoids
    Galuteolin, gossypitrin, herbacetrin,
      isoquercitrin, luteolin, kaempferol
  Alkaloids
    Nicotine, palustrine, and others

Nutrients of Note

Water when fresh: 78.6%
Water when air dried: 7.6%

Hydrangea root
Hydrangea arborescens (Saxifragaceae)

Properties: bitter, diuretic, laxative, cathartic

Systems Affected: urinary, digestive

Common Names: wild hydrangea, seven barks, gravel root, stone root

Folk History and Use

Hydrangea is a hardy perennial native to the eastern half of the United States. In the late 18th century, the leaves of the plant were used in place of tobacco to allegedly produce euphoria. It was given to women to eliminate wild dreams.

The root is often called gravel root and stone root. It is most noted in folk medicine for its ability to help one eliminate kidney stones. The Cherokee Indians introduced it to the European settlers for this purpose. They called it stone root not only because it was said to remove stones but also because the root is hard like a stone.

Herbalists also use the root to **break up all lumps and tumors**. Its use has spread to include most **imbalances of the urinary system including kidney stone, bladderstone, incontinence, dysuria** and **benign prostatic hypertrophy.**

Medicinal Properties

   Probable action
      Diuretic (flavonoids)
      Laxative (?)
   Possible action
      Antitumor(?)
      Anti renal calculus (?)

Hydrangea contains bitter principles that qualify it as a **blood purifier**. These compounds **increase the production of urine** and provide a **laxative** effect. This herb **enhances the elimination process** especially in the urinary system.

Its use in **eliminating kidney stones** has not been proven scientifically, but the root has a long list of testimonials from those who have employed it. It is quite a harsh herb and not generally used on a daily basis. It is one of the minority of herbs used in acute situations such as when a kidney stone begins to move down the urinary tract.

Hydrangea contains several flavonoids including quercetin and rutin. These compounds are said to **inhibit**

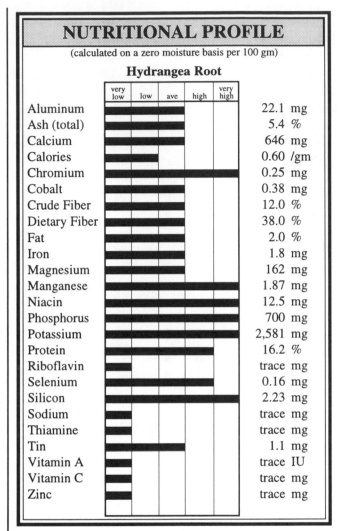

NUTRITIONAL PROFILE
(calculated on a zero moisture basis per 100 gm)

Hydrangea Root

	very low	low	ave	high	very high		
Aluminum						22.1	mg
Ash (total)						5.4	%
Calcium						646	mg
Calories						0.60	/gm
Chromium						0.25	mg
Cobalt						0.38	mg
Crude Fiber						12.0	%
Dietary Fiber						38.0	%
Fat						2.0	%
Iron						1.8	mg
Magnesium						162	mg
Manganese						1.87	mg
Niacin						12.5	mg
Phosphorus						700	mg
Potassium						2,581	mg
Protein						16.2	%
Riboflavin						trace	mg
Selenium						0.16	mg
Silicon						2.23	mg
Sodium						trace	mg
Thiamine						trace	mg
Tin						1.1	mg
Vitamin A						trace	IU
Vitamin C						trace	mg
Zinc						trace	mg

tumor formation and **reduce inflammation** and have a **diuretic** effect. They are likely responsible for much of its action. In addition, the root contains other bitter principles including hygangein whose action has not yet been determined.

Typical Daily Usage

   Fresh root: 1 tablespoon
   Dried root: 1.5 gm
   Extract: 1.5 gm, 7 ml alcohol, 8 ml water

Traditional Formulas

   Alfalfa and Yucca combination

Chemical Constituents

   Aromatic compounds
      Resin

Bitter compounds
    Saponins
        Hydrangin and others
    Flavonoids
        Rutin, quercetin, kaempferol and others
    Mucilaginous compounds
        Polysaccharides

Gum: 9%

Nutrients of Note

Water when fresh: 65%
Water when air dried: 5.2%
Sugars: 6% (sucrose)

Juniper berry
Juniperus communis (Pinaceae)

Properties: aromatic, diuretic, antiseptic, blood purifier, antirheumatic

Systems Affected: urinary, glandular

Common Names: juniper bush

Folk History and Use

Juniper berry is the fruit of one of the most common species of the pine family. The plant is an aromatic evergreen with blue green berries. Junipers are widely used as ornamental trees and cultivated for their berries. Most of the commercial production occurs in eastern Europe where the plant is indigenous. The berries' oil is the principle flavor of the alcoholic beverage gin. It is also used in perfumery and in cosmetics. The tree itself is the source of cade oil, a tarry substance similar to pine tar.

Juniper berry oil is chemically similar to turpentine and Australian tea tree oil. In fact, the most prominent component of juniper berry oil is terpinen-4-ol, also the most prominent component of tea tree oil.

Juniper berries are most often used in folk medicine as a **diuretic**. The oil is thought to **increase the production of urine** by irritating the kidney's filtration glomerulae. The oil is also irritating to microbes, so much so that it kills many of them.

Its use as an **antiseptic** both topically for **psoriasis** and internally for treating **infections** is well documented in the popular literature. It is especially noted for **eliminating chronic infections of the prostate and urinary tract** in males suffering from benign **prostatic hypertrophy.**

Medicinal Properties

Definite action
    Diuretic (volatile oil)
    Antiseptic (volatile oil)

Juniper is a **blood purifier** in the sense that its volatile oil helps the body eliminate impurites from the blood

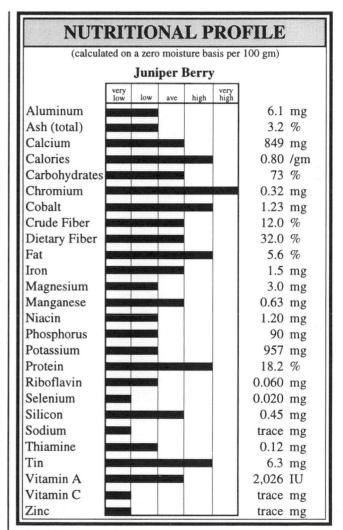

NUTRITIONAL PROFILE
(calculated on a zero moisture basis per 100 gm)

Juniper Berry

	very low	low	ave	high	very high	
Aluminum						6.1 mg
Ash (total)						3.2 %
Calcium						849 mg
Calories						0.80 /gm
Carbohydrates						73 %
Chromium						0.32 mg
Cobalt						1.23 mg
Crude Fiber						12.0 %
Dietary Fiber						32.0 %
Fat						5.6 %
Iron						1.5 mg
Magnesium						3.0 mg
Manganese						0.63 mg
Niacin						1.20 mg
Phosphorus						90 mg
Potassium						957 mg
Protein						18.2 %
Riboflavin						0.060 mg
Selenium						0.020 mg
Silicon						0.45 mg
Sodium						trace mg
Thiamine						0.12 mg
Tin						6.3 mg
Vitamin A						2,026 IU
Vitamin C						trace mg
Zinc						trace mg

through the urinary tract. The diuresis is accomplished by irritating the filtering tissues of the kidneys and causing them to increase the quantity of fluid they release. One note on cleansing the blood in this manner: all serum constituents are discharged by this process. Essential nutrients as well as toxins are lost. The essential nutrients must be replaced if ones homeostasis is to be maintained.

Juniper berry is an excellent **antiseptic** that works best on contact. Its **disinfectant** action is similar to that of pine cleaners. Topically, juniper oil can be applied to cuts and scrapes just like tea tree oil. Ingesting the berries or its oil will help to **overcome bacterial and yeast infections**. Its extract can be used as a gargle.

Its use in treating benign prostatic hypertrophy requires increasing large amounts of the berry and some allergic reactions have been reported. This application is only a superficial treatment since these types of infections are only outgrowths of the primary inflammation in the prostate.

The irritating nature of the oil makes it potentially dangerous to those with impaired kidney function since inflammation often accompanies irritation.

Typical Daily Usage

Fresh berry: 1 teaspoon
Dried berry: 0.5-1 gm
Extract: 1 gm dried berry, 5 ml alcohol, 5 ml water

Traditional Formulas

Ginger and Dong Quai combination
Goldenseal and Juniper combination
Uva Ursi combination

Chemical Constituents

Aromatic compounds
Volatile oil: 2-4%
Terpenes
pinene, cadinene, camphene, terpinin-4-ol
Fixed oil and resin: 7-12%
Astringent compounds
Gallotannin

Nutrients of Note

Water when fresh: 69%
Water when air dried: 6%
Sugars: 8% (fructose, glucose)
Fruit acids: 1% (formic, fumaric)

Kelp herb
Fucus vesiculosis (Fucaceae)

Properties: mucilaginous, demulcent, emollient, iodine source

Systems Affected: digestive, glandular

Folk History and Use

Kelp is a group of brown algae with large, flat, leaf-like fronds that are usually attached to rocks in 10-150 foot seas. Kelp, native to the Pacific Ocean, includes species of Macrocystis and Nereocystis; while species of Larminaria are native to the Atlantic coast of North America.

The great Pacific sea kelp used by herbalists is Fucus vesiculosis and gets its name from the Greek "phykos" which is a derivative of "phytein" meaning to grow, in reference to the plant's remarkable length. The species name vesiculosis is from the Latin "vesicula" meaning a little vesicle, referring to the air blisters found in the frond.

Kelp is employed by herbalists as a mineral supplement. It is especially prized for its iodine content, for which it is used to treat **hypothyroidism** and **obesity**.

Kelp has also been used as a **blood purifier** and to treat **atherosclerosis** and **rheumatism**. It functions in

NUTRITIONAL PROFILE
(calculated on a zero moisture basis per 100 gm)

Kelp Herb

Nutrient	very low	low	ave	high	very high	Value
Aluminum						63.1 mg
Ash (total)						25.0 %
Calcium						3,040 mg
Calories						0.50 /gm
Carbohydrates						65.5 %
Chromium						0.07 mg
Cobalt						0.16 mg
Crude Fiber						9.8 %
Dietary Fiber						48.2 %
Fat						3.0 %
Iron						1.6 mg
Magnesium						867 mg
Manganese						0.76 mg
Niacin						4.70 mg
Phosphorus						249 mg
Potassium						2,110 mg
Protein						6.5 %
Riboflavin						0 mg
Selenium						0.17 mg
Silicon						0.76 mg
Sodium						5,610 mg
Thiamine						0 mg
Tin						2.4 mg
Vitamin A						6,600 IU
Vitamin C						25.8 mg
Zinc						0.06 mg

these conditions by absorbing toxins from the bowel. It is especially effective at absorbing the metabolic products produced by yeasts.

Kelp is most famous for its use in foods. In the Orient, it is used to flavor soups and suishi. In North America, it is popular as a cattle feed.

The pharmaceutical and confectionary industries use the purified mucilage of kelp (algin) in virtually all classes of products. Algin is found in lozenges as a demulcent, in tablets as a disintegrating agent, in peel-off facial masks as a thickener and in many creams and lotions. Calcium salts of algin form fibers suitable for surgery, and dentists make irreversible dental impressions with it. Nearly every gelatin, pudding condiment, ice cream and processed cheese product contain algin, as it produces a smooth mouth feel and rich texture.

Medicinal Properties

Definite Actions
The benefits of viscous fiber
Lowers bowel transit time
Absorbs toxins from the bowel
Regulates intestinal flora
Demulcent to digestive tract
Iodine source

The medicinal virtues of kelp are primarily related to its content of viscous fiber called algin. Algin is responsible for the use of kelp in the treatment of **obesity, atherosclerosis** and as a **blood purifier**. Algin absorbs most nutrients as well as toxins from the digestive tract in much the same way that a water softener removes the "hardness" from tap water. This results in less toxins entering the circulatory system. It also reduces caloric intake.

Kelp is primarily employed by herbalists as a natural source of minerals, and while it does contain significant quantities of iodine, calcium and potassium, its benefits as a mineral supplement are diminished by its high content of sodium and heavy metals such as arsenic, lead and mercury. The fact that its mineral content is virtually inorganic (a result of saturation in a saline brine), and the fact that algin forms insoluble salts with all but the electrolyte minerals, makes most of the trace minerals unavailable for absorption.

By using the purified form of kelp (i.e. algin), especially the potassium salt of algin, the herb is useful as a toxin scavenger for the digestive tract and as a demulcent and source of viscous fiber. Recent studies have shown potassium alginate to be a hypotensive agent since it releases potassium as it scavenges toxins from the digestive tract.

The raw form of kelp performs the duties of a water softener for the oceans. It helps to cleanse the sea of heavy metals and other products of man-made pollution. When it washes up on the beach or is harvested, it is a water softener that needs regenerating.

Typical Daily Usage

Fresh herb: 1/4-1/2 cup
Dried herb: 2-4 teaspoon
Extract: 3 teaspoon dried herb, 75 ml alcohol, 75 ml water

Traditional Formulas

Black Cohosh combination
Irish Moss and Kelp combination
Kelp combination
Alfalfa and Dandelion combination
Pollen and Ginseng combination

Chemical Constituents

Aromatic compounds
Fixed Oils and Resins
Saturated fatty acids
palmitic, stearic, myristic, squalane
Unsaturated fatty acids
oleic, arachidonic
Bitter compounds
Saponins
Cholesterol, fucosterol, beta sitosterol
Mucilaginous compounds
Algin: 35-50%

Nutrients of Note

Water when fresh: 88.2%
Water when air dried: 4.3%
Sugars: 2% (mannitol)
Iodine 540 ppm

Licorice root
Glycyrrhiza glabra (Leguminoseae)

Properties: bitter, expectorant, laxative, anti-inflammatory, antispasmodic, demulcent, antiulcer

Systems Affected: glandular, digestive, repiratory

Common Names: sweetwood

Folk History and Use

If you think licorice is just candy, think again. Licorice is also a useful herb. Although some licorice candy does contain an extract of the root of licorice herb, most licorice flavor comes from anise oil or a combination of licorice and anise. There are 14 species of licorice which are natives of warmer temperate countries in both the New and Old World. About ten species have sweet roots.

Licorice is a member of the pea family, and is a large sweet pea-like plant. The plants are graceful with light, spreading pinnate foliage, presenting an almost feathery appearance from a distance. Taproots may sink three or four feet and should be harvested in the fall. The genus name, Glycyrrhiza, is derived from the root words "glukus" meaning sweet and "riza" meaning root, alluding to the fact that the dried roots can be chewed like a confection because of their sweet flavor.

The use of licorice has been known since ancient times. It was introduced to the Greeks by the Scythians. It was also used by the Chinese and the Hindus. Hippocrates, Pliny, Culpepper and numerous other herbalists have made use of it.

Great quantities of licorice were found with the fabulous treasures of King Tut and other Egyptian rulers. The Egyptians believed that the licorice could be used to prepare a sweet drink, "maisus," in the next world.

Hippocrates and others living in hot climates praised licorice for its ability to provide sweetness and still alleviate thirst, a unique property among sweet substances.

The Brahmans of India, the Hindus, Greeks, Romans, Babylonians and Chinese all knew of the value of lico-

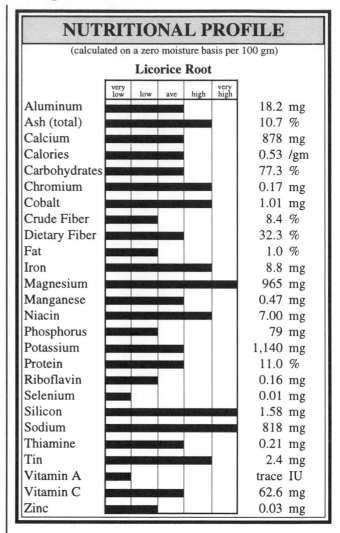

NUTRITIONAL PROFILE
(calculated on a zero moisture basis per 100 gm)

Licorice Root

	very low	low	ave	high	very high		
Aluminum						18.2	mg
Ash (total)						10.7	%
Calcium						878	mg
Calories						0.53	/gm
Carbohydrates						77.3	%
Chromium						0.17	mg
Cobalt						1.01	mg
Crude Fiber						8.4	%
Dietary Fiber						32.3	%
Fat						1.0	%
Iron						8.8	mg
Magnesium						965	mg
Manganese						0.47	mg
Niacin						7.00	mg
Phosphorus						79	mg
Potassium						1,140	mg
Protein						11.0	%
Riboflavin						0.16	mg
Selenium						0.01	mg
Silicon						1.58	mg
Sodium						818	mg
Thiamine						0.21	mg
Tin						2.4	mg
Vitamin A						trace	IU
Vitamin C						62.6	mg
Zinc						0.03	mg

rice. In ancient Greece and Rome, licorice was employed as a tonic and also as a remedy for **colds, coughs** and **sore throat**. The ancient Hindus believed it increased sexual vigor when prepared as a beverage with milk and sugar. The Chinese maintained that eating the root would give them strength and endurance and also prepared a special tea of it for use as a medicine.

Indeed, licorice holds a prominent place in Chinese herbology. It is the most often used herb in Chinese herbal combinations and is thought to harmonize the action of all other herbs.

In North American folk medicine, licorice is used as a **cough suppressant, expectorant, laxative** and to treat **various cancers**. Early pharmacists used it as a flavoring and sweetening agent in many of their syrups and lozenges. Today, licorice extracts are popular sweeteners in confections for diabetics and those suffering from hypoglycemia.

In India, licorice has been used as a **sweetener, aphrodisiac, emmenagogue** and **galactogogue.**

The South Koreans use it along with ginseng in an oral contraceptive preparation for women.

Licorice extracts have been used in China in the clinical treatment of numerous illnesses including **gastric and duodenal ulcers, bronchial asthma, infectious hepatitis, malaria, diabetes insipidus** and **contact dermatitis**.

Presently, licorice extracts are used extensively as ingredients in **cough drops and syrups, tonics, laxatives, antismoking lozenges** and other preparations. They are also used as flavoring agents to mask bitter, nauseous or other undesirable tastes in certain medicines.

Medicinal Properties

Definite Actions
Expectorant (glycyrhizin)
Antispasmodic (flavonoids)
Anti-inflammatory (glycyrrhizin)
Laxative (glycyrrhizin)
Hypertensive (glycyrrhizin)
Antiulcer (flavonoids)
Estrogenic (glycyrrhizin)
Mineralocorticoid properties (glycyrrhizin)
Emmenagogue (glycyrrhizin)
Antibacterial (flavonoids)
Antifungal (flavonoids)
Immune stimulant (?)

The most famous active principle in licorice root is a saponin-like glycoside called glycyrrhizin which is 50 times as sweet as sugar. Its use as a non-caloric sweetener is limited, however, because of the strong taste it imparts to food. It is most often employed to mask the taste of bitter medicines like cascara.

The large quantity of saponin-like substances in licorice possess a surfactant property that may facilitate the absorption of poorly absorbed drugs. This explains, in part, its traditional use as a harmonizing herb in Chinese herbology.

Glycyrrhizin and its aglycones, including glycyrrhetinic acid, exhibit mineralocortoid-type properties. These properties include increasing extracellular fluid and plasma volume, sodium retention and loss of potassium, which leads to hypertension. Licorice has been used in desert regions to prevent extreme thirst on low water intake.

Glycyrrhizin is also responsible for the anti-inflammatory and antitussive properties which make it useful in treating coughs and congestions. The anti-inflammatory properties of the herb are employed as dermatological agents in middle eastern countries. Glycyrrhetenic acid is also used in the treatment of chronic adrenocorticoid insufficiency (Addison's disease).

Glycyrrhizin increases fluid and sodium retention and promotes potassium depletion. Persons with cardiac problems and hypertension should avoid consumption of significant quantities of licorice.

Many other properties of licorice can be attributed to its flavonoids and coumarin derivatives. These substances produce the **antispasmodic, anti-ulcer** and **antimicrobial** effects of the herb.

Most of the toxicity exhibited by licorice is due to the glycyrrhizin (edema, hypocalemia, etc.) and when deglycyrrhizinized licorice is used to treat gastric and duodenal ulcers. The size of the ulcer can be reduced by 70-90% after one month. Healing occurs in patients who are not confined to bed and many who continue to work during the treatment.

Typical Daily Usage

Fresh root: 2-4 tablespoon
Dried root: 3-6 gm
Extract: 4.5 gm dried root, 22 ml alcohol, 23 ml
water

Traditional Formulas

Agastache and Shengu combination
Cascara combination
Chickweed and Cascara combination
Ginger combination
Ginger and Licorice combination
Psyllium combination
Black Cohosh combination

Black Cohosh and Blessed Thistle combination
Licorice combination
Raspberry and Dong Quai combination
Rehmannia and Ophiopogon combination
Ginseng combination
Golden Seal and Juniper combination
Licorice and Red Beet combination
Bupleurum and Peony combination
Astragalus and Ganoderma combination
Dandelion and Purslane combination
Fushen and Dragon Bone combination
Pollen and Ginseng combination
Bupleurum and Cyperus combination
Pinellia and Citrus combination
Forsythia and Schizonepeta combination
Alisma and Hoelen combination

Chemical Constituents

Aromatic compounds
 Volatile Oils
  Terpenes
   Acetol, heranol, 2-acetyl furan,
    thujone, fenchone and others
 Fixed Oils and Resins
  Saturated fatty acids
   Caprylic, hexanoic, palmitic
  Unsaturated fatty acids
   Linoleic, linolenic
Astringent compounds
 Salicylic acid
Bitter compounds
 Triterpenoids and glycosides (7-15%)-11
  glycyrrhizin
  glycyrrhizic Acid
  glycyrrhetic acid
  liquiritc acid
 Flavonoids
  Licoflavonol, liquiritin, quercitin, apigenin
   and others
 Coumarins
  umbelliferone, herniarin, liqcoumarin
 Alkaloids
  Tryptamine, Pryrazine and Pyrrolidine type
Mucilaginous compounds
 Pectin: 9%

Nutrients of Note

Water when fresh: 84.3%
Water when air dried: 6.7%
Starch: 5-20%
Sugars: 8-12% (glucose, sucrose)

Lobelia leaves
Lobelia inflata (Lobeliaceae)

Properties: bitter, nervine, antispasmodic, emetic, expectorant

Systems Affected: respiratory, nervous, circulatory, digestive

Common Names: Indian tobacco, emetic weed, poke week, asthma weed, gagroot, wild tobacco

Folk History and Use

The medicinal virtues of lobelia are said to have been discovered by Samuel Thompson in the early 1800's. The story of this discovery says that he convinced a friend to partake of this bitter herb. The friend did so and became "deadly sick" and "greatly relaxed." Upon drinking some water, he vomited and "felt better afterwards than he did before." Thus began a controversy over the toxicity of lobelia that continues to this day. Most scientists who have studied lobelia have proclaimed it a potentially harmful drug, while the folk uses of lobelia point to its built-in overdose preventers: nausea and emesis.

In Western herbology, lobelia is recommended for nearly every complaint. It is used as a balancing herb in herbal combinations much as licorice root is used in Chinese herbology.

Lobelia is native to North America. Its range extends from Labador, Canada to the state of Georgia and west to Arkansas. It is cultivated in North Carolina, Virginia, Tennessee and Hollánd.

The genus Lobelia, was named in honor of Matthias de L'Obel, a Flemish botanist; the specific species (inflata) refers to the fruit which is hollow and distended. Lobelia was used as an emetic, purgative and tobacco substitute by the eastern North American Indian tribes. White men first observed lobelia's emetic properties in 1785, and the drug was introduced into medicine in 1807. Lobelia was recommended for use in the treatment of asthma by Cutler in 1813, and introduced to the English medical profession by Reece in 1829. Historically, lobelia has also been employed for its supposed **anti-syphilitic, blood cleansing** and **sudorific properties.**

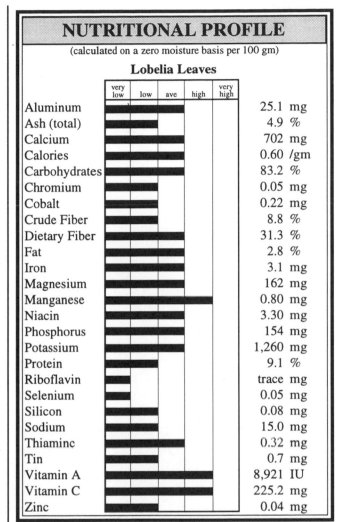

NUTRITIONAL PROFILE
(calculated on a zero moisture basis per 100 gm)

Lobelia Leaves

	very low	low	ave	high	very high	
Aluminum						25.1 mg
Ash (total)						4.9 %
Calcium						702 mg
Calories						0.60 /gm
Carbohydrates						83.2 %
Chromium						0.05 mg
Cobalt						0.22 mg
Crude Fiber						8.8 %
Dietary Fiber						31.3 %
Fat						2.8 %
Iron						3.1 mg
Magnesium						162 mg
Manganese						0.80 mg
Niacin						3.30 mg
Phosphorus						154 mg
Potassium						1,260 mg
Protein						9.1 %
Riboflavin						trace mg
Selenium						0.05 mg
Silicon						0.08 mg
Sodium						15.0 mg
Thiamine						0.32 mg
Tin						0.7 mg
Vitamin A						8,921 IU
Vitamin C						225.2 mg
Zinc						0.04 mg

Lobelia has traditionally been used as an **antispasmodic, antiasthmatic, diaphoretic, expectorant, emetic** and **sedative**. It has been utilized in the treatment of **asthma, whooping cough, bruises, ulcers, inflammations, sprains, ringworm, swelling, insect bites** and **poison ivy symptoms.**

Medicinal Properties

Definite Action
  Antispasmodic (alkaloids)
  Emetic--in overdoses(alkaloids)
  Nervine (alkaloids)
  Diuretic (alkaloids)
  Laxative (alkaloids)
  Expectorant (alkaloids)

Lobelia has been utilized as a **respiratory stimulant, an antiasthmatic,** an **expectorant** (in cases of laryngitis and bronchitis)**,** a **spasmolytic** and an **emetic**. Lobelia is used topically in the treatment of **myositis** and **rheumatic nodules**. It is used in emergency situations to revive patients who have taken an overdose of a narcotic, as lobelia's action is much like that of nicotine.

Lobeline salts are commonly used as a tobacco substitute in many over-the-counter stop smoking preparations. Lobelia and its extracts are used as ingredients in cough preparations and in counter-irritant preparations. In large doses it acts as a **purgative** and a **diuretic.**

The pharmacological action of lobelia is dose dependent and since natural products are notorious for their variations in active constituent concentrations, doctors and scientists always worry about the potential safety hazards associated with the lay use of the plant. Untrained practitioners are not considered prepared for the potential severe reactions to therapeutic doses which include nausea, vomiting, diarrhea, coughing, headache, tremors and dizziness. Symptoms of an overdose include vomiting, profuse diaphoresis, hypotension (manifested as low blood pressure), paresis, tachycardia, hypothermia (depressed body temperatures), stupor, paralysis, respiratory depression and convulsions.

In spite of the potential for dosing errors, lobelia remains a mainstay of Western herbal therapies. In small doses (0.2-0.6 gm dried powdered herb), the effects are activating and energizing (expectorant, spasmolytic). In moderate doses (0.4-1.5 gm dried powdered herb) the effects are powerful and relaxant. In large doses (2.5-4 gm dried powdered herb) the effects are emetic and relaxant.

Typical Daily Usage

Fresh leaf: 2-6 teaspoon
Dried leaf: 1-3 gm
Extract: 2 gm dried leaf, 10 ml alcohol, 10 ml water

Traditional Formulas

Cascara combination
Ephedra and Senega combination

Chemical constituents

Bitter compounds
Alkaloids
Pyridine type: 0.4 - 0.5%
Lobeline, lobelanine, lobelanidine and others

Nutrients of Note

Water when fresh: 88.7%
Water when air dried: 6.8%

Milk Thistle leaf
Silybum marianum (Compositae)

Properties: bitter, liver protectant, antioxidant, liver reguvenator

Systems Affected: digestive, circulatory

Common Names: emetic root, snake milk, milk ipecac

Folk History and Use

Milk thistle derives its name from the milky sap that comes from its stems and leaves. It is a persistent annual that grows up to ten feet high. Like most thistles, it has prickly leaves. It is also identified by its spine-ridged, reddish purple flowers. Milk thistle is native to the Middle East but now grows all over the temperate regions of North America.

Most commercially available milk thistle is a concentrated extract of the sap. Processing the bitter latex in this manner allows the flavonoids to be standardized (usually to 80% silymarin) and the prickles and spines of the plant to be avoided by the consumer.

Milk thistle has a long folk history of successfully treating **liver disorders** which have been confirmed by scientific study. The plant is also used to increase the production of milk in nursing mothers. Most importantly is its ability to **prevent liver damage** by inhibiting the production of enzymes that lead to free radical and leucotriene formation. It is an effective **antioxidant** that functions mainly in the liver. In this regard, it is useful in treating **cirrosis, chronic hepatitis, fatty liver deposits, inflammatory skin conditions** and **jaundice.** Standardized extracts of milk thistle are widely used pharmaceuticals in Europe. There they are employed not only as cures for disease conditions but also as a daily form of liver protection. The plant appears to have no toxic effects even when used for months at a time.

Medicinal Properties

Definite action
Antioxidant (silymarin)
Liver protectant (silymarin)
Liver cell proliferant (silymarin)

The flavonoids in milk thistle are responsible for its actions. They have the ability to prevent liver destruction and enhance liver function.

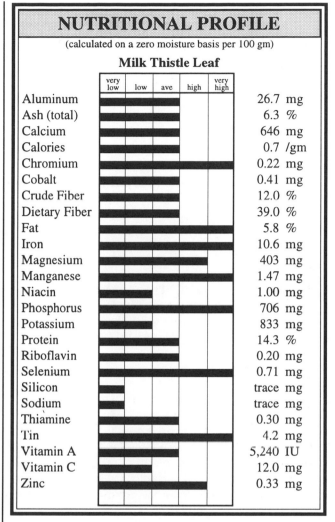

NUTRITIONAL PROFILE
(calculated on a zero moisture basis per 100 gm)

Milk Thistle Leaf

	very low	low	ave	high	very high	Amount
Aluminum						26.7 mg
Ash (total)						6.3 %
Calcium						646 mg
Calories						0.7 /gm
Chromium						0.22 mg
Cobalt						0.41 mg
Crude Fiber						12.0 %
Dietary Fiber						39.0 %
Fat						5.8 %
Iron						10.6 mg
Magnesium						403 mg
Manganese						1.47 mg
Niacin						1.00 mg
Phosphorus						706 mg
Potassium						833 mg
Protein						14.3 %
Riboflavin						0.20 mg
Selenium						0.71 mg
Silicon						trace mg
Sodium						trace mg
Thiamine						0.30 mg
Tin						4.2 mg
Vitamin A						5,240 IU
Vitamin C						12.0 mg
Zinc						0.33 mg

These bitter compounds protect the liver by inhibiting the enzymes responsible for the production of leucotrienes and prostaglandins. These compounds are often involved in inflammatory conditions of the liver and skin. In addition, the group of silymarin flavonoids are more powerful antioxidants than vitamin E which makes them useful in preventing free radical damage.

These compounds also help **regenerate liver cells** by stimulating protein synthesis. This results in an increase in the rate at which new liver cells are produced to replace damaged old ones. However, this cell proliferant stimulus does not affect malignant liver tissue.

In summary, milk thistle is very useful in treating all **inflammatory conditions of the liver** and **skin.**

Typical Daily Usage

Fresh leaf: 2-3 teaspoon

Dried leaf: 1-3 gm
Extract: 175 mg 80% silymarin standard
 concentrate

Traditional Formulas

Dandelion and Barberry combination
Dandelion and Parsley combination

Chemical Constituents

Aromatic compounds
 Resin
Bitter compounds
 Flavonoids
  Silymarin
   Silybin, silydianin, silychristine and
    others

Nutrients of Note

Water when fresh: 78%
Water when air dried: 5.6%

Mullein leaf

Verbascum thapsus (Scrophulariaceae)

Properties: mucilaginous, expectorant, diuretic, astringent, antispasmodic

Systems affected: respiratory, digestive

Common Names: moth mullein, white mullein, verbascum flowers, woollen blanket herb, flannel flower, cow's lungwort, velvet leaf

Folk History and Use

Mullein is a common plant in most parts of the United States. It has a distinctive wooly leaf that forms a rosette near the ground. It is a biennial producing a tall stem that often reaches more than three feet high. The stem produces a yellow flowering seed pod with copious quantities of seed. The seeds are wind blown and easily germinate in any disturbed ground or waste place.

Mullein has a folk history of use that focuses on respiratory ailments. It has traditionally been used to treat **coughs, colds, croup, bronchitis** and **asthma.** Because of its soothing nature, it has also been used to treat **hemorrhoids, ulcers** and **inflammatory skin disorders.** The flowers and seeds contain an essential oil used to treat **earache.** Mullein is considered the herb of choice for **lung ailments**.

Medicinal Properties

Definite action
 The benefits of viscous fiber (mucilage)
  Lowers bowel transit time
  Regulates colonic flora
  Soothes inflamed tissues
 Expectorant (mucilage)
 Astringent (tannin)
Probable action
 Diuretic (?)

NUTRITIONAL PROFILE

(calculated on a zero moisture basis per 100 gm)

Mullein Leaf

Nutrient	Value	
Aluminum	109	mg
Ash (total)	8.6	%
Calcium	1,330	mg
Calories	0.50	/gm
Carbohydrates	80.3	%
Chromium	0.14	mg
Cobalt	1.28	mg
Crude Fiber	11.1	%
Dietary Fiber	35.0	%
Fat	1.3	%
Iron	23.6	mg
Magnesium	323	mg
Manganese	1.20	mg
Niacin	9.50	mg
Phosphorus	570	mg
Potassium	1,320	mg
Protein	10.8	%
Riboflavin	0.11	mg
Selenium	0.05	mg
Silicon	0.74	mg
Sodium	76.0	mg
Thiamine	trace	mg
Tin	1.2	mg
Vitamin A	7,230	IU
Vitamin C	77.6	mg
Zinc	0.04	mg

Mullein is a mucilaginous herb that has many properties similar to marshmallow root. Its mucilage content is probably responsible for most of its medicinal properties. The saponins and tannin contribute to its soothing effects but little else is known about it scientifically.

Typical Daily Usage

Fresh leaf: 1-2 tablespoon
Dried leaf: 2-3 gm
Extract: 2 gm in a cup of boiling water

Traditional Formulas

Pumpkin and Cascara combination
Goldenseal and Juniper combination
Red Beet and Yellow Dock combination
Fenugreek combination
Ephedra and Passionflower combination

Chemical Constituents

Astringent compounds
   Tannin
Bitter compounds
   Saponins
Mucilaginous compounds
   Polysaccharides
     Mucilage

Nutrients of Note

Water when fresh: 56%
Water when air dried: 6.9%

Nettle leaf
Urtica dioica (Urticaceae)

Properties: bitter, diuretic, hemostatic, antitumor, antiseptic, emmenogogue, expectorant, vermifuge, antispasmodic

Systems Affected: urinary, respiratory, glandular, digestive

Common Names: stinging nettle

Folk History and Use

Stinging nettle is the common name for this herb. Much to the chagrin of recreational hikers, it grows in thick patches along stream banks and in shaded areas of most temperate climates of the world. It is reported in the traditional medical literature of Europe, China and North America.

The plant has dark green leaves with bristles that transfer irritating chemicals on contact. When the plant is cut at ground level and air dried, its stinging principles degrade substantially rendering it useful as animal feed and in traditional medicine with diminished chance of allergic reaction.

Extracts of nettle have been included in hair tonics for centuries due to its purported ability to stimulate hair growth. Like many bitter herbs, nettle is a **blood purifier**. Its long list of traditional uses can be summed up in its ability to increase the **production of urine**, its mild **laxative** effect and its ability to increase the efficiency of **liver** and **kidney** function. Besides these general effects, folk use points to the herb's affinity for

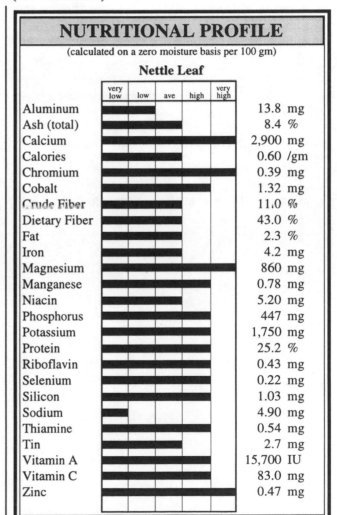

NUTRITIONAL PROFILE						
(calculated on a zero moisture basis per 100 gm)						
Nettle Leaf						
	very low	low	ave	high	very high	
Aluminum						13.8 mg
Ash (total)						8.4 %
Calcium						2,900 mg
Calories						0.60 /gm
Chromium						0.39 mg
Cobalt						1.32 mg
Crude Fiber						11.0 %
Dietary Fiber						43.0 %
Fat						2.3 %
Iron						4.2 mg
Magnesium						860 mg
Manganese						0.78 mg
Niacin						5.20 mg
Phosphorus						447 mg
Potassium						1,750 mg
Protein						25.2 %
Riboflavin						0.43 mg
Selenium						0.22 mg
Silicon						1.03 mg
Sodium						4.90 mg
Thiamine						0.54 mg
Tin						2.7 mg
Vitamin A						15,700 IU
Vitamin C						83.0 mg
Zinc						0.47 mg

treating imbalances of the mucous membranes. It has traditionally been used to treat **asthma, ulcers, bronchits, jaundice, nephritis, hemorrhoids** and **spasmodic dysmenorrhea**

Medicinal Properties

Probable action
Diuretic (?)
Emmenogogue (?)
Counterirritant to mucous membranes (?)

Scientists have only studied the sting of nettle leaf but little else. The sting is due to the action of histamine, acetylcholine and serotonin present in the leaf bristles. When taken orally, its action may be much like capsicum. The compounds in nettle irritate the mucous membranes of the digestive system, the membranes then counter the irritation by producing protective mucous. This, in turn, produces sympathetic responses in other mucous membranes of the body. These sympathetic responses would be centered on the **reproductive, respiratory** and **urinary systems** of the body, resulting in the long list of folk uses attributed to nettle.

A note of caution should accompany the use of nettle as it has been known to produce allergic reactions in some people.

Typical Daily Usage

Dried leaf: 3-6 gm
Extract: 4.5 gm dried leaf, 22 ml alcohol, 23 ml
water

Traditional Formulas

Red Beet and Yellow Dock combination

Chemical Constituents

Astringent compounds
Tannin
Bitter compounds
Saponins
Lignans
Sitosterol
Flavonoids
(uncharacterized)
Histamine
Acetylcholine
Serotonin

Nutrients of note

Water when fresh: 80%
Water when air dried: 6%
Chlorophyllins: 0.02%

Oatgrass (straw)
Avena sativa (Graminae)

Properties: mucilaginous, antidepressant, diuretic, nutrient source

Systems Affected: nervous, structural

Folk History and Use

Oatgrass, or oatstraw as it is popularly known, is the young shoots of the grain plant Avena sativa. Much has been written about the seed of this plant and especially about the effect of oat bran on serum cholesterol. To herbalists, however, oatmeal is for breakfast while oatgrass tea is for dinner. The young shoots of the oat plant can be sprouted like alfalfa and eaten as a rich source of minerals. The shoots and even the straw remaining after the grain has been harvested are excellent sources of the major minerals used in the structure of the body including magnesium and calcium.

A tea or extract of this herbal product is the most effective way of obtaining its virtues. The dried plant material is too fibrous to be eaten directly. Oatgrass tea is said to **relieve hysteria** and **balance the menstrual cycle of females**. Further, it is touted as a prevention for **osteoporosis** and a quick **cure of urinary tract infections.**

One word of warning: commercially available oatstraw is much less expensive than oatgrass. The quality of oatgrass is determined much like it is for barleygrass or wheatgrass, i.e. by its green color and characteristic odor.

Medicinal Properties

    Definite action
        Source of minerals
    Probable action
        Diuretic (?)
        Sedative (?)

Little is known about the chemistry of oatgrass. We performed a nutritional analysis on it for this work but little else is available. It ranks as the best terrestrial source of magnesium in our study. **Magnesium deficiency** has been linked to **menstrual disorders, irritability** and **poor calcium absorption**. This may contribute to its folk uses.

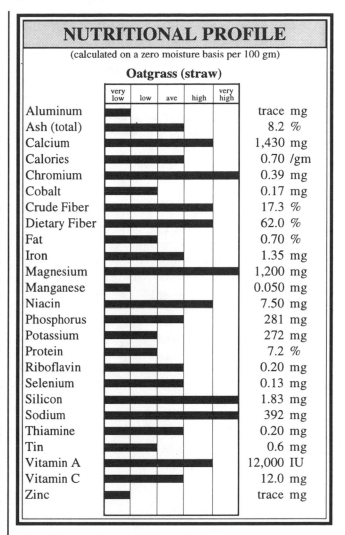

NUTRITIONAL PROFILE
(calculated on a zero moisture basis per 100 gm)
Oatgrass (straw)

Nutrient	Value	Unit
Aluminum	trace	mg
Ash (total)	8.2	%
Calcium	1,430	mg
Calories	0.70	/gm
Chromium	0.39	mg
Cobalt	0.17	mg
Crude Fiber	17.3	%
Dietary Fiber	62.0	%
Fat	0.70	%
Iron	1.35	mg
Magnesium	1,200	mg
Manganese	0.050	mg
Niacin	7.50	mg
Phosphorus	281	mg
Potassium	272	mg
Protein	7.2	%
Riboflavin	0.20	mg
Selenium	0.13	mg
Silicon	1.83	mg
Sodium	392	mg
Thiamine	0.20	mg
Tin	0.6	mg
Vitamin A	12,000	IU
Vitamin C	12.0	mg
Zinc	trace	mg

Typical Daily Usage

Fresh grass: 1-2 tablespoon
Dried grass: 2-3 gm
Extract: 2.5 gm dried grass in a cup of boiling water

Traditional Formulas

Marshmallow and Plantain combination

Nutrients of Note
Water when fresh: 78%
Water when air dried: 6.7%

Panax Ginseng root
Panax ginseng (Aralaceae)

Properties: bitter, adaptogen, circulatory stimulant, cardiac tonic, liver tonic, alterative

Systems Affected: immune, circulatory, glandular

Common Names: five finger root, American ginseng, sang, ninsin, panax, pannag, red berry

Folk History and Use

Ginseng has a worldwide reputation for maintaining good health, increasing one's resistance to fatigue, stress and disease, postponing old age symptoms and otherwise making healthier people out of those who take it regularly. The Chinese do not use it to cure a disease. For this reason, it has been difficult for Western pharmacologists and physicians to understand the benefits of ginseng.

Ginseng is the only plant used routinely by so great a number of more or less healthy individuals for stimulation, added energy and a sense of well-being. It is considered a panacea for those who want to increase longevity and health.

Ginseng has been an important part of the medicine of China and Tibet for thousands of years. In Shen Nung's <u>Materia medica</u> (196 A.D.), it was described as;

> a tonic to the five viscera: quieting the spirits, establishing the soul, allaying fear, expelling evil effluvia, brightening the eyes, opening the heart, benefiting the understanding and, if taken for some time, invigorating the body and prolonging life.

These folk claims are now being vindicated by modern research.

Three members of the Araliaceae family are marketed as ginseng: Chinese ginseng (Panax ginseng), American ginseng (Panax quinquefolium) and Siberian ginseng (Eleuthrococcus senticosus). To each of these are attributed the adaptogenic properties of ginseng. Eleuthrococcus is described separately in this work.

Panax has developed a folk reputation as a male herb that somehow increases testosterone production. Some females have avoided it for this reason. There is no scientific basis for this reputation and it has been included in many formulas designed to balance the female reproductive system. Eleuthrococcus, on the other

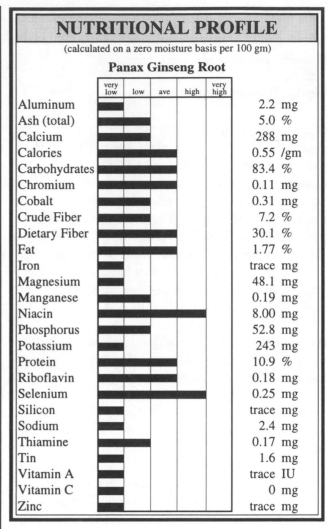

NUTRITIONAL PROFILE
(calculated on a zero moisture basis per 100 gm)

Panax Ginseng Root

Nutrient	very low	low	ave	high	very high	Value	Unit
Aluminum	■					2.2	mg
Ash (total)		■				5.0	%
Calcium		■				288	mg
Calories			■			0.55	/gm
Carbohydrates			■			83.4	%
Chromium			■			0.11	mg
Cobalt			■			0.31	mg
Crude Fiber			■			7.2	%
Dietary Fiber			■			30.1	%
Fat		■				1.77	%
Iron	■					trace	mg
Magnesium		■				48.1	mg
Manganese		■				0.19	mg
Niacin				■		8.00	mg
Phosphorus		■				52.8	mg
Potassium		■				243	mg
Protein			■			10.9	%
Riboflavin			■			0.18	mg
Selenium				■		0.25	mg
Silicon	■					trace	mg
Sodium	■					2.4	mg
Thiamine		■				0.17	mg
Tin		■				1.6	mg
Vitamin A		■				trace	IU
Vitamin C	■					0	mg
Zinc	■					trace	mg

hand, has become popular because it is less expensive and is considered to be without hormonal effect except to regulate blood sugar imbalances.

Panax derives its name from the Greek word "panacea" meaning all healing. The species name ginseng is Chinese for man plant, in reference to the shape of the root. The species name, "quinquefolium," is Latin for five fingered root, also in reference to its shape. The roots most resembling the human form are the most in demand. This is because the Doctrine of Signatures classifies ginseng as a tonic to the entire body and specifically the male body parts.

Ginseng has been used in Chinese medicines as an alterative to modify favorably the course of a disease or difficulty, specifically **tuberculosis, coughs, nausea, diabetes, indigestion, diarrhea, kidney degeneration, gout, rheumatism, suppurating sores, carbuncles, enuresis, insomnia, leprosy, radiation poisoning,** weakness of the spleen, longevity, sexual indifference and impotence. Many believe that ginseng also has aphrodisiac properties maintaining sexual potency in the male.

Medicinal Properties

Definite action
Adaptogen (saponins)
Cardiotonic (saponins)
Immune stimulant (saponins)
Increases endurance (saponins)
Liver enzyme stimulant (saponins)

Pharmacologically speaking, ginseng is classified as an adaptogen because some studies in animals suggest that it may help the body to adapt to stress and to correct adrenal and thyroid dysfunctions. Such effects, if real, are quite subtle, but are apparently a function of the panaxoside saponin glycosides contained in the root.

An adaptogen is a non-toxic substance that increases the body's resistance to adverse physical, chemical and biological factors.

Ginseng appears to have little effect in the absence of stress, but when stress occurs, it encourages a faster response of stress hormone and a more rapid return to normalcy. The action of ginseng is distinct from that of synthetic stimulants such as the amphetamines, for ginseng neither provokes excitation nor disturbs normal sleep. Administration may be prolonged and repeated without side effects. A generalized tonic effect is usually demonstrated after about two weeks and peaks after a month of treatment.

The root stimulates immune function by increasing natural killer cell activity. It also increases the rate at which liver cells are generated. Part of its anti-aging properties may be due to the fact that ginseng makes oxygen uptake and usage more efficient.

Panax ginseng contains a complex mixture of triterpenoid saponins. These glycosides have been categorized into three series: the panaxosides, the ginsenosides and the chikusetsusaponins. Their properties include (1) panaxin, a stimulant for the midbrain, heart, and vessels; (2) panax acid, a stimulant for the heart and general metabolism; (3) panaquilin, a stimulant for internal secretions; (4) panacin, a volatile oil that stimulates the central nervous system; and (5) ginsenin, which lowers blood sugar.

Since the effectiveness of ginseng appears to be useful mostly to counteract stress, it has come into general use for those who suffer from chronic diseases: anemia, depression, any chronic and debilitating disease especially of the heart and blood vessels, also after surgery, during convalescence, chronic infections such as tuberculosis and simply old age.

Scientific studies on ginseng will always yield conflicting results because of the balancing effect of the saponins. One study will show hypoglycemic effects while another will show hyperglycemic effects and yet another will yield no effect on blood sugar. This is not because ginseng isn't working, but because the nature of the test is wrong. Remember, an adaptogen only works in response to stress. Unstressed control groups will always yield negative results.

Typical Daily Usage

Fresh root: 1 tablespoon
Dried root: 1-2 gm
Extract: 2 gm dried root, 10 m; alcohol, 10 ml water

Traditional Formulas

Garlic combination
Biota and Zizyphus combination
Agastache and Shengu combination
Ginseng and Licorice combination
Dong Quai and Peony combination
Ginseng combination
Ginseng and Saw Palmetto combination
Bupleurum and Peony combination
Astragalus and Ganoderma combination
Dandelion and Purslane combination
Ginseng and Phaffia combination
Fushen and Dragon Bone combination
Bupleurum and Cyperus combination
Eucommia and Achyranthes combination

Chemical Constituents

Aromatic compounds
Essential oil
Panacene
Bitter compounds
Triterpenoid Saponins
Ginsenosides (11 identified)
Panaxosides (6 identified)
Mucilaginous compounds
Polysaccharides
Gum: 13%

Nutrients of Note

Water when fresh: 78.8%
Water when air dried: 7.8%
Sugars: 9% (glucose, sucrose, fructose, maltose)
Starch: 12%

Papaya fruit
Carica papaya (Caricaceae)

Properties: bitter, digestive aid, vermifuge

Systems Affected: digestive

Folk History and Use

Papaya fruit comes from a small tree that is native to the tropical regions of the American hemisphere. The fruits are smooth skinned and melon shaped, they are prized for their unique flavor and used fresh, in ice cream and tropical juice drinks.

Perhaps most importantly is the fruit's use as a source of the proteolytic enzyme papain. For this use, the green fruits are slit like opium poppy bulbs and a milky, enzyme-rich crude papain is scaped off.

Papaya is used as a food supplement to help digest proteins into peptides and amino acids. It also digests carbohydrates and fats into useful compounds which can then be absorbed through the intestines. Pepsin is also used for this purpose but suffers in popularity because it comes from animals and has a higher allergic rate than does papain and papaya.

Papain is also sold commercially as a meat tenderizer and has been used in a novel nonsurgical method of correcting herniated discs.

Papaya is used in folk medicine to treat **hypo–chlorhydria** and to **eliminate parasites and microbes** whose protein rich cell membranes may be susceptible to these proteolytic enzymes.

Medicinal Properties

Definite action
    Aids protein digestion (papain)
    Aids fat digestion (papain)
    Aids carbohydrate digestion (papain)
Probable action
    Vermifuge (papain)

Papain is a mixture of food digesting enzymes. These enzymes cut proteins which are long chains of amino acids into smaller chains and even into individual amino acids while in the digestive tract. Papain also helps digest fats and carbohydrates into compounds that the body in turn manufactures into useful molecules or metabolizes.

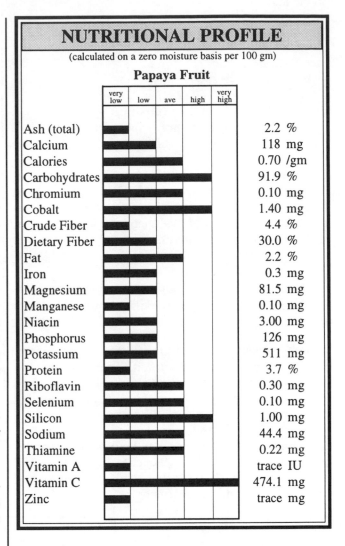

NUTRITIONAL PROFILE
(calculated on a zero moisture basis per 100 gm)

Papaya Fruit

	very low	low	ave	high	very high	
Ash (total)	■					2.2 %
Calcium		■				118 mg
Calories			■			0.70 /gm
Carbohydrates				■		91.9 %
Chromium				■		0.10 mg
Cobalt				■		1.40 mg
Crude Fiber		■				4.4 %
Dietary Fiber			■			30.0 %
Fat			■			2.2 %
Iron		■				0.3 mg
Magnesium			■			81.5 mg
Manganese		■				0.10 mg
Niacin			■			3.00 mg
Phosphorus			■			126 mg
Potassium			■			511 mg
Protein	■					3.7 %
Riboflavin			■			0.30 mg
Selenium		■				0.10 mg
Silicon				■		1.00 mg
Sodium		■				44.4 mg
Thiamine		■				0.22 mg
Vitamin A	■					trace IU
Vitamin C					■	474.1 mg
Zinc	■					trace mg

One note of caution when using any digestive enzyme: your body is made of the kinds of compounds that papain digests and overuse of them can lead to local inflammation of tissue, holes in one's digestive tract and allergic reactions.

Typical Daily Usage

Fresh fruit: 1-2 tablespoon
Dried fruit: 1.5-3 gm

Traditional Formulas

Chickweed and Cascara combination
Papaya and Peppermint combination

Chemical Constituents

Aromatic compounds
    Volatile oil
    Resin
Bitter compounds
    Digestive enzymes
        Papain, chymopapain, lysozyme, lipase
Mucilaginous compounds
    Polysaccharides
        Pectin

Nutrients of Note

Water when fresh: 86.5%
Water when air dried: 7.6%
Sugars: 18: (fructose, glucose)
Fruit acids: 7% (tartaric, malic, fumaric)

Parsley herb
Petroselinum crispum (Umbelliferae)

Properties: aromatic, diuretic, urinary tonic, carminative

Systems Affected: urinary, digestive

Common Names: parsley breakstone, garden parsley, rock parsley

Folk History and Use

Parsley is known as a plate garnish whose use is not only ornamental, but is also used as an after dinner breath mint to reduce mouth odor. Chlorophyll, abundant in fresh parsley, does indeed absorb odors and is the basis for this use. Parsley is also used as a **diuretic**, **laxative** and **emmenagogue**.

Parsley is a small, herbaceous plant with dark green, curly divided leaves. Native to the eastern Mediterranean countries, it is now well established in many countries, including the United States and Great Britain.

Dioscorides first assigned parsley its name by distinguishing between two "selinons," celery and parsley. Celery was called "helioselinon" or marsh selinon, and parsley was called "petroselinon" or rock selinon. Dioscorides' name for the plant has since been revised to petroselinum.

In Greek mythology, parsley was used as a garland for the head of Hercules after he successfully performed his 12 labors. The Greeks planted parsley near graves and the Greek expression "to be in need of parsley" referred to anyone who was near death.

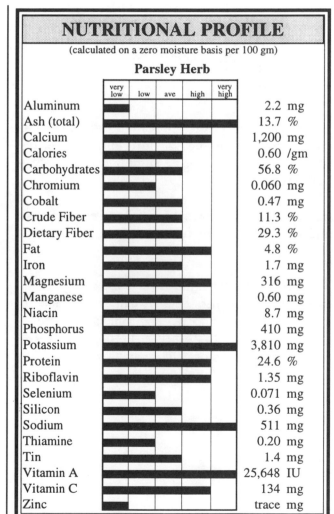

NUTRITIONAL PROFILE
(calculated on a zero moisture basis per 100 gm)

Parsley Herb

Nutrient	very low	low	ave	high	very high	Value
Aluminum						2.2 mg
Ash (total)						13.7 %
Calcium						1,200 mg
Calories						0.60 /gm
Carbohydrates						56.8 %
Chromium						0.060 mg
Cobalt						0.47 mg
Crude Fiber						11.3 %
Dietary Fiber						29.3 %
Fat						4.8 %
Iron						1.7 mg
Magnesium						316 mg
Manganese						0.60 mg
Niacin						8.7 mg
Phosphorus						410 mg
Potassium						3,810 mg
Protein						24.6 %
Riboflavin						1.35 mg
Selenium						0.071 mg
Silicon						0.36 mg
Sodium						511 mg
Thiamine						0.20 mg
Tin						1.4 mg
Vitamin A						25,648 IU
Vitamin C						134 mg
Zinc						trace mg

At Roman banquets, parsley leaves were hung around the necks of indulgers in alcoholic spirits, because it was believed that the leaves would absorb the alcohol fumes of the wine and prevent total drunkenness. The Romans also believed that one should eat parsley after indulging in garlic because it would act as a deodorant and absorb the smell.

Parsley has been used as a **tonic for the urinary system.** It is good for **difficult urination** and is an old folk remedy for **kidney stones** and **gallstones**. It is used to treat **jaundice, menstrual difficulties, asthma, coughs, indigestion** and **dropsy.**

Medicinal Properties
Definite Actions
    Antimicrobial (essential oil and flavonoids)
    Hypotensive (essential oils)
    Antipyretic (apiole)
    Carminative (essential oil)
    Emmenagogue (essential oil)
Probable Actions
    Laxative (?)
    Diuretic (flavonoids)
Possible Actions
    Liver stimulant (?)

The essential oil is responsible for the **diuretic, laxative, hypotensive** and **antimicrobial** properties. Myristicin is also a **uterine stimulant** and apiol has **antipyretic** properties.

Furocoumarins present in the volatile oil are phototoxic and may cause skin inflammations and contact dermatitis.

Many of its folk claims are as yet unproven. The chlorophyll content in parsley is partially responsible for its deodorant characteristics and complements the essential oil as a breath freshener. Fresh parsley is best suited for this use since chlorophyll oxidizes rapidly upon drying (See alfalfa).

Typical Daily Usage

Fresh herb: 2-4 tablespoon
Dried herb: 3-6 gm
Extract: 4.5 gm dried herb, 22 ml alcohol, 23 ml
    water

Traditional Formulas

Garlic combination
Capsicum and Garlic combination
Ginger and Dong Quai combination
Irish Moss and Kelp combination
Kelp combination
Dandelion and Barberry combination
Dandelion and Parsley combination
Rose Hips and Broccoli combination
Parsley and Senega combination
Ginseng and Parsley combination
Uva Ursi combination

Chemical Constituents

Aromatic compounds
    Volatile Oils: 0.05-.3%
        Terpenes
        Myristicin, apiole, beta-phellandrene,
           myrcene and others
    Fixed Oils and Resins: 2-4%
Bitter compounds
    Flavonoids
        Apiin, luteolin, apigenin and others
    Coumarins
        Bergapten, xanthotoxin, isopimpinellin
           and others

Nutrients of Note
Water when fresh: 92.1%
Water when air dried: 8.6%
Sugars: 9% (glucose, fructose)

Parthenium root
Parthenium integrifolia (Compositae)

Properties: mucilaginous, immune stimulant, antimicrobial

Systems Affected: immune, respiratory, digestive

Folk History and Use

Parthenium integrifolia is a perennial herb native to Missouri and grows over much of the eastern United States. It grows to a height of about three feet and has long hairy leaves that are often over a foot in length. It has white flowers and a dark brown root.

The Native Americans were discovered by the European settlers of the midwest of the United States to be chewing the root of this plant to cure coughs and sore throats.

It is a cousin to the echinacea species and shares many of their folk uses. During the late 19th century, it became regular practice to substitute parthenium for echinacea since most of the echinacea was being sent to German markets. Without the flowers to distinguish the plants as parthenium, this substitution became commonplace. Besides the botanical similarities, parthenium worked as well as echinacea to combat coughs, colds and other infectious ailments. During the past fifty years most of the echinacea of commerce was probably parthenium.

Parthenium has traditionally been used to treat **debility, fatigue, resiratory infection, gastrointestinal infection** and **venereal diseases.**

Medicinal Properties

Definite action
     Immune stimulant (?)
Probable action
     Antimicrobial (?)

Parthenium has been shown to both **mobilize and activate natural killer cells** and other **immune cells**. This effect is most pronounced when oral supplements are combined with anerobic exercise. Not only are the immune cells released into the blood stream, but their **killing power and longevity improved tenfold**.

This plant's nutritional profile matches very well with the nutrients one would like to find in an immune stimulating herb. It is relatively high in zinc and vitamin A, both very useful to one's immune system.

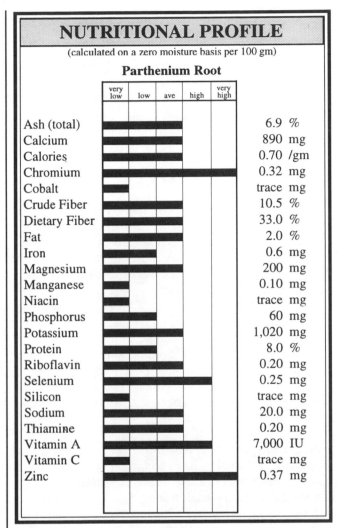

NUTRITIONAL PROFILE
(calculated on a zero moisture basis per 100 gm)

Parthenium Root

	very low	low	ave	high	very high		
Ash (total)						6.9	%
Calcium						890	mg
Calories						0.70	/gm
Chromium						0.32	mg
Cobalt						trace	mg
Crude Fiber						10.5	%
Dietary Fiber						33.0	%
Fat						2.0	%
Iron						0.6	mg
Magnesium						200	mg
Manganese						0.10	mg
Niacin						trace	mg
Phosphorus						60	mg
Potassium						1,020	mg
Protein						8.0	%
Riboflavin						0.20	mg
Selenium						0.25	mg
Silicon						trace	mg
Sodium						20.0	mg
Thiamine						0.20	mg
Vitamin A						7,000	IU
Vitamin C						trace	mg
Zinc						0.37	mg

The mode of action for this plant has not been studied or determined. It is possibly due to polysaccharides but these have not been characterized.

Typical Daily Usage

Fresh root: 1 tablespoon
Dried root: 1.5 gm
Extract: 1.5 gm dried root, 8 ml alcohol, 7 ml water

Traditional Formulas

Parthenium and Goldenseal combination
Parthenuim and Myrrh combination

Chemical Constituents

Aromatic compounds
     Essential oil
     Resin

Bitter compounds
Flavonoids
Mucilaginous compounds
Polysaccharides
Gum: 9%
Inulin: 15%

Nutrients of Note

Water when fresh: 84%
Water when air dried: 5%
Starch: 12%

Passionflower
Passiflora incarnata (Passifloraceae)

Properties: bitter, CNS depressant, antispasmodic

Systems Affected: nervous, skeletal

Folk History and Use

Passionflower is a viney plant named for its fruit and flowers. It is native to the subtropical regions of the American hemisphere. Passion fruit juice is often included in exotic drinks for its unique taste and color. The fruit itself is edible but many seeds and a pulpy texture diminish its popularity.

Early Spanish explorers saw this plant as a sign of God's favor since the flowers contained the elements of the crucifixion of Christ: the corona appearing to represent the crown of thorns, the petals representing ten true apostles, etc. Both its common and scientific name are derived from the plant being a living symbol of Christ's suffering or passion.

Homeopaths have used passionflower to treat **pain** and **insomnia**. Herbalists have had great success using it to treat **imbalances of the nervous system** including **insomnia, nervous tension** and **stress headaches**. Besides being an excellent herbal sedative, passionflower **relieves smooth muscle spasms**. This makes it useful for treating **spasmodic dysmenorrhea, colic, diarrhea, hemorrhoids, blood pressure,** and **epilepsy**.

Medicinal Properties

Definite action
CNS depressant (alkaloids, flavonoids)
Antispasmodic (alkaloids, flavonoids)
Hypotensive (alkaloids)
Antifungal (passicol)
Narcotic (alkaloids)

The medicinal properties of passionflower are attributed primarily to its alkaloids and flavonoids. Like many plant extracts, when the alkaloids and flavonoids are separated they lose their original effect. Indeed, the alkaloids in passionflower have little activity by themselves, but show the sedative and narcotic effects when a crude extract containing both the flavonoids and alkaloids is administered.

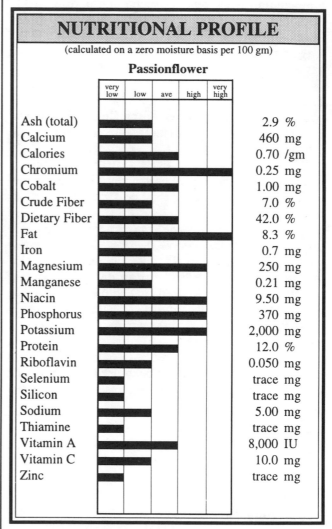

NUTRITIONAL PROFILE
(calculated on a zero moisture basis per 100 gm)
Passionflower

Nutrient	very low	low	ave	high	very high	Value
Ash (total)						2.9 %
Calcium						460 mg
Calories						0.70 /gm
Chromium						0.25 mg
Cobalt						1.00 mg
Crude Fiber						7.0 %
Dietary Fiber						42.0 %
Fat						8.3 %
Iron						0.7 mg
Magnesium						250 mg
Manganese						0.21 mg
Niacin						9.50 mg
Phosphorus						370 mg
Potassium						2,000 mg
Protein						12.0 %
Riboflavin						0.050 mg
Selenium						trace mg
Silicon						trace mg
Sodium						5.00 mg
Thiamine						trace mg
Vitamin A						8,000 IU
Vitamin C						10.0 mg
Zinc						trace mg

There are two families of alkaloids in passionflower, the harman group and the harmala group. The harman group produces effects similar to coffee. The harmala group produces drowsiness, inhibits the enzyme monoamine oxidase and relieves smooth muscle spasms.

The flavonoids of passionflower work in tandem with the alkaloids to enhance the overall effect of the herb. Passionflower also has an antifungal principle called passicol that shows intermediate killing power on candida species.

Typical Daily Usage

Fresh herb: 1-2 tablespoon
Dried herb: 1-3 gm
Extract: 2 gm dried herb, 10 ml alcohol, 10 ml
water

Traditional Formulas

Chamomile and Passionflower combination
Valerian and Black Cohosh combination
Ephedra and Passionflower combination

Chemical Constituents

Astringent compounds
Tannin

Bitter compounds
Alkaloids
Harman group
harman, harmol, harmine and others
Harmala group
harmala, harmaline and others
Flavonoids
Vitexin, saponarin and others

Nutrients of Note

Water when fresh: 89%
Water when air dried: 5.8%

Pau D' Arco inner bark

Tabebuia heptaphylla (Bignoniaceae)

Properties: astringent, antifungal, antitumor

Systems Affected: digestive, circulatory, structural

Common Names: taheebo

Folk History and Use

Pau d'arco is a hardy, deciduous tree that withstands severe winds and weather and reaches a height up to 30 meters. It resists fungal growth, even in its native rain forests.

Its purple colored inner bark was one of the major healing plants of the Incas and continues to be used today by the Callaway tribe of Indians. It is known by many names. In Argentina, it is called "lapacho" and in Brazil, "ipe." Here in the United States, however, the herb is known most frequently as pau d'arco or taheebo.

More pau d' arco trees are found in Argentina and Brazil than in any other country. The plant also grows in other parts of South America, Central America, Mexico and the Bahamas. It has also been found in other tropical areas, such as India, where it has been used as a medicinal herb.

Pau d'arco is as new to Western herbalists as capsicum was to Europeans in the early 1500's. Today, much confusion exists about its identification and use not only among herbalists, but also among taxonomists as well.

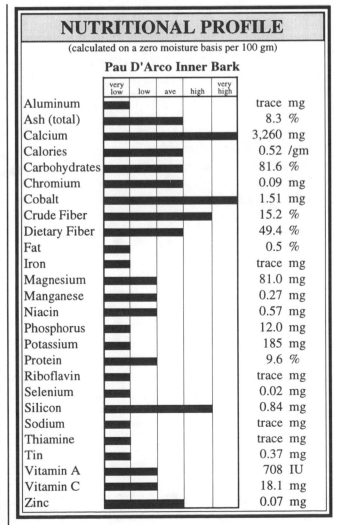

NUTRITIONAL PROFILE

(calculated on a zero moisture basis per 100 gm)

Pau D'Arco Inner Bark

	very low	low	ave	high	very high		
Aluminum						trace	mg
Ash (total)						8.3	%
Calcium						3,260	mg
Calories						0.52	/gm
Carbohydrates						81.6	%
Chromium						0.09	mg
Cobalt						1.51	mg
Crude Fiber						15.2	%
Dietary Fiber						49.4	%
Fat						0.5	%
Iron						trace	mg
Magnesium						81.0	mg
Manganese						0.27	mg
Niacin						0.57	mg
Phosphorus						12.0	mg
Potassium						185	mg
Protein						9.6	%
Riboflavin						trace	mg
Selenium						0.02	mg
Silicon						0.84	mg
Sodium						trace	mg
Thiamine						trace	mg
Tin						0.37	mg
Vitamin A						708	IU
Vitamin C						18.1	mg
Zinc						0.07	mg

There are dozens of different species of pau d'arco. They can be identified by their leaf configuration and flower color including pink, red, yellow and violet-flowered species. The trees with red, violet and pink flowers are preferred for medicinals, while the yellow-flowered species are considered to be an inferior product. The best pau d'arco is reported to be the violet-flowered Tabebuia heptaphylla, which grows mainly in Argentina. Argentina is also a large supplier of the violet-flowered species, while Brazil is the largest supplier of the yellow and red-flowered species.

The herb is harvested by peeling the bark from the tree in vertical strips from the ground up to the height of man. Only the inner bark is used for medicinal purposes and this must be painstakingly separated from the outer bark.

The Incas and native tribes of South America use pau d'arco bark externally as a poultice or decoction for treating **skin diseases** including **eczema, psoriasis, fungal infections, hemorrhoids** and **skin cancers.**

A tea made from the bark is used as a **blood purifier**, to treat **ulcers** and **rheumatism** and is said to cure **leukemia**. It is also **diuretic** and **antipyretic**.

The recent popularity of pau d'arco in Western herbology is attributed to its **antifungal** activity in treating **systemic yeast infections** like **candida albicans.**

Medicinal Properties

Definite Actions
    Astringent (tannins)
    Antifungal (tannins)
Possible Actions
    Antitumor activity (lapachol)

Pau d'arco has been studied extensively for its potential use as an antitumor agent. The studies, including those sponsored by the American Cancer Society at the National Institute of Health, have shown the purified individual napthaquinones to have little antitumor activity in vitro. These initial findings have essentially closed the book on conventional anticancer research with this herb.

However, the folk remedies for pau d'arco used a crude, boiling water extract (tea) that included all 16 known naphthaquinones and other, as yet unknown factors, to produce the antitumor effect. No one has yet proven or disproven the antitumor effects of pau d'arco as used by the South American Indians.

Other less controversial claims for pau d'arco include its astringency due to the tannins present and its antifungal action due to the naphthaquinones and tannins.

Yeast infections often accompany or follow antibiotic therapy and can be especially resistant to conventional treatment. The antifungal action of pau d'arco is used to combat these infections by drinking the tea thrice daily.

Typical Daily Usage

Fresh inner bark: 1/4-1/2 cup
Dried inner bark: 6-12 gm
Extract: 9 gm dried inner bark, 45 ml alcohol, 45
    ml water

Traditional Formulas

Pau D' Arco and Yellow Dock combination

Chemical Constituents

Aromatic compounds
    Volatile Oils - trace
    Fixed Oils and Resins
Astringent compounds
    Tannins
    Pseudo tannins
        Chrysophanic acid
Bitter compounds
    Naphthoquinones
        Lapachol, dehydrotectol, dehydro alpha
        Lapachine, dehydroisolapachone and
            others
    Saponins
        Sitosterol and others

Nutrients of Note

Water when fresh: 82.1%
Water when air dried: 7.8%

Peppermint leaf
Mentha piperita (Labiatae)

Properties: aromatic, stimulant, antispasmodic, carminative, antimicrobial, astringent

Systems Affected: digestive, circulatory, respiratory

Folk History and Use

Peppermint is a universally loved and widely used flavoring found in everything from toothpaste to liquor and medicine. Nearly one million cups of peppermint tea are consumed daily, making it the third most popular tea flavor in the world (behind black tea and chamomile tea).

The popularity of peppermint is based on its volatile oil, which contains an abundance of menthol, a time-honored and clinically proven aid to **digestion**. Menthol is also a mild **antispasmodic** which makes it useful for relieving **menstrual cramps** and **nausea**. It is also a mild **vasodilator**, creating a warm or flushed feeling by **stimulating circulation.**

The generic name for mint (i.e. mentha) is derived from the Greek, "Mintha," who in Greek mythology was the daughter of Cocytus. She was supposed to have been embodied in this plant by Prosperpine in a fit of jealousy. The species name "piperita" has reference to the peppery or pungent qualities of the plant.

There are three species of mint in cultivation and general use: spearmint, peppermint and pennyroyal, the first two being popular flavorings used in cooking.

Peppermint is a native of Europe, but has escaped cultivation in most temperate regions. In the United States, peppermint is more common then spearmint in waste places. Peppermint was first cultivated in England in 1750 and in Europe in 1771. Peppermint oil is an important European product and several varieties of peppermint have been developed, the chief ones being black and white. The black peppermint has high yields of lower quality oil (based on menthol content), while the white peppermint produces high quality oil in smaller amounts. American peppermint is of the black variety containing less than 50% menthol.

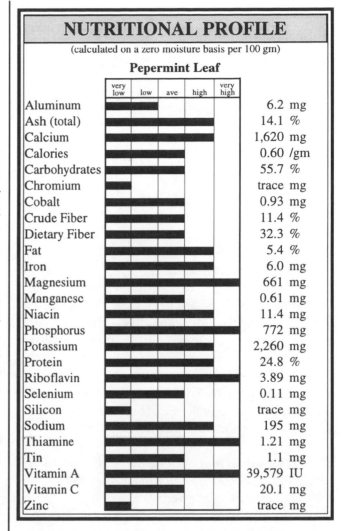

NUTRITIONAL PROFILE
(calculated on a zero moisture basis per 100 gm)

Pepermint Leaf

	very low	low	ave	high	very high	Value
Aluminum		■				6.2 mg
Ash (total)				■		14.1 %
Calcium				■		1,620 mg
Calories			■			0.60 /gm
Carbohydrates				■		55.7 %
Chromium	■					trace mg
Cobalt				■		0.93 mg
Crude Fiber			■			11.4 %
Dietary Fiber				■		32.3 %
Fat				■		5.4 %
Iron			■			6.0 mg
Magnesium					■	661 mg
Manganese			■			0.61 mg
Niacin				■		11.4 mg
Phosphorus				■		772 mg
Potassium				■		2,260 mg
Protein				■		24.8 %
Riboflavin					■	3.89 mg
Selenium				■		0.11 mg
Silicon	■					trace mg
Sodium				■		195 mg
Thiamine				■		1.21 mg
Tin				■		1.1 mg
Vitamin A				■		39,579 IU
Vitamin C		■				20.1 mg
Zinc	■					trace mg

Japanese farms produce the best quality oil because of their unique climate. Japanese oil contains up to 85% menthol. However, much of the Japanese oil in commerce has been dementholized and is at best, only a substitute for flavoring agents in toothpaste, etc. It is not uncommon for American peppermint oil to be adulterated with dementholized oil or with camphor oil, cedar oil or other volatile oils.

There is some doubt that the ancient Greeks used peppermint, although two species were known to them. The Romans used peppermint for flavoring and adornment. The ancient Egyptians cultivated peppermint and a 13th century Icelandic pharmacopoea includes it.

Peppermint oil is used in the food industry for flavoring. The herb and oil is used in the culinary arts because of its stimulating, **stomachic** and **carminative** properties. In medicine, peppermint has been useful as an **antispasmodic, expectorant** and **irritant**. It is used in alleviating the symptoms of **colds, flu** and **general fevers, nervous disorders, flatulent colic, rheumatism,** as a **local anesthetic** and to cover the taste or quality of the nauseating or griping effects of other medicines.

Medicinal Properties

Definite Actions
Antimicrobial (volatile oil)
Antispasmodic (volatile oil)
Vasodilator (volatile oil)
Astringent (tannin)
Probable Actions
Expectorant
Diaphoretic (volatile oil)

The oil of peppermint has been shown to be **antimicrobial** and **antiviral** against **Newcastle disease, herpes simplex, vaccinia, Semliki Forest** and **West Nile viruses.**

It also exhibits **spasmolytic** activity on smooth muscles and stimulates the production of digestive fluids which account for its carminative action.

The flavonoids in peppermint also add to the **spasmolytic** effects, **vasodilating** effects and **antimicrobial** properties of the herb.

The azulenes (See chamomile) show **anti-inflammatory** and **anti-ulcer** properties and the tannins provide the **astringency.**

One note of warning about peppermint is that the concentrated oils are very potent and may cause contact dermatitis, flushing and headache if rubbed on large portions of the skin or inhaled profusely. The whole leaf contains large quantities of astringent tannins that can damage the liver and intestine with prolonged use.

Typical Daily Uasge

Fresh leaf: 1/4-1/2 cup
Dried leaf: 6-12 gm
Extract: 9 gm dried leaf, 45 ml alcohol, 45 ml water

Traditional Formulas

Ginger and Barberry combination
Papaya and Peppermint combination
Ginseng combination
Chamomile and Rose Hips combination

Chemical Constituents

Aromatic compounds
Volatile Oil: 2-3%
Terpenes
Menthol, menthone, menthofuran, cineole and others
Azulenes
bisabolene
Fixed Oils and Resins
Astringent compounds
Tannin
Bitter compounds
Flavonoids
Rutin, menthoside, isorhoifolin, hesperetin and others

Nutrients of Note
Water when fresh: 85.1%
Water when air dried: 7.1%

Plantain seed

Plantago major (Plantaginaceae)

Properties: mucilaginous, antidiarrheal, antitumor, anti-inflammatory, antirheumatic, candidistatic

Systems Affected: digestive, immune

Common Names: broadleaved plantain, ripple grass, wagbread, white man's foot

Folk History and Use

Plantain seed is of the same genus of grainseed producing weeds that includes psyllium seed. Plantain is so common that it was once used as bird seed, but folk literature notes it as a cure for cancers of the digestive system and soft tissues. Like psyllium, plantain contains much mucilage that swells when placed in water. This makes it useful for giving bulk to the stool and for soothing inflamed mucous membranes.

In addition to its bulking effects, plantain has a reputation for **stimulating the immune system**. This property is not well defined since plantain is usually used in combination with other herbs and these effects may be attributable to them.

Plantain has traditionally been used to treat **diarrhea, dyssentary, inflammatory bowel conditions, hemmorhoids, breast cancer, thrush** and **colon cancer**.

Medicinal Properties

Definite action
    The benefits of viscous fiber
        Lowers bowel transit time
        Regulates colonic flora
        Absorbs toxins form bowel
    Diuretic (?)
Probable action
    Expectorant (mucilage)
Possible action
    Immune stimulant (?)

Plantain differs from most of the other mucilaginous herbs because of its reputed immune stimulating prop-

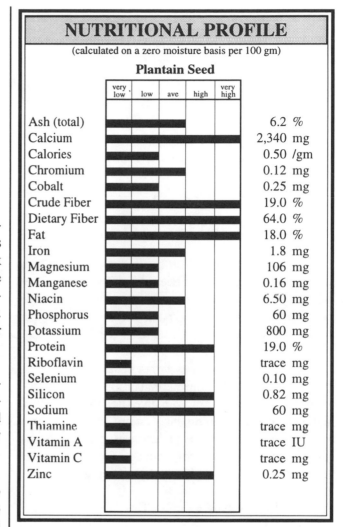

NUTRITIONAL PROFILE						
(calculated on a zero moisture basis per 100 gm)						
Plantain Seed						
	very low	low	ave	high	very high	
Ash (total)						6.2 %
Calcium						2,340 mg
Calories						0.50 /gm
Chromium						0.12 mg
Cobalt						0.25 mg
Crude Fiber						19.0 %
Dietary Fiber						64.0 %
Fat						18.0 %
Iron						1.8 mg
Magnesium						106 mg
Manganese						0.16 mg
Niacin						6.50 mg
Phosphorus						60 mg
Potassium						800 mg
Protein						19.0 %
Riboflavin						trace mg
Selenium						0.10 mg
Silicon						0.82 mg
Sodium						60 mg
Thiamine						trace mg
Vitamin A						trace IU
Vitamin C						trace mg
Zinc						0.25 mg

erties. As with other mucilaginous herbs like marshmallow root, the mucilage may trigger a sympathetic response in all mucous membranes of the body. Most of its reputation comes from topical application either to the surface tissues of the body or in the digestive tract.

Typical Daily Usage

Fresh seed: 2-4 teaspoon
Dried seed: 5-15 gm
Extract: 1-2 teaspoon in a glass of water

Traditional Formulas

Plantain combination
Goldenseal and Bugleweed combination

Marshmallow and Plantain combination

Chemical Constituents

Astringent compounds
  Tannin
Mucilaginous compounds
  Polysaccharides

Gum: 10 %
Mucilage: 25%

Nutrients of Note

Water when fresh: 70%
Water when air dried: 6%
Fixed oil: 18% (oleic, linoleic, linolenic)

Pollen

Properties: nutrient source, immune stimulant

Systems Affected: digestive, immune

Common Names: bee pollen

Folk History and Use

Pollen consists of plant pollens gathered by worker bees and mixed with nectar and bee saliva. The worker bees then pack this conglomerate into a granule that sticks to its back leg. It is carried back to the hive and fed to the male drones.

The types of pollen the bees gather naturally varies with their locale, but large commercial crops like citrus fruit or alfalfa can lend a predominant pollen to the product. In the nutritional supplement industry, pollen gathered from desert climates are prized most highly. Many people use pollen as a folk remedy for allergies and desert climates are considered hypoallergenic.

Commercially, pollen is gathered by forcing the worker bees through a small wire mesh placed at the opening of the hive. This mesh rubs the pollen off their legs. Recently, pollen has been gathered without bees where machines pass through fields of wind pollenated plants. This method of gathering pollen is favored by those who want a microbiologically cleaner product, but avoided by those who like the randomness of a natural product.

Pollen has traditionally been used to treat **allergies,** to **improve stamina** and add **longevity.**

Medicinal Properties

Definite action
  Nutrient source
Possible action
  Allergy hyposensitization

NUTRITIONAL PROFILE
(calculated on a zero moisture basis per 100 gm)

Pollen

	very low	low	ave	high	very high		
Aluminum	■					trace	mg
Ash (total)		■				3.4	%
Calcium	■					44.8	mg
Calories				■		0.80	/gm
Carbohydrates	■					44.8	%
Chromium					■	0.32	mg
Cobalt				■		1.45	mg
Crude Fiber	■					3.0	%
Dietary Fiber	■					13.0	%
Fat			■			1.8	%
Iron	■					trace	mg
Magnesium	■					59.0	mg
Manganese		■				0.12	mg
Niacin				■		7.20	mg
Phosphorus	■					251	mg
Potassium	■					555	mg
Protein					■	30.0	%
Riboflavin		■				0.10	mg
Selenium	■					0.07	mg
Silicon		■				trace	mg
Sodium	■					3.70	mg
Thiamine	■					0.29	mg
Tin			■			1.2	mg
Vitamin A				■		7,012	IU
Vitamin C		■				23.5	mg
Zinc		■				0.13	mg

Pollen is a good source of food for bees. It contains about 30% protein and over 50% carbohydrates. Its folk use as a concentrated, complete energy source is derived from the fact that bees produce lots of energy for their size. Hence, the term "busy as a bee."

Pollen grains have a protective coat that makes them very durable. 200 million year old intact pollen grains have been identified in rock samples. Bee saliva provides enzymes to dissolve this coat and free up the contents of the pollen grains. The human digestive system can also provide these enzymes, but pollen gathered by bees is more bioavailable.

The type of pollen seems to be important only to those who are trying to desensitize themselves from allergies. Allergic reactions to pollen gathered by bees is unusual but does occur.

Typical Daily Usage

Dried Pollen granules: 1-2 teaspoon

Traditional Formulas

Ginseng combination
Pollen and Ginseng combination

Chemical Constituents

Aromatic compounds
Essential oil
Waxes

Nutrients of Note

Water when fresh: 55%
Water when air dried: 4%
Sugars: 20% (fructose, glucose)
Starch: 18%

Psyllium seed or hull
Plantago psyllium (Plantaginaceae)

Properties: mucilaginous, demulcent, laxative

Systems Affected: digestive

Folk History and Use

Psyllium is the most popular mucilaginous herb in use today. Its hulls are well known as **bulk laxatives**. Psyllium is an annual herb, native to the Mediterranean regions of southern Europe, the Canary Islands, northern Africa and as far east as west Pakistan. In west Pakistan, northern and western India, and parts of Europe it is cultivated. It has also been planted on an experimental basis in the southwest United States.

Psyllium grows low to the ground and produces small, white flowers. The seeds, which are the part used, are smooth, dull ovals, varying from 1/16 to 1/8 inch long and are colored pinkish-gray-brown or pinkish-white. Each seed is enveloped in a husk (a white, thin, translucent membrane). The seeds do not have taste or odor, but when soaked in water, they will increase from eight to fourteen times their original size. This is due to the presence of mucilage, complex carbohydrates which attract and hold water. When alcohol is added to the water, however, the seeds will contract back to their original size.

Psyllium derives its name from the Greek word "psylla" meaning a flea because of the resemblance of the seed to a flea. Various forms of psyllium seeds appear in popular over-the-counter bulk laxatives such as Metamucil (G.D. Searle Co.), Naturacil (Mead Johnson), Perdium granules (Rorer), Prompt (G.D. Searle Co.), Syllact (Wallace), Effersyllium (Stuart), Fiberall (Rydelle) and Hydrocil (Howell). The husk mucilage is also used as a thickener or stabilizer in certain frozen dairy desserts.

The written history of the medicinal use of psyllium is surprisingly sketchy. More references refer to its use as a food or cattle fodder than as a medicinal herb. All references agree, however, on its medicinal use as a **bulk laxative**.

In India, psyllium is used as a **diuretic**, and in China, related species are used to treat **bloody urine, coughing** and **high blood pressure.**

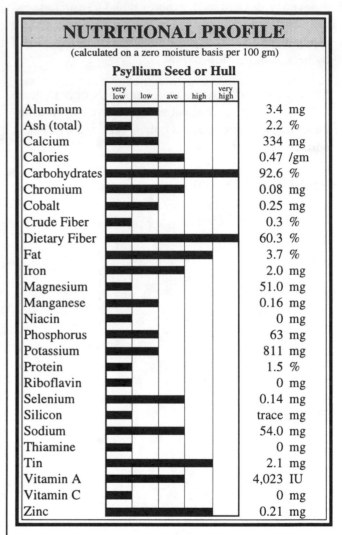

NUTRITIONAL PROFILE						
(calculated on a zero moisture basis per 100 gm)						
Psyllium Seed or Hull						
	very low	low	ave	high	very high	
Aluminum						3.4 mg
Ash (total)						2.2 %
Calcium						334 mg
Calories						0.47 /gm
Carbohydrates						92.6 %
Chromium						0.08 mg
Cobalt						0.25 mg
Crude Fiber						0.3 %
Dietary Fiber						60.3 %
Fat						3.7 %
Iron						2.0 mg
Magnesium						51.0 mg
Manganese						0.16 mg
Niacin						0 mg
Phosphorus						63 mg
Potassium						811 mg
Protein						1.5 %
Riboflavin						0 mg
Selenium						0.14 mg
Silicon						trace mg
Sodium						54.0 mg
Thiamine						0 mg
Tin						2.1 mg
Vitamin A						4,023 IU
Vitamin C						0 mg
Zinc						0.21 mg

Medicinal Properties

Definite Actions
 The benefits of viscous fiber
 Lowers bowel transit time
 Absorbs toxins from blower
 Regulates intestinal flora
 Demulcent on digestive tract
Probable Actions
 Diuretic (tannins)

Psyllium is a bulk laxative that increases the volume of the intestinal contents. This stretching action on the wall of the intestine encourages **peristaltic** activity in the bowel. The indigestible mucilage (active principle) is found both in the whole seed and the husk and swells when it comes in contact with water. The husks are most often employed since the seed germ contains oils and tannins which are undesirable in bulk laxative preparations.

Bulk laxatives are most popular with people over 50 years old who lead sedentary lives and need to stimulate the normal reflex activity of the bowel. Most of the popular psyllium preparations on the market today are predispersed liquids for convenience.

Today, there is a popular usage for psyllium and indeed for many mucilaginous herbs in the area of chronic yeast infections. **Candida infections** can be eradicated with harsh antibiotics and very restrictive diets, but psyllium can be employed to prevent the systemic absorption of the yeast's metabolic wastes that many individuals are sensitive to.

In their efforts to survive in one's colon, these yeasts produce toxins that can cause many allergic reactions. It is difficult at best to try and kill them all and only a few remaining candida yeasts can cause the sensitive reactions in some individuals. Psyllium is proving more beneficial and practical for many individuals who suffer from **chonic yeast infections.**

Typical Daily Usage

Fresh seed or hull: 1/2 cup
Dried seed or hull: 1-2 tablespoon
Extract: 1 tablespoon dried seed or hull in a cup of water

Traditional Formulas

Gymnema combination
Psyllium combination

Chemical Costituents

Aromatic compounds
Fixed Oils and Resins
Saturated fatty acids
Caprylic, stearic, palmitic, butyric and others
Unsaturated fatty acids
Linoleic, oleic
Astringent compounds
Tannin
Bitter compounds
Saponins
Sitosterol, stigmasterol, campesterol
Alkaloids
Indicain, plantagonine
Flavonoids
Aucubin
Mucilaginous compounds
Mucilage: 30-40%

Nutrients of Note

Water when fresh: 78.2%
Water when air dried: 6.9%

Red Clover flower
Trifolium pratense (Fabaceae)

Properties: bitter, diuretic, expectorant, cholagogue, antispasmodic, antirheumatic, estrogenic

Systems Affected: digestive, urinary, respiratory, glandular

Common Names: purple clover, trefoil, cleaver grass, cow grass

Folk History and Use

Red clover is extensively grown on pasture land. It is widely used as a forage crop for cattle and poultry. The plant itself is a legume so it fixes nitrogen and prevents erosion. It is often compared to alfalfa both for its nutritional value and appearance. It has many branched stems with groups of three leaves at the end of each stem. It is distinguished botanically and medicinally by its red flower.

The flowers are used in folk medicine as a cure for any lump or tumor. They are reported to have **diuretic, expectorant, antispasmodic and estrogenic** properties.

Red clover is a **blood purifier** that **increases the body's production of urine and mucous** and **promotes menstrual flow**. It is most often combined with chapparal as a folk remedy for cancer.

Red clover has been used to treat **cancer, rheumatism, jaundice, inflammatory skin conditions, spasmodic dysmenorrhea** and **bronchitis.**

Medicinal Properties

Definite action
   Diuretic (flavonoids)
   Expectorant (bitter principles)
   Cholagogue (bitter principles)
   Estrogenic (flavonoids)
   Antispasmodic (flavonoids)
Probable action
   Antitumor (?)
   Antirheumatic (?)

Red clover has a long folk history for curing **cancers** and **purifiying the blood** but has been studied as a cattle feed. The bitter principles in the flowers are probably responsible for its action. Its function as a blood purifier is easy to account for since an increase in urine and

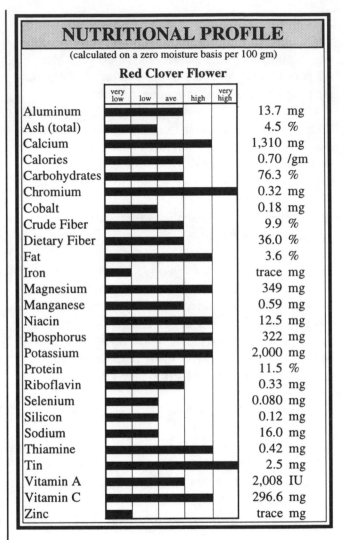

NUTRITIONAL PROFILE
(calculated on a zero moisture basis per 100 gm)

Red Clover Flower

	very low	low	ave	high	very high		
Aluminum						13.7	mg
Ash (total)						4.5	%
Calcium						1,310	mg
Calories						0.70	/gm
Carbohydrates						76.3	%
Chromium						0.32	mg
Cobalt						0.18	mg
Crude Fiber						9.9	%
Dietary Fiber						36.0	%
Fat						3.6	%
Iron						trace	mg
Magnesium						349	mg
Manganese						0.59	mg
Niacin						12.5	mg
Phosphorus						322	mg
Potassium						2,000	mg
Protein						11.5	%
Riboflavin						0.33	mg
Selenium						0.080	mg
Silicon						0.12	mg
Sodium						16.0	mg
Thiamine						0.42	mg
Tin						2.5	mg
Vitamin A						2,008	IU
Vitamin C						296.6	mg
Zinc						trace	mg

mucous output are relatively easy to measure. Its reputation for **eliminating lumps and tumors** has not been studied scientifically, but many testimonials have been logged in popular literature.

The flowers are difficult to harvest mechanically without getting a fair amount of the hay. Before the fall of communism, inexpensive labor was employed to harvest red clover flowers by hand. Recently, the price for good quality material has increased and inferior hay is often substituted.

Typical Daily Usage

Fresh flower: 1-2 tablespoon
Dried flower: 2-3 gm
Extract: 3 gm dried flower, 15 ml alcohol, 15 ml water

Traditional Formulas

Cascara combination
Pau D' Arco and Yellow Dock combination
Rose Hips and Broccoli combination

Chemical Constituents

Aromatic compounds
　Essential oil
　Resin
Bitter compounds
　Salicylates
　　Salicylic acid

Coumarins
　Coumaric acid, coumestrol
Saponins
　Trifolianol and others
Flavonoids
　Formononetin, trifolin and others
Mucilaginous compounds
　Polysaccharides
　　Gum: 5%

Nutrients of Note

Water when fresh: 82%
Water when air dried: 5%
Sugars: 12% (fructose, glucose, rhamnose)

Red Raspberry leaf
Rubus idaeus (Rosaceae)

Properties: astringent, antispasmodic, stimulant

Systems Affected: digestive, urinary, circulatory

Common Names: American raspberry, wild red raspberry

Folk History and Use

Red raspberry leaf tea is one of the most renowned herbal teas. It has a wide reputation as a **female tonic for relieving excessive menstrual bleeding**. For pregnant women, it is used to relieve **nausea, prevent nausea, prevent spotting, to tone the uterus in preparation for childbirth and to reduce the pain of childbirth.**

Because of its widespread availability in pleasantly flavored teas, the astringent leaves are administered to children to treat **diarrhea, flu** and **vomiting**.

Red raspberry is a member of the rose family and is native to England, where the plants grow on graveled road sides and hedgebarks. They are called ramps after Rampion, from the Latin "Rapunculus", a derivative of "rapa" meaning turnip. The roots were formerly boiled and eaten like turnips. It is now cultivated widely in all temperate climates of the world.

The generic name "rubus" comes from the Latin meaning red, and idaeus from the Latin "ida", the name of a mountain in Phrygia where the plant grew in abundance.

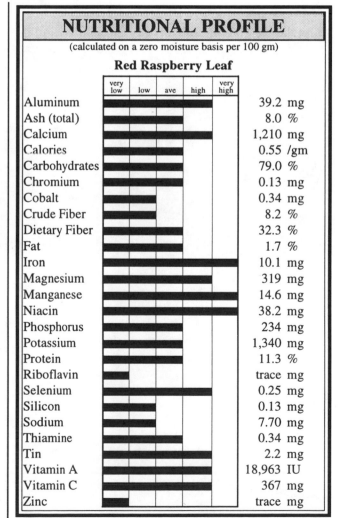

NUTRITIONAL PROFILE
(calculated on a zero moisture basis per 100 gm)
Red Raspberry Leaf

	very low	low	ave	high	very high		
Aluminum						39.2	mg
Ash (total)						8.0	%
Calcium						1,210	mg
Calories						0.55	/gm
Carbohydrates						79.0	%
Chromium						0.13	mg
Cobalt						0.34	mg
Crude Fiber						8.2	%
Dietary Fiber						32.3	%
Fat						1.7	%
Iron						10.1	mg
Magnesium						319	mg
Manganese						14.6	mg
Niacin						38.2	mg
Phosphorus						234	mg
Potassium						1,340	mg
Protein						11.3	%
Riboflavin						trace	mg
Selenium						0.25	mg
Silicon						0.13	mg
Sodium						7.70	mg
Thiamine						0.34	mg
Tin						2.2	mg
Vitamin A						18,963	IU
Vitamin C						367	mg
Zinc						trace	mg

Medicinal Properties

Definite Action
  Astringent (tannin)
  Antidiarrheal (tannin)
Probable Action
  Antiseptic (tannin)
  Antispasmodic (tannin)

Red raspberry leaf possess the classic properties of **astringent** herbs. The organic acids, especially the tannins and fruit acids (i.e. citric and malic), are responsible for these properties. The nutritional profile of red raspberry leaves shows a manganese content twice as high as any other herb making it the richest source of manganese in our study. The author speculates that manganese complexes may play a role in the red color of the fruit.

Typical Daily Usage

Fresh leaf: 1/4-1/2 cup
Dried leaf: 6-12 gm
Extract: 9 gm dried leaf, 45 ml alcohol, 45 ml water

Traditional Formulas

Cascara and Dong Quai combination
Black Cohosh and Golden Seal combination
Black Cohosh and Raspberry combination
False Unicorn and Golden Seal combination
Eyebright combination

Chemical Constituents

Aromatic compounds
  Volatile Oil
  Fixed Oil and Resin
Astringent compounds
  Tannin: 10-12%
  Organic Acids
    Citric and malic
Bitter compounds
  Flavonoids
Mucilaginous compounds
  Pectin: 5%

Nutrients of Note

Water when fresh: 83.1%
Water when air dried: 6.7%
Sugars: 6% (sucrose, fructose, glucose

Rosehips fruit

Rosa canina (Rosaceae)

Properties: astringent, nutrient source, antiseptic, antispasmodic

Systems Affected: immune, structural

Folk History and Use

Roses are thorny shrubs native to Europe and North America. The word rosa comes from the Greek word "rodon" meaning red, since the rose of the ancient Greeks was deep crimson. This is probably the source for the fable of the rose springing from the blood of Adonis.

Rosehips, the dried fruit of roses, are most famous as a natural source of vitamins and minerals, especially vitamin C. They also contain bioflavonoids and tannins that make the herb popular in treating **stress, infection, diarrhea, thirst** and **gastritis.**

Medicinal Properties

Definite Actions
Antiscorbutic (vitamin C)
Antimicrobial (flavonoids)
Antispasmodic (flavonoids)
Astringent (tannin)
Diuretic (?)

Vitamin C has **antiscorbutic** activity and is an essential nutrient most famous for its ability to **strengthen capillary fragility and connective tissue** (See vitamin C).

The bioflavonoids derive their name from the Latin world "flavus" meaning yellow. For more than 150 years, the dyeing industry used polyphenolic compounds (chemically similar to bioflavonoids) to dye linen, cotton and silk yellow. Not until a year later did scientists discover serendipitously that these yellow dyes worked synergistically with vitamin C.

The common dyes were called flavones, so scientists now refer to flavones with nutritive value as bioflavones or bioflavonoids.

Experiments with bioflavonoids have shown that they effect the heart and circulatory system and strengthen the capillaries. Generally, they are used as spasmolytics and diuretics. Most good sources of bioflavonoids are also good sources of vitamin C.

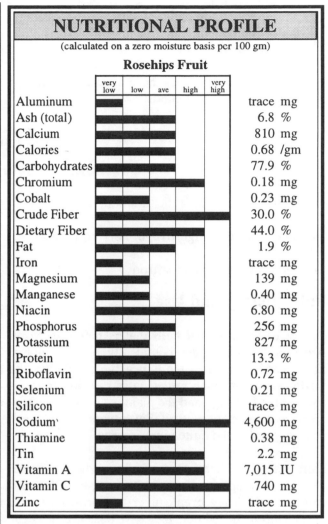

NUTRITIONAL PROFILE
(calculated on a zero moisture basis per 100 gm)

Rosehips Fruit

	very low	low	ave	high	very high		
Aluminum						trace	mg
Ash (total)						6.8	%
Calcium						810	mg
Calories						0.68	/gm
Carbohydrates						77.9	%
Chromium						0.18	mg
Cobalt						0.23	mg
Crude Fiber						30.0	%
Dietary Fiber						44.0	%
Fat						1.9	%
Iron						trace	mg
Magnesium						139	mg
Manganese						0.40	mg
Niacin						6.80	mg
Phosphorus						256	mg
Potassium						827	mg
Protein						13.3	%
Riboflavin						0.72	mg
Selenium						0.21	mg
Silicon						trace	mg
Sodium						4,600	mg
Thiamine						0.38	mg
Tin						2.2	mg
Vitamin A						7,015	IU
Vitamin C						740	mg
Zinc						trace	mg

Typical Daily Usage

Fresh fruit: 1/4-1/2 cup
Dried fruit: 6-12 gm
Extract: 9 gm dried fruit in a cup of boiling water

Traditional Formulas

Plantain combination
Dandelion and Barberry combination
Rose Hips and Broccoli combination
Pollen and Ginseng combination
Chamomile and Rose Hips combination

Chemical Constituents

Aromatic compounds
Volatile Oils
Fixed Oils and Resins

Astringent compounds
Tannin: 2%
Catechin
Organic acids
Citric and malic
Bitter compounds
Saponins
Flavonoids: 0.25%
Quercitin, rutin, hesperidin and others
Mucilaginous compounds
Pectin: 14%

Nutrients of Note

Water when fresh: 81.3%
Water when air dried: 7.3%
Sugars: 15% (fructose, sucrose, glucose)
Starch: 18%

Safflower
Carthamus tinctorius (Compositae)

Properties: bitter, diaporetic, diuretic, laxative

Systems affected: digestive, urinary, respiratory

Common Names: false saffron

Folk History and Use

Safflower is an annual herb that is native to North America. It is not related botanically, but the color of its flower is similar to the expensive saffron, so the safflower is commonly called false saffron. It grows about three feet high and the plant is cultivated extensively as a source of seed oil. Safflowers are yellowish orange in color and quite bitter in taste.

Safflowers have been used in folk medicine to treat children's complaints including **fever, measles and chicken pox.** They **break fever** and **produce much perspiration**. In addition, they have been used to **regulate menstrual disorders** and **calm the nerves.**

Medicinal Properties

Definite action
Diaphoretic (bitter principles)
Diuretic (bitter principles)
Laxative (bitter principles)
Antipyretic (bitter principles)

Safflowers are widely used in folk medicine and easily obtained as a by-product of the oilseed production. They are an excellent source of essential fatty acids. Their medicinal action has not been studied but many testimonials persist about their use in treating **spasmodic dysmenorrhea, liver disorders** and **fevers.**

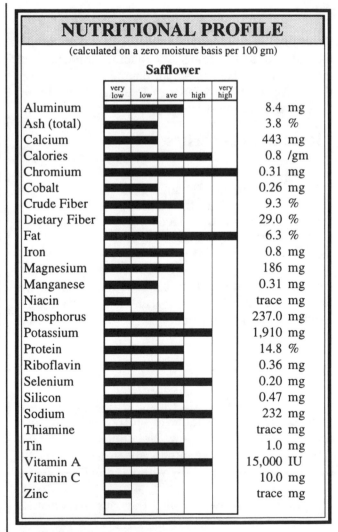

NUTRITIONAL PROFILE
(calculated on a zero moisture basis per 100 gm)

Safflower

	very low	low	ave	high	very high		
Aluminum						8.4	mg
Ash (total)						3.8	%
Calcium						443	mg
Calories						0.8	/gm
Chromium						0.31	mg
Cobalt						0.26	mg
Crude Fiber						9.3	%
Dietary Fiber						29.0	%
Fat						6.3	%
Iron						0.8	mg
Magnesium						186	mg
Manganese						0.31	mg
Niacin						trace	mg
Phosphorus						237.0	mg
Potassium						1,910	mg
Protein						14.8	%
Riboflavin						0.36	mg
Selenium						0.20	mg
Silicon						0.47	mg
Sodium						232	mg
Thiamine						trace	mg
Tin						1.0	mg
Vitamin A						15,000	IU
Vitamin C						10.0	mg
Zinc						trace	mg

Typical Daily Usage

Fresh flower: 1-2 tablespoon
Dried flower: 2-3 gm
Extract: 3 gm dried flower, 15 ml alcohol, 15 ml water

Traditional Formulas

Chickweed and Cascara combination
Gentain and Cascara combination
Licorice combination
Ginseng combination

Chemical Constituents

Aromatic compounds
  Fixed oil and resin: 6-10%
    Essential fatty acids
      Linoleic, linolenic and others
  Carotenes
  Xanthophylls
Astringent compounds
  Tannin
Bitter compounds
  Flavonoids
    Quercitin and others

Nutrients of note
  Water when fresh: 86%
  Water when air dried: 6.1%
  Sugars: 9% (glucose)
  Starch : 10%

Sage leaf
Salvia officinalis (Labiatae

Properties: aromatic, stimulant, carminative, antispasmodic, antiseptic, immune stimulant

Systems Affected: digestive, nervous, lymphatic

Common Names: garden sage, wild sage

Folk History and Use

"He that would live for aye, must eat sage in May." (English Proverb)

The Latin name for sage, "salvia," means saviour. This species was formerly thought of as the herbal saviour of mankind. English herbalists believed that in the garden, this plant would prosper or wane as the owners business prospered or failed. It was also said that the plant grows vigorously in any garden where the wife rules the house. It was common, therefore, for the husband to prune the garden ruthlessly to destroy the evidence of his subservience. There are folk tales of sage being used against the bitings of serpents, to cure palsy and to improve memory. In France, it was displayed in cemeteries to mitigate grief. The Italians eat sage to preserve their health.

"Why should a man die whilst sage grows in his garden?" (English Proverb)

Sage is native to the Mediterranean region and is now found in kitchen gardens worldwide. It is a small, evergreen shrub that is moderately winter-hardy. It flowers in August, giving rise to whorls of purple flowers. All parts of the plant are strongly scented.

NUTRITIONAL PROFILE
(calculated on a zero moisture basis per 100 gm)

Sage Leaf

	very low	low	ave	high	very high	Value
Aluminum						11.5 mg
Ash (total)						8.7 %
Calcium						1,080 mg
Calories						0.68 /gm
Carbohydrates						66.0 %
Chromium						0.030 mg
Cobalt						trace mg
Crude Fiber						19.6 %
Dietary Fiber						28.9 %
Fat						13.8 %
Iron						1.5 mg
Magnesium						283 mg
Manganese						0.30 mg
Niacin						6.20 mg
Phosphorus						128 mg
Potassium						2,470 mg
Protein						11.5 %
Riboflavin						0.36 mg
Selenium						trace mg
Silicon						0.31 mg
Sodium						108 mg
Thiamine						0.82 mg
Tin						0.8 mg
Vitamin A						6,413 IU
Vitamin C						35.0 mg
Zinc						0.59 mg

Sage is a common culinary herb, being used to flavor wines, preserves, cheeses, poultry and meats. There is no more wholesome way of taking it than to eat the leaves with bread and butter. It is used in domestic medicine for **mouthwash, gargles, fevers** and **upset stomach.**

Sage extracts have strong **antioxidant** activity due to the presence of labiatic acid and carnosic acid. This property is employed to cure meats, to preserve other foods and to suppress the odor of fish.

Sage is a **stimulant, astringent and carminative**. It has been used in **dyspepsia, to treat sore throats, tonsillitis, stomatitis, gingivitis, headaches** and **night sweats**.

The Chinese value it in treating yin (cold) conditions such as **weakness of the stomach, nerves and digestive system**. Sage also has the ability to **decrease perspiration (antihydrotic)** which makes it useful to desert peoples and in deodorant preparations.

Medicinal Properties

Definite Action
  Antimicrobial (volatile oil and flavonoids)
  Antispasmodic (flavonoids)
  Astringent (tannins)
  Antioxidant (phenolic acids)
Probable Action
  Digestive aid (volatile oil)
  Immune stimulant (?)

Sage is a member of the labiatae or mint family. Most mints, including sage, are aromatic herbs whose volatile oils are the desired medicinal principle.

Thujone, camphor, cineole (eucalyptus fragrance) and borneol are the major constituents of the essential oil in sage. These compounds are **antimicrobial** and **antispasmodic**. Sage oil helps protect against **acetylcholine spasms**. The **carminative** property of the oil results from its ability to **stimulate the production of digestive fluids** and **relax smooth muscles**.

The flavonoids present also contribute to the **antimicrobial** action of sage.

The phenolic acids, especially labiatic and carnosic acids, are powerful **antioxidants** and account for sage's ability to preserve meat products.

The **astringent** effects of sage are due in part to the tannins present.

Typical Daily Usage

Fresh leaf: 2-4 tablespoon
Dried leaf: 3-6 gm
Extract: 4.5 gm dried herb, 22 ml alcohol, 23 ml
  water

Traditional Formulas

Chamomile and Rose Hips combination
Horsetail and Gelatin combination

Chemical Constituents
Aromatic compounds
  Volatile Oils: 1-2.5%
    Terpenes
      Thujone, cineole, borneol and others
      borneol
  Fixed Oil and Resin: 3-5%
Astringent compounds
  Tannins: 0.5-1.0%
    Salviatannin
  Phenolic Acids (anti-oxidants)
    Salvin, rosmarinic and others
Bitter compounds
  Flavonoids-8
    Genkwanin, luteolin, hispidulin, salvigenin
      and others
  Bitter resin
    Picrosalvin and carnosol

Nutrients of Note

Water when fresh: 84.3%
Water when air dried: 8.0%

Sarsaparilla root
Smilax officinalis (Liliaceae)

Properties: bitter, antirheumatic, antiseptic, digestive aid, antipyretic, blood purifier

Systems Affected: immune, digestive

Common Names: red sarsaparilla, small spikenard, spignet, quay, quill

Folk History and Use

Sarsaparilla root comes from a perennial vine that grows in the tropical climates of Central and South America. It is a major flavor ingredient of root beer, and along with yucca root, gives the soft drink its foaming properties. The bitter saponins that foam in aqueous solution also give the root its medicinal action.

Sarsaparilla was originally brought to Europe in the 15th century by Spanish explorers as a cure for syphillis. It gained popularity again after a century and a half of mercury torture proved useless for the treatment of venereal disease. It found widespread use in the snake oils of the 19th century, later as a spring tonic for treating rheumatism and today as a beverage flavor. Root extracts I have tasted are only slightly bitter. It appears that sarsaparilla is included in root beers more for its color and foaming contributions than flavor.

Sarsparilla is essentially a **blood purifier** that acts mainly in the colon. It controls the balance of colonic flora and binds the toxins produced by the resident yeasts and bacteria. Most of the bitter principles in the root are not absorbed appreciably into the blood. They are activated only in alkaline solutions like the environment of the colon. This prevents them from interfering with the processes of digestion and absorption in the upper digestive tract. In the lower bowel, they react with the alkaline media and **bind to a variety of toxins.**

Toxin in this sense means allergen. It is any compound that elicits an immune response. For example, some people are very sensitive (allergic) to the metabolic waste of yeasts such as candida. In some individuals even a minute quantity of these compounds produces a syndrome of symptoms. Individuals with these sensitivities go to great lengths to eliminate the yeasts through antibiotics and dietary control. Others have

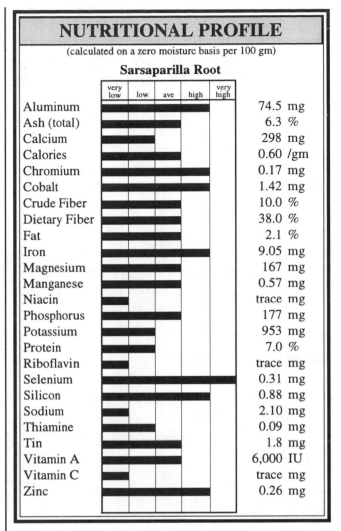

NUTRITIONAL PROFILE
(calculated on a zero moisture basis per 100 gm)

Sarsaparilla Root

	very low	low	ave	high	very high	
Aluminum						74.5 mg
Ash (total)						6.3 %
Calcium						298 mg
Calories						0.60 /gm
Chromium						0.17 mg
Cobalt						1.42 mg
Crude Fiber						10.0 %
Dietary Fiber						38.0 %
Fat						2.1 %
Iron						9.05 mg
Magnesium						167 mg
Manganese						0.57 mg
Niacin						trace mg
Phosphorus						177 mg
Potassium						953 mg
Protein						7.0 %
Riboflavin						trace mg
Selenium						0.31 mg
Silicon						0.88 mg
Sodium						2.10 mg
Thiamine						0.09 mg
Tin						1.8 mg
Vitamin A						6,000 IU
Vitamin C						trace mg
Zinc						0.26 mg

an apparent immunity to these toxins and suffer no ill effects. Sarsaparilla, like yucca, binds to these toxins and causes them to be eliminated from the bowel.

Many of the allergic reactions to colonic flora metabolites are manifested as inflammations. This probably accounts for the popular history of sarsaparilla in the treatment of **rheumatism, arthritis, inflammatory bowel conditions** and **skin inflammations including psoriasis.**

Medicinal Properties

Definite action
    Binds endotoxins (steroidal saponins)
Probable action
    Antiseptic (?)
    Blood Purifier (?)

Sarsaparilla has shown some **antibiotic** activity. A Chinese study showed the root to be 90% effective in treating acute cases and 50% effective in treating chronic cases. Its action is due to its content of steroidal saponins.

You can demonstrate the pH reaction of these saponins by performing a simple test. First, mix a little of the root in some vinegar and note its color. Then add slowly a weak solution of baking soda to the vinegar until you see the color darken noticably. This crudely imitates what happens in your own digestive tract and shows how smart nature is in protecting our digestion from these binding chemicals by allowing their protective release in the colon.

The steroidal saponins are also used by body builders as a dietary supplement of the building blocks required by the body to manufacture steroidal hormones. Remember, these compounds are not absorbed appreciably from the bowel and are not very effective for this application.

Typical Daily Usage

Fresh root: 2-4 tablespoon
Dried root: 3-6 gm
Extract: 4.5 gm dried root, 22 ml alcohol, 23 ml water

Traditional Formulas

Black Cohosh and Blessed Thistle combination
Ginseng and Saw Palmetto combination
Irish Moss and Kelp combination
Alfalfa and Yucca combination
Pau D' Arco and Yellow Dock combination

Chemical Constituents

Aromatic compounds
    Volatile oil
Bitter compounds
    Saponins
        Sarsaponin
        Smilasaponin
        Sarsaparilloside

Nutrients of Note

Water when fresh: 79%
Water when air dried: 6.2%
Starch: 25%

Saw Palmetto berry
Serenoa repens (Palmae)

Properties: bitter, antiandrogenic, anti-inflammatory, antihistamine

Systems Affected: urinary, structural

Folk History and Use

Saw palmetto is a fan palm that grows in thick groups in the southeast portion of the United States. It has large leaf fans that can be up to two feet long. The berries are dark brown and are harvested in late September.

The berries have a rich tradition as a sexual stimulant and aphrodisiac. They are said to make **infertile males fertile** and **increase breast size in women**. Scientists have found steroidal precursors in saw palmetto berries, but these sitosterols are not absorbed well in the intestines. Even though saw palmetto won't improve your sex life to any great extent or give greater definition to your musculature, it has been shown to help men **reduce their enlarged prostates**. The ability of the berries to **relieve the inflammation and pain of benign prostatic hypertrophy** qualifies it as a sexual stimulant, relatively speaking, since the absence of pain is pleasure.

Medicinal Properties

Definite action
    Antiandrogenic (bitter principle)
    Diuretic (bitter principle)
    Urinary antisepic (bitter principle)
Possible action
    Aphrodisiac (?)

Recently, the berries have been shown to **reduce prostatic enlargement** by inhibiting the enzyme testosterone-5-alpha reductase. Some as yet unidentified compound has a direct action on estrogen receptors in the body and inhibits the production of this enzyme. Its identity is probably being withheld because of the potential profits that will come from a drug derivative of this plant extract. Perhaps a billion dollars in sales are at stake and the naturally occurring compounds in this plant cannot be protected by patents.

Typical Daily Usage

Fresh berry: 2-3 teaspoon
Dried berry: 1-1.5 gm
Extract: 1.5 gm dried berry, 8 ml alcohol, 7 ml
    water

Traditional Formulas
Ginseng and Saw Palmetto combination

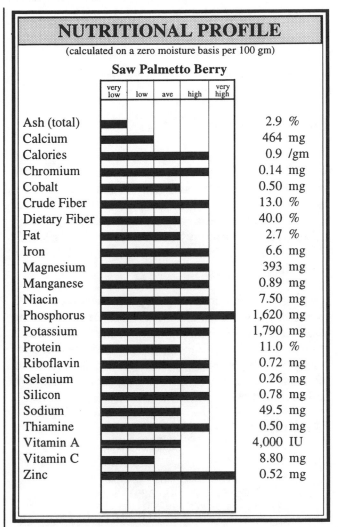

NUTRITIONAL PROFILE
(calculated on a zero moisture basis per 100 gm)

Saw Palmetto Berry

	very low	low	ave	high	very high		
Ash (total)						2.9	%
Calcium						464	mg
Calories						0.9	/gm
Chromium						0.14	mg
Cobalt						0.50	mg
Crude Fiber						13.0	%
Dietary Fiber						40.0	%
Fat						2.7	%
Iron						6.6	mg
Magnesium						393	mg
Manganese						0.89	mg
Niacin						7.50	mg
Phosphorus						1,620	mg
Potassium						1,790	mg
Protein						11.0	%
Riboflavin						0.72	mg
Selenium						0.26	mg
Silicon						0.78	mg
Sodium						49.5	mg
Thiamine						0.50	mg
Vitamin A						4,000	IU
Vitamin C						8.80	mg
Zinc						0.52	mg

Chemical Constituents

Aromatic compounds
    Volatile oil
    Resin
Bitter compounds
    Saponins
        Sitosterols
    Unidentified compounds with antiandrogenic
        activity
Mucilaginous compounds
    Pectin: 6%

Nutrients of Note

Water when fresh: 87%
Water when air dried: 8.3%
Sugars: 10% (fructose, glucose, sorbitol)

Schizandra fruit
Schizandra chinensis (Schizandraceae)

Properties: bitter, adaptogen, expectorant, antitussive, CNS depressant, antihepatotoxic

Systems Affected: immune, nervous, respiratory, digestive

Folk History and Use

Schizandra fruit comes from aromatic trees that are native to China and Russia. It has been traditionally used by the Chinese to suppress **coughs** and to protect against more serious respiratory conditions. Besides its calming effects on coughs, it also has a **calming effect on the nervous system**. It is reported to be similar in action to alcohol; first, stimulating the CNS, then depressing it.

It has been shown to have a **hepatoprotectant** effect, **increasing the enzymatic metabolism of toxins in the liver**. This action is thought to be similar in mechanism to milk thistle. Schizandra also **increases the production of digestive enzymes** and, for this reason, is often used to catalyze or increase the bioavailability of herbal remedies.

Medicinal Properties

Definite action
  Hepatoprotectant (lignans)
  CNS depressant (lignans)
  Digestive aid (lignans)
Probable action
  Adaptogen (?)
  Antitussive (lignans)
Possible action
  Antiseptic (?)

Schizandra fruit has been shown to **increase the production of enzymes in the liver and the organs of digestion, especially the bowel**. This increases the ability of the body to **metabolize and eliminate toxins**. Its reputation as an **adaptogen** is probably linked to these protecting qualities.

Its reported **antitussive** and **pulmonary protecting** properties have not been scientifically confirmed, but its effective use in this manner is widely documented.

Schizandra is most often found in formulas used to **relieve stress**. The fruit can be a profound CNS depressant. It is rarely sold by itself since those who wish to achieve calmness don't usually want to be depressed.

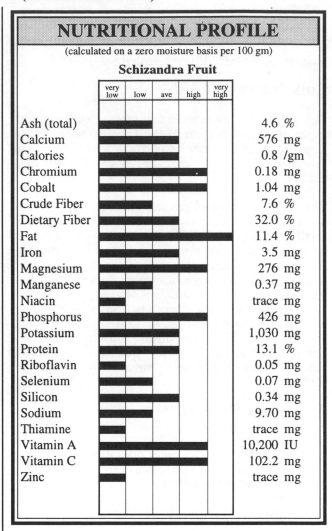

NUTRITIONAL PROFILE
(calculated on a zero moisture basis per 100 gm)

Schizandra Fruit

	very low	low	ave	high	very high		
Ash (total)						4.6	%
Calcium						576	mg
Calories						0.8	/gm
Chromium						0.18	mg
Cobalt						1.04	mg
Crude Fiber						7.6	%
Dietary Fiber						32.0	%
Fat						11.4	%
Iron						3.5	mg
Magnesium						276	mg
Manganese						0.37	mg
Niacin						trace	mg
Phosphorus						426	mg
Potassium						1,030	mg
Protein						13.1	%
Riboflavin						0.05	mg
Selenium						0.07	mg
Silicon						0.34	mg
Sodium						9.70	mg
Thiamine						trace	mg
Vitamin A						10,200	IU
Vitamin C						102.2	mg
Zinc						trace	mg

Therefore, it is often combined with ginseng, gotu kola or pollen, which are herbal products used to increase one's stamina.

Typical Daily Usage

Fresh fruit: 1 teaspoon
Dried fruit: 0.5 gm
Extract: 0.5 gm dried fruit, 3 ml alcohol, 2 ml water

Traditional Formulas

Biota and Zizyphus combination
Rehmannia and Ophiopogon combination
Astragalus and Ganoderma combination
Pollen and Ginseng combination
Pinellia and Citrus combination
Anemarrhena and Astragalus combination

Chemical Constituents

Aromatic compounds
  Volatile oil
Bitter compounds
  Lignans: 2%
    Schizandrin and related compounds

Nutrients of note

Water when fresh: 85%
Water when air dried: 7.7%
Sugars: 12% (fructose, glucose)
Fruit acids: 10% (malic, citric, tartaric)

Scullcap herb
Scutellaria lateriflora (Labiatae)

Properties: aromatic, anticonvulsive, antispasmodic, antibacterial, sedative

Systems Affected: nervous, structural

Common Names: blue scullcap, blue pimpernel, hoodwort, mad-dog weed, side flower, scullcap helmet flower, American scullcap

Folk History and Use

The scullcaps are a group of herbaceous plants scattered over the temperate climates of the world. The American species, lateriflora, is used as a **nervine**. The herb is found along the banks of rivers and lakes and in other moist places.

Its popular and generic names are derived from the Latin "scutella" meaning a small dish in reference to the shape of the appendage to the flower, which resembles a cap in appearance.

American scullcap was formerly called mad dog scullcap or madweed, for having the reputation of curing hydrophobia (canine rabies).

Scullcap has been reported to be both **tonic** and **antispasmodic**. It has been recommended for almost every ailment of the nervous system. Specific uses have been as treatment for **chorea, convulsions, tetanus, tremors, delirium tremens, insomnia, hysteria, nervous tension, St. Vitus dance, muscular twitching, hyperesthesia, neuralgia, anuresis** and **paralysis agitans**. A popular cold treatment uses a tea made of scullcap combined with boneset.

The French call the plant toque. The Chinese use the root of scuttelaria baicalensis as a cooling antipyretic herb that has diuretic and laxative properties.

Medicinal Properties

Definite Action
  Antibacterial (flavonoids)

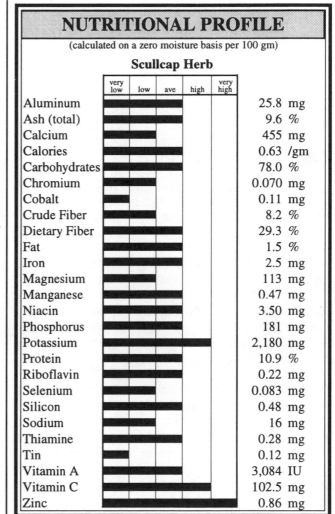

NUTRITIONAL PROFILE
(calculated on a zero moisture basis per 100 gm)

Scullcap Herb

	very low	low	ave	high	very high	
Aluminum						25.8 mg
Ash (total)						9.6 %
Calcium						455 mg
Calories						0.63 /gm
Carbohydrates						78.0 %
Chromium						0.070 mg
Cobalt						0.11 mg
Crude Fiber						8.2 %
Dietary Fiber						29.3 %
Fat						1.5 %
Iron						2.5 mg
Magnesium						113 mg
Manganese						0.47 mg
Niacin						3.50 mg
Phosphorus						181 mg
Potassium						2,180 mg
Protein						10.9 %
Riboflavin						0.22 mg
Selenium						0.083 mg
Silicon						0.48 mg
Sodium						16 mg
Thiamine						0.28 mg
Tin						0.12 mg
Vitamin A						3,084 IU
Vitamin C						102.5 mg
Zinc						0.86 mg

Probable Action
  Sedative (?)
  Antispasmodic (flavonoids)

The use of scullcap still rests mainly on folk reputation. The only studies on this plant show it to possess **antibacterial** principles. However, it is known to contain flavonoids which possess **antispasmodic** action and may be responsible for its **sedative action.**

Typical Daily Usage

Fresh herb: 2-4 tablespoon
Dried herb: 3-6 gm
Extract: 4.5 gm dried herb, 22 ml alcohol, 23 ml water

Traditional Formulas

Scullcap combination
Valerian and Black Cohosh combination
Yerba Santa combination

Chemical Constituents

Aromatic compounds

Volatile oil: 0.3%
Fixed oil and resin: 2-4%
Astringent compounds
  Tannin
Bitter compounds
  Flavonoids
    Scutellarin and others
Mucilaginous compounds
  Gum: 8-12%

Nutrients of Note

Water when fresh: 86.3%
Water when air dried: 8.9%

Senna leaf
Cassia senna (Leguminoseae)

Properties: bitter, laxative

Systems Affected: digestive

Common Names: wild senna, locust plant

Folk History and Use

Senna is a small shrub that grows in the upper Nile regions of Africa and the Arabian peninsula.

Senna was first used as a medicine by the Arabians. It was first noticed in the writing of the Arabian physicians, Serapion and Mesue, as early as the 9th century A.D. The name senna itself is Arabian.

It is a prompt, efficient and safe purgative formerly used to **reduce fevers** and **febrile complaints** and in other cases where a moderate **laxative** was needed. Senna leaves have the disadvantage of producing severe griping when used alone. Herbalists and physicians alike overcome this difficulty by combining it with various aromatic herbs and alkaline salts, especially epsom salts (magnesium sulfate).

Senna is popular today both as a crude herb and in over-the-counter and prescription **laxatives**, such as Senokot (Purdue Fredrick) and Perdiem (Rover).

Medicinal Properties

Definite Action
  Stimulates peristalsis (anthraquinones)
Probable Actions
  Antispasmodic (flavonoids)

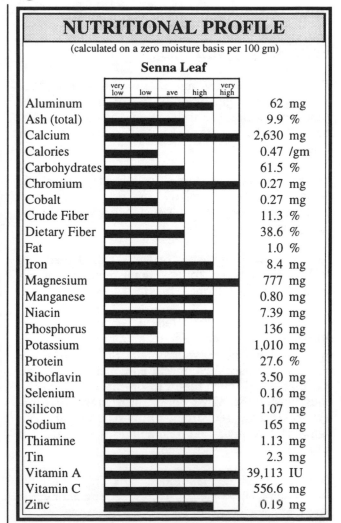

NUTRITIONAL PROFILE
(calculated on a zero moisture basis per 100 gm)

Senna Leaf

	very low	low	ave	high	very high	Value	
Aluminum				■		62	mg
Ash (total)		■				9.9	%
Calcium					■	2,630	mg
Calories		■				0.47	/gm
Carbohydrates			■			61.5	%
Chromium		■				0.27	mg
Cobalt		■				0.27	mg
Crude Fiber			■			11.3	%
Dietary Fiber				■		38.6	%
Fat		■				1.0	%
Iron			■			8.4	mg
Magnesium					■	777	mg
Manganese			■			0.80	mg
Niacin				■		7.39	mg
Phosphorus		■				136	mg
Potassium				■		1,010	mg
Protein			■			27.6	%
Riboflavin					■	3.50	mg
Selenium				■		0.16	mg
Silicon				■		1.07	mg
Sodium				■		165	mg
Thiamine				■		1.13	mg
Tin				■		2.3	mg
Vitamin A					■	39,113	IU
Vitamin C				■		556.6	mg
Zinc				■		0.19	mg

The primary active properties are anthraquinone compounds consisting mostly of the dianthrone glycosides called sennosides A and B (rhein-dianthrone glycosides). There are also minor amounts of sennosides C and D (rhein-aloe emodin hetero dianthrone glycosides) that show activity. The sennosides are only present in the dried leaves and pods of the plant, being formed by enzymatic processes after picking and during drying.

These constituents have a cathartic effect through stimulating peristalsis of the large intestine and bring about their action in 6-8 hours.

They are absorbed from the small intestine to act on the nerves of the large intestine to stimulate motor propulsion in the colon. Because the anthraquinones are absorbed, the laxative effect can be transmitted to nursing infants of mothers taking senna.

Senna causes gripping unless taken in combination with carminative herbs such as ginger, cloves or various mint species. Although generally recognized as safe, senna is somewhat more habit forming than cascara.

Typical Daily Usage

Fresh leaf: Do not eat
Dried leaf: 1-2 gm
Extract: 1 gm dried leaf, 5 ml alcohol, 5 ml water

Traditional Formulas

Senna Combination

Chemcial Constituents

Astringent compounds
Salicylic acid
Pseudotannins
Chrysophanic acid
Bitter compounds
Anthraquinones
Sennosides A,B,C,D; rhein, aloe emodin, chysophanol
Flavonoids
Kaempferol and others
Saponins
Sitosterol: 0.33%

Nutrients of Note

Water when fresh: 79.7%
Water when air dried: 5.6%
Sugars: 13% (glucose, fructose, sucrose, pinitol,mannitol)

Siberian Ginseng root
Eleuthrococcus senticosus (Araliaceae)

Properties: bitter, adaptogen, immune stimulant,
hypoglycemic, circulatory stimulant

Systems Affected: immune, circulatory, glandular

Folk History and Use

Siberian ginseng is a cousin of panax ginseng. These two ginsengs differ in effect more from a folk medicine basis than from a scientific basis.

Siberian ginseng is said to lack the hormonal-like side effects of panax but, in fact, has estrogenic activity just as panax does. Siberian ginseng is used primarily to enhance endurance, to regulate blood sugar and to stimulate immune function.

The Eleuthrococcus plant is a spiny shrub that grows to about six feet in height. It has a carrot shaped taproot that provides the herb of commerce. The leaves of Eleuthrococcus have medicinal value as well as the bark, but are not used extensively by herbalists. It grows abundantly in most of the Far East and takes its common name from its native genesis.

It has traditionally been used to treat **hypoclycemia, lethargy, immune deficiency and improve memory, appetite** and **general health.**

Medicinal Properties

Definite action
Immunostimulant (saponins)
Hypoglycemic (saponins)
Adaptogen (saponins)

Siberian ginseng contains saponins called eleuthrosides that are similar chemically to the saponins in panax. These chemicals have become known as adaptogens. An **adaptogen** is a non toxic compound that increases resistance to physical, chemical and emotional stresses. These compounds seem only to be activated when one is under stress. They then work to increase the activity of natural killer cells and other immune cells and chemicals. They also increase the efficiency with which oxygen is delivered to individual cells. These compounds also have a broad effect on the glandular system. **Blood sugar and pressure are said to be normalized** and **adrenal and thyroid hormones are stimulated.**

When siberian ginseng is taken in combination with aerobic exercise, **natural killer cells are mobilized and activated**. Indeed, the activation comtinues for up

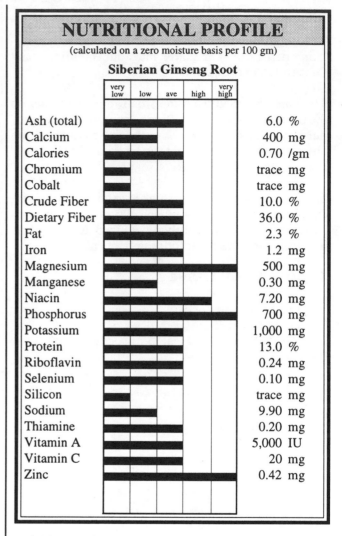

NUTRITIONAL PROFILE
(calculated on a zero moisture basis per 100 gm)

Siberian Ginseng Root

	very low	low	ave	high	very high		
Ash (total)						6.0	%
Calcium						400	mg
Calories						0.70	/gm
Chromium						trace	mg
Cobalt						trace	mg
Crude Fiber						10.0	%
Dietary Fiber						36.0	%
Fat						2.3	%
Iron						1.2	mg
Magnesium						500	mg
Manganese						0.30	mg
Niacin						7.20	mg
Phosphorus						700	mg
Potassium						1,000	mg
Protein						13.0	%
Riboflavin						0.24	mg
Selenium						0.10	mg
Silicon						trace	mg
Sodium						9.90	mg
Thiamine						0.20	mg
Vitamin A						5,000	IU
Vitamin C						20	mg
Zinc						0.42	mg

to 24 hours after the exercise program. With exercise alone natural killer cell mobilization only lasts two hours and activation of these cells never does occur. This fact may explain many of the longevity and antiaging claims proposed for the herb.

Typical Daily Usage

Fresh root: 1-2 teaspoon
Dried root: 0.5-1 gm
Extract: 1 gm dried root, 5 ml alcohol, 5 ml water

Traditional Formulas

Garlic combination
Black Cohosh and Blessed Thistle combination
Ginseng combination
Ginseng and Saw palmetto combination
Ginseng and Phaffia combination
Rosehips and Broccoli combination

Ginseng and Gotu Kola combination
Pollen and Ginseng combination
Cedar Berry combination
Ginseng and Parsley combination

Eleuthrosides (13 identified)
Mucilaginous compounds
Polysaccharides
Gum:7%

Chemical Constituents

Aromatic compounds
    Essential oil
Bitter compounds
    Saponins

Nutrients of Note

Water when fresh: 79%
Water when air dried: 6.9%
Sugars: 9% (glucose, sucrose, galactose, maltose)

Slippery Elm inner bark
Ulmus fulva (Ulmaceae)

Properties: mucilaginous, demulcent, nutritient source, emollient, astringent

Systems Affected: digestive, structural, respiratory

Common Names: red elm, Indian elm, American elm, moose elm

Folk History and Use

Slippery elm has a white and slightly aromatic inner bark which has long been used as a survival health food. It helped keep George Washington's army alive during the bitter winter at Valley Forge. Many pioneer families utilized it as food when nothing else was available to save themselves from starvation.

Slippery elm is a deciduous tree that grows to a height of 50 feet or more with rough, dark brown and deeply furrowed outer bark. The inner bark (cambium) of the slippery elm tree is tough and flexible with a fine fibrous texture. It has an odor somewhat like fenugreek and has a mucilaginous, insipid taste. When ground to a fine powder, this bark makes an excellent flour extender and can be used in a variety of recipes. Some writers claim that it has a food value equal to that of oatmeal and have recommended it as a wholesome and nourishing food for invalids and children.

Slippery elm is native to the United States and Canada, especially north of the Carolina's and west of the Appalachians. Much of the bark of commerce is harvested in the state of Michigan.

The generic name Ulmus is from the Celtic "ulm" or elm meaning trunk. Fulva is from the Latin "fulvus," meaning deep yellow or tawny and referring to the color of the inner bark.

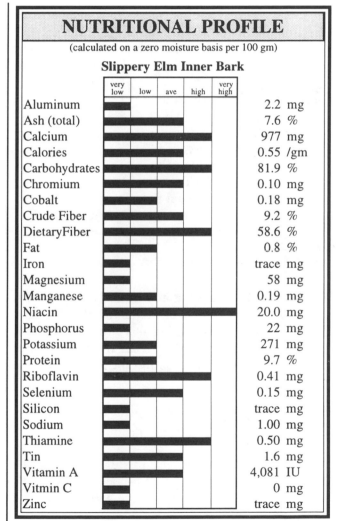

NUTRITIONAL PROFILE
(calculated on a zero moisture basis per 100 gm)

Slippery Elm Inner Bark

	very low	low	ave	high	very high		
Aluminum						2.2	mg
Ash (total)						7.6	%
Calcium						977	mg
Calories						0.55	/gm
Carbohydrates						81.9	%
Chromium						0.10	mg
Cobalt						0.18	mg
Crude Fiber						9.2	%
DietaryFiber						58.6	%
Fat						0.8	%
Iron						trace	mg
Magnesium						58	mg
Manganese						0.19	mg
Niacin						20.0	mg
Phosphorus						22	mg
Potassium						271	mg
Protein						9.7	%
Riboflavin						0.41	mg
Selenium						0.15	mg
Silicon						trace	mg
Sodium						1.00	mg
Thiamine						0.50	mg
Tin						1.6	mg
Vitamin A						4,081	IU
Vitmin C						0	mg
Zinc						trace	mg

The color of slippery elm is important to note since the outer bark contains much tannin and crude fiber and often contaminates the herb of commerce. Be sure to avoid dark colored material as this is more astringent and fibrous than pure inner bark.

The early white settlers of America found the Native Americans using the inner bark of slippery elm to retard rancidity in fatty substances. The Indians prepared bear's fat by melting it with the bark, in the proportion of an ounce of the bark to a pound of the fat, keeping them heated together for a few minutes and then straining off the fat. The settlers with success tried the same process with butter and lard.

As a healing agent, the Indians applied slippery elm bark in the form of a **poultice for wounds, burns**, etc. Internally, it was used as a tea, so that its soothing properties could reach the membranes of the throat, stomach and intestines. It has also been used in **cutaneous eruptions** and as a food.

Modern herbalists have also used slippery elm to treat affections of the **respiratory tract**. However, slippery elm is only effective on the respiratory tract when used topically so that it may contact the lining of the throat.

Medicinal Properties

Definite Action
    The benefits of viscous fiber
        Lowers bowel transit time
        Absorbs toxins from bowel
        Regulates intestinal flora
        Demulcent action on digestive tract
    Astringent (tannin)
Probable Action
    Expectorant (mucilage)

The **demulcent, emollient and wound healing properties** of slippery elm are due to its mucilage content. The mucilage is viscous fiber that **lowers the bowel transit time, absorbs toxins from the bowel, regulates intestinal flora** and **soothes the lining of the digestive tract.**

The **demulcent** effects are also active when the herb is used externally as a poultice or in an ointment.

The most popular modern use of slippery elm is as a **demulcent expectorant**. This property is explained by the ability of tannins to combine with mucous and precipitate it.

Slippery elm decoctions are drank hourly to coat the throat and allow the tannins to congeal the mucous build-ups, thus facilitating the expulsion of excess mucous.

Beware of respiratory formulas based on slippery elm that are in capsules or tablets to be swallowed as this negates any demulcent action on the throat.

Typical Daily Usage

Fresh inner bark: 1/4-1/2 cup
Dried inner bark: 2-4 teaspoon
Extract: 3 teaspoon dried bark in 4 cups of boiling
    water

Traditional Formulas

Pumpkin and Cascara combination
Comfrey combination
Plantain combination
Slippery Elm combination
Ginseng combination
Alfalfa and Yucca combination
Chamomile and Rose Hips combination
Ephedra and Passionflower combination
Marshmallow and Plantain combination

Nutritional Profile

Aromatic compounds
    Volatile oil
    Fixed oil and resin
Astringent compounds
    Tannin
Mucilaginous compounds
    Mucilage: 25-35%

Nutrients of Note

Water when fresh: 83.6%
Water when air dried: 8.9%
Starch: 8-21%
Sugars: 9% (glucose, sucrose)

Spirulina algae

Spirulina spp. (Oscillatoriaceae)

Properties: nutrient source

Systems Affected: digestive

Folk History and Use

Spirulina is the name of a genus of blue-green algae. Spirulina grows in fresh water and has been harvested for at least four centuries as an animal feed and more rarely as food for human consumption.

Today, spirulina is consumed as a health food and nutritional supplement. It is a highly concentrated source of protein, vitamins and minerals but its price is commensurately high. It contains high quantities of bioavailable iron and all minerals generally. Care must be taken to ensure the quality of spirulina supplements. If the water the algae is grown in is contaminated with heavy metals, the spirulina will concentrate them and pass them on to the human consumer. Insect contamination can also be a problem if the ponds are not properly covered. Inclement weather can also stir up mud which often becomes inseparable from the algae.

The drawback of spirulina supplements is that you have to consume 10 or more grams daily to get a reasonable amount of nutrients. Ten grams is only two teaspoonsful, which makes spirulina a very concentrated food source.

Spirulina is popularly held to be an **appetite suppressant.** This stems from the idea that the algae are two thirds protein by weight and that the protein has a disproportionate amount of the amino acid phenylalanine in it. This folk claim is not supported by scientific study but makes great promotional copy.

Medicinal Properties

  Definite action
    Nutritional supplement

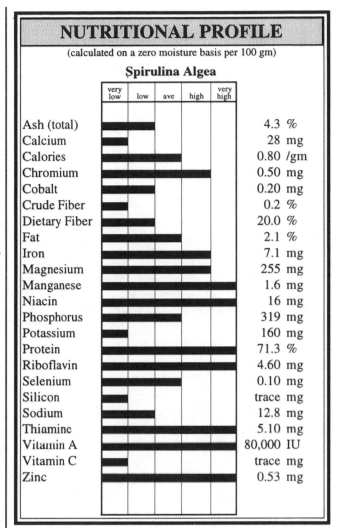

NUTRITIONAL PROFILE

(calculated on a zero moisture basis per 100 gm)

Spirulina Algea

	very low	low	ave	high	very high	
Ash (total)						4.3 %
Calcium						28 mg
Calories						0.80 /gm
Chromium						0.50 mg
Cobalt						0.20 mg
Crude Fiber						0.2 %
Dietary Fiber						20.0 %
Fat						2.1 %
Iron						7.1 mg
Magnesium						255 mg
Manganese						1.6 mg
Niacin						16 mg
Phosphorus						319 mg
Potassium						160 mg
Protein						71.3 %
Riboflavin						4.60 mg
Selenium						0.10 mg
Silicon						trace mg
Sodium						12.8 mg
Thiamine						5.10 mg
Vitamin A						80,000 IU
Vitamin C						trace mg
Zinc						0.53 mg

Typical Daily Usage

  Dried algae: 5-10 gm

Tea Tree oil
Melaleuca alternifolia (Myrtaceae)

Properties: aromatic, antiseptic

Systems Affected: structural, digestive

Folk History and Use

Tea tree oil has a rich folklore. It was first praised by the European explorer Captain James Cook as a topical antiseptic. It was used widely until penicillin was discovered. Clinical studies were performed on tea tree oil over 60 years ago to develop its **antiseptic** properties. It is much like turpentine but is thought by folk practicioners to be less caustic to skin and hair.

Tea tree oil is extracted by steam distillation of the leaves of the Australian tea tree. The tree is native to swampy areas of New South Wales in Australia. It has been used to treat **all kinds of skin ailments, cuts, burns, acne, cold sores and irritations of the mouth** and **throat.**

Medicinal Properties

Definite action
Antiseptic (volatile oil)

Tea tree oil is the steam distillate of the leaves of the tea tree. The oil is similar chemically to turpentine (the steam distillate of pine trees). It contains a variety of terpenes and sesquiterpenes, terpinen-4-ol being the most prized. The oil is **antiseptic** and makes tea tree oil useful for various topical applications.

Typical Daily Usage

Oil: Apply liberally to affected area

Traditional Formulas
Generally used in soothing ointment bases

Chemical Constituents

Aromatic compounds
Volatile oil
Terpenes
Sesquiterpenes (terpinen-4-ol)

Thyme leaf

Thymus vulgaris (Labiatae)

Properties: aromatic, antiseptic, antihelmintic, astringent, carminative, antispasmodic

Systems Affected: digestive, structural, circulatory

Common Names: garden or common thyme, tomillo, mother of thyme, serpyllum

Folk History and Use

In ancient Greece, thyme was a symbol of bravery. It was a great compliment to tell a person he smelled of thyme. The generic name, thymus, comes from the Greek word, "thymos," meaning strength, in reference to its invigorating odor. The species name, vulgaris, is Latin for "common, ordinary" and was obviously applied by taxonomists who did not understand its use as a symbol of bravery.

Thyme is an erect, evergreen shrub native to the Mediterranean region and extensively cultivated in southern Europe and California.

Thyme is widely known as a common culinary herb used in baked goods, meat, condiments and vegetables. Thyme oil is used to flavor alcoholic beverages. The oil possesses **antioxidant** properties that make it effective in curing pork.

It is used in pharmaceuticals as an **antispasmodic, carminative, counterirritant** and in **mouth washes**. It is also used as an **anthelmintic, sedative, diaphoretic** and **expectorant.**

Thymol is also used in the feminine hygiene products; Bo Caral, PMC Douche powder, Stomaseptine and Zonite, in the Otic products, Auro Ear Drops and Stall Otic drops, in the external analgesics, Vicks Vaporub, Zemo liquid and in Listerine mouthwash.

Thymol is most often used in antifungal creams, lotions and ointments, in concentrations ranging from 0.1-1.0%.

Medicinal Properties

Definite Actions
Carminative (thymol)
Antioxidant (thymol)
Antibacterial (thymol)
Anthelmintic (thymol)
Astringent (tannin)

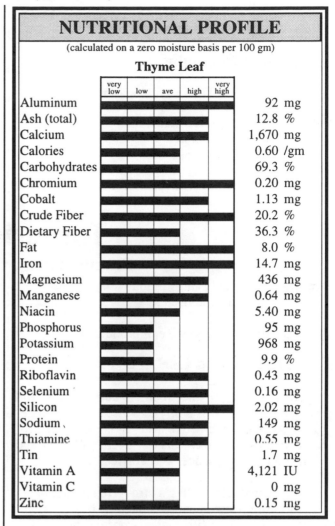

NUTRITIONAL PROFILE
(calculated on a zero moisture basis per 100 gm)

Thyme Leaf

	very low	low	ave	high	very high		
Aluminum					■	92	mg
Ash (total)			■			12.8	%
Calcium				■		1,670	mg
Calories			■			0.60	/gm
Carbohydrates			■			69.3	%
Chromium				■		0.20	mg
Cobalt					■	1.13	mg
Crude Fiber				■		20.2	%
Dietary Fiber				■		36.3	%
Fat					■	8.0	%
Iron					■	14.7	mg
Magnesium				■		436	mg
Manganese			■			0.64	mg
Niacin			■			5.40	mg
Phosphorus		■				95	mg
Potassium		■				968	mg
Protein		■				9.9	%
Riboflavin				■		0.43	mg
Selenium			■			0.16	mg
Silicon					■	2.02	mg
Sodium			■			149	mg
Thiamine				■		0.55	mg
Tin			■			1.7	mg
Vitamin A			■			4,121	IU
Vitamin C	■					0	mg
Zinc		■				0.15	mg

Probable Actions
Expectorant (thymol)
Antispasmodic (thymol)
Digestive aid (thymol)

The action of thyme is attributed to two groups of chemicals (1) the volatile phenolic compounds–thymol and carvacrol and (2) the tannins.

Thymol is **carminative, antioxidant, antibacterial and anthelmintic**. Its **carminative** properties are attributed to its volatile oils which irritate the gastrointestinal lining thus **stimulating the production of gastric fluids.**

Thymol is also quite toxic in large doses. Toxic symptoms include nausea, vomiting, gastric pain, headache, dizziness, convulsions, coma, cardiac and respiratory collapse.

Typical Daily Usage

Fresh leaf: 2-4 tablespoon
Dried leaf: 3-6 gm
Extract: 4.5 gm dried herb, 22 ml alcohol, 23 ml
water

Traditional Formulas

Fenugreek and Thyme combination

Chemical Constituents
Aromatic compounds
Volatile Oils: 0.8-2.6%
Terpenes
Cymene, terpineol, linalool, thujanol
and others
Fixed oil and resin: 3-5%
Thymol and carvacrol
Astringent compounds
Tannin: 10%
Pseudotannins
Caffeic acid, labiatic acid, ursolic acid
Flavonoids
Quercitin and others

Nutrients of Note

Water when fresh: 83.2%
Water when air dried: 7.8%

Tumeric herb
Curcuma longa (Zingiberaceae)

Properties: aromatic, anti-inflammatory, anti-arthritic, antiseptic

Systems Affected: digestive, reproductive

Folk History and Use

Tumeric is the major spice found in curry powder and prepared mustard. It is easily identified by its orange-yellow color and distinctive taste. It is most noted for its use in flavoring meat dishes, as a condiment and relish and in soups, sauces and gravies.

As a medicinal herb it has a strong reputation as an **anti-inflammatory** agent. As such, it has been employed to treat **hepatitis, inflammatory bowel diseases, bruises, colic** and **spasmodic dysmenorrhea**. The herb is also **astringent** and is used to treat **ulcers** and **hemmorhages.**

It has been known for some time that the herb has **antiseptic** properties, but it was formerly too pricey to be used in that manner. Today, however, it is becoming popular as a cleansing agent to rid one's colon of **parasites** and **yeast infections.**

Medicinal Properties

Definite action
Anti-inflammatory (volatile oil)
Antiseptic (volatile oil)
Possible action
Antiarthritic (?)

Tumeric has been shown to exhibit **antiseptic, anti-inflammatory** and **antihepatotoxic effects.** It relies

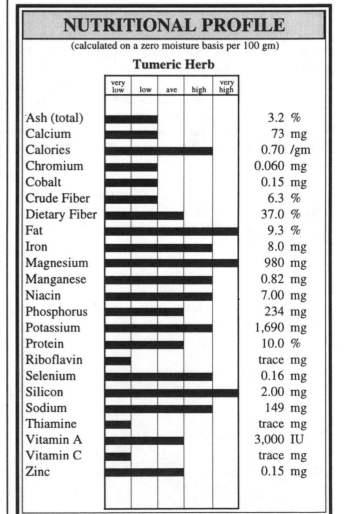

NUTRITIONAL PROFILE
(calculated on a zero moisture basis per 100 gm)

Tumeric Herb

	very low	low	ave	high	very high		
Ash (total)						3.2	%
Calcium						73	mg
Calories						0.70	/gm
Chromium						0.060	mg
Cobalt						0.15	mg
Crude Fiber						6.3	%
Dietary Fiber						37.0	%
Fat						9.3	%
Iron						8.0	mg
Magnesium						980	mg
Manganese						0.82	mg
Niacin						7.00	mg
Phosphorus						234	mg
Potassium						1,690	mg
Protein						10.0	%
Riboflavin						trace	mg
Selenium						0.16	mg
Silicon						2.00	mg
Sodium						149	mg
Thiamine						trace	mg
Vitamin A						3,000	IU
Vitamin C						trace	mg
Zinc						0.15	mg

on its volatile oil for its actions. It is noted for its ability to treat **inflammations of the digestive system** and the **reproductive system**. This makes it useful in folk remedies for **hepatitis, flatulence** and **spasmodic dysmenorrhea**. It **increases the production of enzymes in the liver** that metabolize toxins in a manner similar to schizandra, licorice and milk thistle. This may also explain its anti-inflammatory effects.

The volatile oil has also been shown to be **antiseptic**. It effectively kills many gram(+) and gram(-) **bacteria** as well as many **yeasts** and **molds**.

Typical Daily Usage

Fresh herb: 3-5 gm
Dried herb: 0.3-0.5 gm
Extract: 0.4 gm dried herb, 2 ml alcohol, 2 ml water

Traditional Formulas

Elecampane combination

Chemical Constituents

Aromatic compounds
 Volatile oil: 5-8%
  Turmerone
  Atlantone
  Zingiberone
  Curcumin (coloring material)
 Resin

Nutrients of Note

Water when fresh: 69%
Water when air dried: 6.6%
Sugars: 35-40% (glucose, fructose)

Uva Ursi leaf

Arctostaphylos Uva Ursi (Ericaeae)

Properties: bitter, diuretic, astringent, urinary antiseptic

Systems Affected: urinary

Folk History and Use

Uva ursi is a bushy, evergreen shrub with small, leathery leaves that is native to the temperate regions of the northern hemisphere.

It derives its name, uva ursi, from the Latin "uva" or grape and "ursus" meaning bear. Arctostaphylos is from the Greek, "arktos," meaning bear and "staphyle," a bunch of grapes. Both names are derivatives of the common name bearberry, since the fruit is rough and unpleasant (i.e. only fit for a bear), and grows in bunches like grapes.

Uva ursi is an **astringent** herb with strong affinity for the **urinary system**. It has been used to help correct **bedwetting, bladder diseases, cystitis, kidney congestion and infections of the kidneys** and **urinary tract**. It is also said to have the ability to **dissolve kidney stones**. Due to the proximity of the prostate to the urinary tract in males, it has also been used in **prostate remedies**.

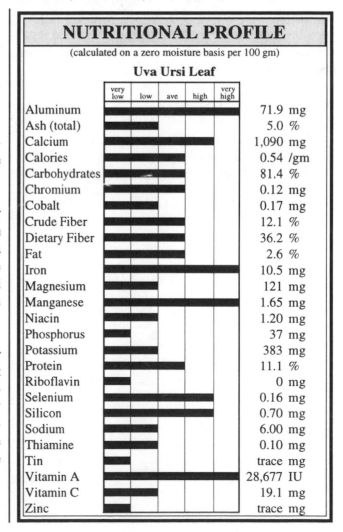

NUTRITIONAL PROFILE
(calculated on a zero moisture basis per 100 gm)

Uva Ursi Leaf

	very low	low	ave	high	very high	
Aluminum						71.9 mg
Ash (total)						5.0 %
Calcium						1,090 mg
Calories						0.54 /gm
Carbohydrates						81.4 %
Chromium						0.12 mg
Cobalt						0.17 mg
Crude Fiber						12.1 %
Dietary Fiber						36.2 %
Fat						2.6 %
Iron						10.5 mg
Magnesium						121 mg
Manganese						1.65 mg
Niacin						1.20 mg
Phosphorus						37 mg
Potassium						383 mg
Protein						11.1 %
Riboflavin						0 mg
Selenium						0.16 mg
Silicon						0.70 mg
Sodium						6.00 mg
Thiamine						0.10 mg
Tin						trace mg
Vitamin A						28,677 IU
Vitamin C						19.1 mg
Zinc						trace mg

Medicinal Properties

Definite Action
Antiseptic on urinary tract (hydroquinone)
Astringent (tannin)
Diuretic (hydroquinone)

Uva ursi contains two groups of known active principles (1) hydroquinone glucosides and (2) tannins. The tannins are so abundant that the Russians formerly used uva ursi for tanning animal hides.

The hydroquinone glycosides are hydrolyzed by alkaline urine and act to **disinfect the urinary tract** and **stimulate the production of urine**. Sodium bicarbonate is often administered with uva ursi to help increase the alkalinity of the urine.

Beta-carotene, present in generous quantities in uva ursi, is known to **stimulate the production of epithelial cells**. Ursolic acid has **antiseptic** properties and the flavonoids have **spasmolytic** properties on the smooth muscles which help reduce reactions to pain stimulus in urinary tract infections and increase renal volume in inflamed renal tubules. The flavonoids are also **antiseptic** and **diuretic** agents.

Typical Daily Usage

Fresh leaf: 2-4 tablespoon
Dried leaf: 3-6 gm
Extract: 4.5 gm dried leaf, 22 ml alcohol, 23 ml
water

Traditional Formulas

False Unicorn and Golden Seal combination
Ginger and Dong Quai combination
Golden Seal and Juniper combination
Ginseng and Parsley combination
Uva Ursi combination

Chemical Constituents

Aromatic compounds
Volatile Oils
Fixed Oils and Resins
Astringent compounds
Tannin: 6-7%
gallic acid and others
Ursolic acid (antiseptic)
Bitter compounds
Hydroquinones: 5-18%
arbutin and others
Flavonoids
Quercitin and others
Allantoin

Nutrients of Note

Water when fresh: 88.4%
Water when air dried: 8.6%

Valerian root
Valeriana officinalis (Valerianaceae)

Properties: aromatic, nervine, antispasmodic

Systems Affected: nervous, structural

Common Names: great wild valerian, setwell, capon's tail

Folk History and Use

Valerian is native to England, Europe and the United States, and is specifically cultivated in Holland, Germany and England. Closely related varieties grow in China and the Far East. Still other varieties are native to South America.

Besides its medicinal virtues, valerian is most famous for its distinct odor which is reminiscent of rotten cheese or dirty socks. Valerian is first mentioned in writings from the 9th and 10th centuries. The drug is mentioned in Anglo-Saxon works of the 11th century. Valerian was formerly used as a drug, a spice and a perfume.

The Romans prepared spikenard ointment from the young shoots of a variety of valerian. Valerian derives its name from the Latin "valene," to be strong, referring to the medicinal virtues of the plant. Dioscorides and Galen called it "Phu" in reference to its offensive odor and prescribed it for headaches and as a diuretic.

Valerian has traditionally been used as a **nervine, antispasmodic** and **stomachic**. The best results have been obtained in cases of **hysteria** and **hypochondriac,** where the primary causes of difficulty are emotional or mental. It has also been helpful for **migraines** and **insomnia,** as well as **depression.** Cats seem to be attracted to valerian and, along with other small mammals, have been known to appear intoxicated after ingesting it.

In centuries past, it was supposedly taken as often as coffee by ladies in Germany, resulting in **lack of nervousness or irritability**. It was used as a condiment during medieval times and as a perfume during the 16th century.

Valerian has also been employed as a sedative in the treatment of **nervousness, hysteria** and **convulsions.** Other afflictions which valerian has been credited with curing include: **bruises, coughs, croup, the plague, hypochondria, migraine headaches, epilepsy,** some

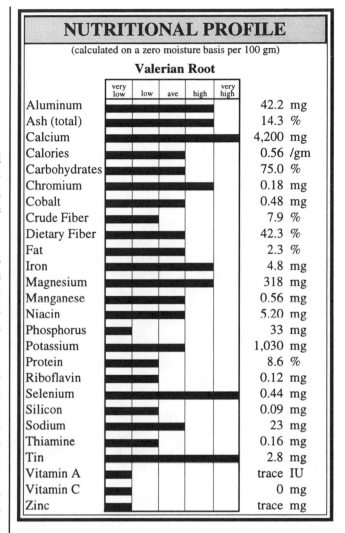

NUTRITIONAL PROFILE
(calculated on a zero moisture basis per 100 gm)

Valerian Root

	very low	low	ave	high	very high		
Aluminum						42.2	mg
Ash (total)						14.3	%
Calcium						4,200	mg
Calories						0.56	/gm
Carbohydrates						75.0	%
Chromium						0.18	mg
Cobalt						0.48	mg
Crude Fiber						7.9	%
Dietary Fiber						42.3	%
Fat						2.3	%
Iron						4.8	mg
Magnesium						318	mg
Manganese						0.56	mg
Niacin						5.20	mg
Phosphorus						33	mg
Potassium						1,030	mg
Protein						8.6	%
Riboflavin						0.12	mg
Selenium						0.44	mg
Silicon						0.09	mg
Sodium						23	mg
Thiamine						0.16	mg
Tin						2.8	mg
Vitamin A						trace	IU
Vitamin C						0	mg
Zinc						trace	mg

forms of **fever** and most diseases of the **nervous system**.

In Indo-China, the root is part of an herbal combination used to treat indigestion and toothache. It is used alone to ease inflammation.

In Guatemala, valerian is mixed with other herbs to lower blood pressure. In Argentina, the roots are steeped into a tea for unruly children.

Today, valerian root is used in many patent medicines, especially in Europe. The virtues of one product called Valamin, a valerian derivative, (tertiary amyl isovaleric acid), has been mistakenly linked to the prescription drug, Valium. Any relationship between the two drugs is strictly phonetic.

Medicinal Properties

Definite Action
    CNS depressant (alkaloids)
    Antispasmodic (alkaloids)
    Analgesic (alkaloids)
    Antibacterial (alkaloids)
Probable Action
    Carminative (?)
    Hypotensive (?)

Valerian acts as a **soother and depressor of the central nervous system**. Several sources indicate that it is not a narcotic, although there is disagreement on that matter. It is a good treatment for the general condition of **nervousness**. It **increases heart action and temperature, causing a feeling of exhilaration, stimulates circulation, secretion and peristalsis for the stomach and intestines**. It is eliminated from the body through the mucous membranes of the kidneys, bronchial tubes and genitourinary tract.

The primary **antispasmodic** component is valerianic acid. This is a thin, oily liquid which has a sour smell similar to rotten cheese.

The tranquilizing effects are provided by the volatile alkaloids called valepotriates. The alkaloids are also **antibacterial**, **antidiuretic** and may help **prevent liver necrosis.**

The dosage form of valerian is important since the active principles are volatile. Alcoholic extracts or extracts fixed in oil are the best way to preserve the herb's essence. The strength of its odor (like dirty socks) is indicative of its activity.

The toxicity of the drug is low, but in large doses it causes headaches, mental excitement, visual illusions, giddiness, restlessness and agitation.

One interesting result of our nutritional study is that valerian root has the highest calcium content of any herb we tested. In fact, valerian farmers find that the plant prefers calcareous soils over shales.

Typical Daily Usage

Fresh root: 2-4 tablespoon
Dried root: 3-6 gm
Extract: 4.5 gm dried root, 22 ml alcohol, 23 ml
    water

Traditional Formulas

Alfalfa and Yucca combination
Scullcap combination
Valerian and Black Cohosh combination
White Willow combination
White Willow and Valerian combination

Chemical Constituents

Aromatic compounds
    Volatile oil: 0.5-2%
        Valerianic acid, bornyl acetate, isovalerate
           and others
Astringent compounds
    Tannin
        Chlorogenic acid and others
Bitter compounds
    Saponins
        Sitosterol and others
    Alkaloids
        Valepotriates
           Valtrate, valerine and others
    Flavonoids
        Quercitin, rutin and others
    Choline: 3%
Mucilaginous compounds
    Gum: 12%

Nutrients of Note

Water when fresh: 88.2%
Water when air dried: 6.9%

White Oak bark
Quercus alba (Fagacea)

Properties: astringent

Systems Affected: structural, digestive

Folk History and Use

White oak is the classic example of an **astringent** herb. It contains high amounts of calcium and tannins that act by precipitating protein to tighten the tissues of the body.

Tannins have been used as **astringents** and **styptics** in cases of anal fissures and **hemorrhoids** and to halt **diarrhea and dysenery**. It is also used in **gargles** and as an **emetic.**

Oaks are common trees in deciduous forests throughout the world. White oaks are native to England and have been naturalized in the United States. Their slow, steady growth and large stature have long been religious and patriotic symbols. The Greeks held it sacred; the Romans dedicated it to Jupiter and the Druids venerated it.

The generic name Quercus is from the Celtic "quer" (handsome) and the "cuez" (tree). Alba refers to the whitish appearance of the bark.

The bark is universally used to tan leather, and the extracted tannin, when mixed with copper sulfate, produces a durable red purple dye.

Medicinal Properties

> Definite Action
> Astringent (tannin)

Tannin, the active principle of white oak bark, are widely distributed in nature. The chemistry of tannins are not fully understood but the mechanism by which they work on protein is quite clear. The term tannin refers to a general group of compounds of plant origin which are able to precipitate the protein of animal hides, prevent their putrification and convert them into leather.

Tannin is best employed only temporarily or more regularly as a gargle, as long-term use can permanently discolor the intestinal mucosa.

Typical Daily Usage

> Fresh bark: 2-4 tablespoon
> Dried bark: 3-6 gm
> Extract: 4.5 gm dried bark, 22 ml alcohol, 23 ml
> water

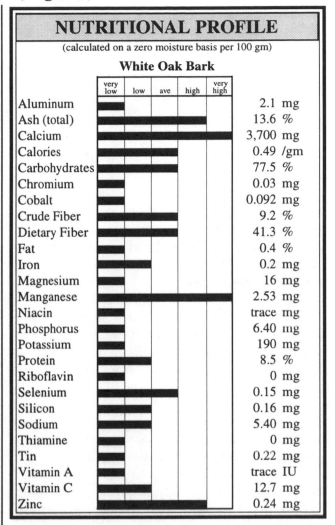

NUTRITIONAL PROFILE
(calculated on a zero moisture basis per 100 gm)

White Oak Bark

	very low	low	ave	high	very high		
Aluminum						2.1	mg
Ash (total)						13.6	%
Calcium						3,700	mg
Calories						0.49	/gm
Carbohydrates						77.5	%
Chromium						0.03	mg
Cobalt						0.092	mg
Crude Fiber						9.2	%
Dietary Fiber						41.3	%
Fat						0.4	%
Iron						0.2	mg
Magnesium						16	mg
Manganese						2.53	mg
Niacin						trace	mg
Phosphorus						6.40	mg
Potassium						190	mg
Protein						8.5	%
Riboflavin						0	mg
Selenium						0.15	mg
Silicon						0.16	mg
Sodium						5.40	mg
Thiamine						0	mg
Tin						0.22	mg
Vitamin A						trace	IU
Vitamin C						12.7	mg
Zinc						0.24	mg

Traditional Formulas

Golden Seal and Juniper combination

Chemical Constituents

> Aromatic compounds
>> Fixed oil and resin
> Astringent compounds
>> Tannin: 15-20%
>>> plobotannin, egallitannin, gallic acid
> Bitter compounds
>> Flavonoids
>>> Quercitin and others

Nutrients of Note

Water when fresh: 77.2%
Water when air dried: 9.9%
Sugars: 3% (glucose)

White Willow bark
Salix alba (Salicaeae)

Properties: bitter, antipyretic, analgesic, anti-inflammatory, astringent, antiseptic

Systems Affected: structural, nervous, circulatory

Folk History and Use

The most used medication in the world, aspirin, is a close relative of the active principle in white willow bark. The bark of various willow and poplar trees have been used throughout recorded history as **antipyretics, analgesics, anti-inflammatory** agents and **astringents** to treat **headache, debility of digestive organs, dandruff, eye problems, malaria, chills, influenza, eczema** and **nosebleed.**

The generic name for white willow, salix, is derived from the Celtic "sal" for near and "lis" for water, referring to its favorite habitat. Salix could also be derived from the Latin "salio" to spring out in reference to its rapid growth.

The Indians of North America decocted willow bark to relieve **headache** and **fever,** and to ease the **aches and pains of sore muscles** and **rheumatism.**

Willow appears frequently in prescriptions on the 4,000-year-old Sumerian tablet from Nippur, in the famous Ebers Papyrus (16th century B.C.) from Egypt, and in ancient Assyrian tablets. Pedanium Dioscorides identified the willow by the Latin name, Salix. He also pointed out its **astringent** qualities in his writings. In addition, he described willow as being beneficial for **earaches, corns** and **gout.**

Claudius Galen, another noted Greek physician used willow bark to treat **inflammations of the eye.**

Hippocrates used willow bark to **relieve pain** and **fever.**

Salicylates have recently been shown to enhance the thermogenic effects of the ephedrine in Chinese ephedra herb. This property makes it useful in weight loss programs that are based on increasing one's body temperature by promoting the burning of brown fat.

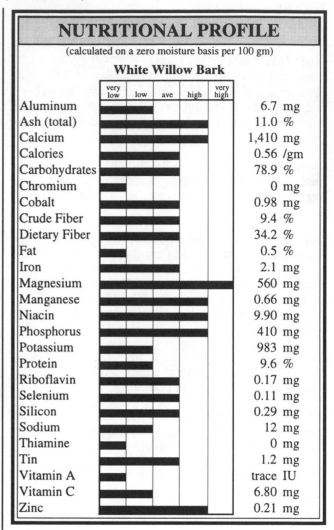

NUTRITIONAL PROFILE
(calculated on a zero moisture basis per 100 gm)

White Willow Bark

	very low	low	ave	high	very high	
Aluminum						6.7 mg
Ash (total)						11.0 %
Calcium						1,410 mg
Calories						0.56 /gm
Carbohydrates						78.9 %
Chromium						0 mg
Cobalt						0.98 mg
Crude Fiber						9.4 %
Dietary Fiber						34.2 %
Fat						0.5 %
Iron						2.1 mg
Magnesium						560 mg
Manganese						0.66 mg
Niacin						9.90 mg
Phosphorus						410 mg
Potassium						983 mg
Protein						9.6 %
Riboflavin						0.17 mg
Selenium						0.11 mg
Silicon						0.29 mg
Sodium						12 mg
Thiamine						0 mg
Tin						1.2 mg
Vitamin A						trace IU
Vitamin C						6.80 mg
Zinc						0.21 mg

Medicinal Properties

Definite Actions
  Antipyretic (salicin)
  Analgesic (salicin)
  Anti-inflammatory (salicin and flavonoids)
  Astringent (tannin)
  Antiseptic (tannin)

In 1827, a French chemist named Leroux extracted the principal active substance in white willow bark that gave relief from pain. He named it Salicin after the willow genus, Salix. Salicin is an intermediate form of salicylic acid. When salicin is taken into the body, it is believed to be converted into salicylic acid, the base molecule of aspirin.

Salicin was listed as an official botanical medicine in the 1955 edition of the National Formulary, and the 1950 edition of the United States Dispensatory and in the U.S. Pharmacopoeia from 1882 through 1926. However, its use in modern medicine has since been discontinued due to the ease and low cost at which synthetic salicylic acid can be produced.

Salicylic acid, the aglycone of salicin, is a caustic phenol that is used topically to **remove warts**. When ingested, it is also caustic to the stomach lining and can cause various side effects including bleeding and ulceration of the stomach lining. Fortunately for humans, white willow bark also contains fiber and tannin which dilute these caustic effects. Fiber slows the release of the salicylate, and tannin tones the irritated membranes and reduces bleeding.

During the 1890's, many chemists searched for relatives of salicylic acid that would not cause so much gastrointestinal irritation. Felix Hofman, a young chemist who worked for Friedrich Bayer and Company, a pharmaceutical company near Cologne, Germany, launched a successful career with the acetyl ester of salicylic acid. He first tested the drug on his arthritic father who couldn't tolerate the harsh action of willow bark on his stomach. In 1899, Bayer company began marketing this product under the name aspirin. (The name comes from acetyl and spireae, meaning a derivative of salicin.)

Salicin is most noted as a **fever-lowering (antipyretic)** agent, facilitating the dissipation of heat through increased peripheral blood flow and sweating; as a **pain-relieving (analgesic)** agent through its depressant action on the central nervous system; and as an **anti-inflammatory** agent for treatment of **rheumatism** and **arthritis**. It also possesses **antithrombotic** properties and in the form of salicylic acid, is **antiseptic**.

The activity of salicylates are due mainly to their ability to produce endorphin like prostaglandins that result in **anti-inflammatory** and **analgesic** effects.

Typical Daily Usage

Fresh bark: 2-4 tablespoon
Dried bark: 3-6 gm
Extract: 4.5 gm dried bark, 22 ml alcohol, 23 ml water

Traditional Formulas

Alfalfa and Yucca combination
White Willow combination
White Willow and Valerian combination

Chemical Constituents

Aromatic compounds
    Fixed oil and resin
Astringent compounds
    Tannin: 12%
Bitter compounds
    Salicin: 2.5-11%
    Flavonoids
        Alboside, apigenin, quercetin, rutin and others
Mucilaginous compounds
    Glucomannan: 8%

Nutrients of Note

Water when fresh: 83.2%
Water when air dried: 7.5%

Wild yam root
Dioscorea villosa (Dioscoreaceae)

Properties: bitter, antispasmodic, antirheumatic, anti-inflammatory, diaphoretic

Systems Affected: glandular, circulatory, digestive

Common Names: colic root, China root, rheumatism root

Folk History and Use

Wild yam root comes from a vine-like herb common to the eastern United States. The root material is very hard and woody. Formerly the virtues of the plant were extracted by soaking it in whisky for up to a month. It has been grown commercially in Mexico since the discovery that it contains steroidal compounds which can be processed into pharmaceutical steroids. This use of the root, coupled with its traditional use as an **antispamodic** and **antirheumatic** gave rise to the saying that wild yam is a natural steroid. Indeed, it contains compounds that are similar in chemical structure to steroids, but these compounds must be digested, absorbed and processed by one's body before becoming steroids or hormones. Eating foods such as wild yam thus provides the building blocks for many complex glandular manufacturing processes.

Wild yam root has traditionally been used to treat any type of **muscle spasm** and **inflammatory condition**. It is especially associated with **relief of inflammatory bowel conditions, arthritis, rheumatism, colic** and **spasmodic dysmenorrhea.**

Recently, the popularity of wild yam has risen greatly due to body builders. These individuals try to enhance their performance by giving their bodies every chance to manufacture its own definition and strength increasing steroids.

The root's reputation as a steroid replacement has led some to use it as a female contraceptive, apparently following the notion that the steroidal effect renders one sterile while taking it regularly.

Its toxicity has not been well explored but mice who are fed the root regularly do not exhibit any unusual effects; however, each succeeding generation becomes slightly smaller in size. For this reason I do not recommend taking this herb to bulk up, or as a natural contraceptive. I have found personal use in small amounts of this root for my own digestive and joint complaints.

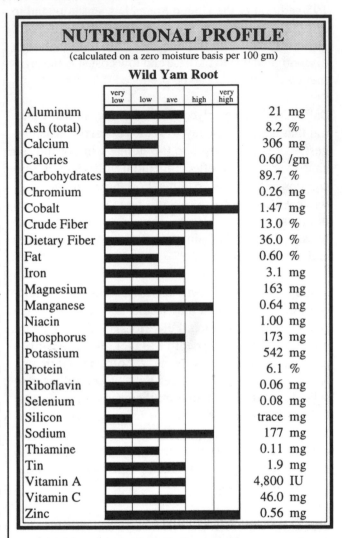

NUTRITIONAL PROFILE
(calculated on a zero moisture basis per 100 gm)

Wild Yam Root

	mg/%
Aluminum	21 mg
Ash (total)	8.2 %
Calcium	306 mg
Calories	0.60 /gm
Carbohydrates	89.7 %
Chromium	0.26 mg
Cobalt	1.47 mg
Crude Fiber	13.0 %
Dietary Fiber	36.0 %
Fat	0.60 %
Iron	3.1 mg
Magnesium	163 mg
Manganese	0.64 mg
Niacin	1.00 mg
Phosphorus	173 mg
Potassium	542 mg
Protein	6.1 %
Riboflavin	0.06 mg
Selenium	0.08 mg
Silicon	trace mg
Sodium	177 mg
Thiamine	0.11 mg
Tin	1.9 mg
Vitamin A	4,800 IU
Vitamin C	46.0 mg
Zinc	0.56 mg

Medicinal Properties

Definite action
   Antispasmodic (steroidal glycocides)
   Anti-inflammatory (steroidal glycocides)
Probable action
   Antirheumatic (steroidal glycocides)
   Emmenogogue (steroidal glycocides)

The action of wild yam is based entirely on it steroidal glycosides. The mechanism of their action is probably quite different for each person that consumes this herb. The body manufactures a wide variety of compounds out of the building blocks provided by wild yam root.

This could explain the balancing effects it has on the digestive and reproductive systems.

Typical Daily Usage

Fresh root: 1-2 teaspoon
Dried root: 2-4 gm
Extract: 3 gm dried root, 15 ml alcohol, 15 ml water

Traditional Formulas

Ginger and Barberry combination
Papaya and Peppermint combination
Slippery Elm combination

Chemical Constituents

Astringent compounds
 Tannin
Bitter compounds
 Saponins
  Sapogenin, yamogenin and others
Mucilaginous compounds
 Polysaccharides
  Mucilage: 15%

Nutrients of Note

Water when fresh: 76.0%
Water when air dried: 6.7%
Starch: 20%

Wood Betony herb
Stachys officinalis (Labiatae)

Properties: astringent, antidiarreal, antidepressant, hypotensive

Systems Affected: nervous, digestive

Folk History and Use

Wood betony is a flowering ornamental plant native to Europe. It has a widespread history of use dating back to the Roman Empire. It has a reputation for being an herbal aspirin and is employed in nearly every self limiting disease. Today it is most useful for treating **diarrhea and headaches**. Additionally, the extract is useful as a gargle for treating **mouth** and **throat irritations.** During the middle ages it obtained a reputation for treating **mental disorders** much more serious than simple headaches. It was reported to magically relieve anxiety and depression.

Medicinal Properties

Definite action
    Astringent (tannin)
    Hypotensive (flavonoids)
    Antidiarreal (tannin)
Possible action
    Antianxiety (?)
    Antidepressant (?)

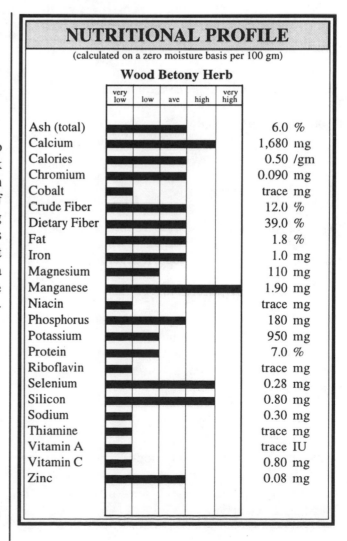

Wood betony contains about 15% tannins, which account for its ability to manage diarrhea. It also contains several flavonoids that have been found to **lower blood pressure**. This probably accounts for the plant's magical powers in treating imbalances of the nervous system ranging from headaches to depression. Wood betony also contains about 0.5% of the digestive enzyme betaine, useful for restoring balance to the digestive system. The plant is not toxic, but overuse could cause irritation of the digestive tract due to the tannins present.

Typical Daily Usage

Fresh herb: 1-2 teaspoon
Dried herb: 0.5-1 gm
Extract: 0.75 gm dried herb, 4 ml alcohol, 4 ml
water

Traditional Formulas

Valerian and Black Cohosh combination
White Willow and Valerian combination

Chemical Constituents

Astringent compounds
Tannin: 15%
Bitter compounds
Flavonoids
Quercitin and others

Nutrients of Note

Water when fresh: 83.2%
Water when air dried: 9.0%
Betaine: 0.5%

Yarrow herb
Achillea millefolium (Compositae)

Properties: astringent, diaphoretic, hemostatic, antibacterial, stimulant, carminative

Systems Affected: digestive, circulatory

Common Names: soldier's woundwart, knight milfoil, staunchwee, herbe militaris

Folk History and Use

The generic name for yarrow, Achillea, was granted this herb in honor of the Greek warrior-god Achilles, who used the herb to stop the bleeding in wounds of his soldiers. It has been extensively used since Achilles' time to **stanch bleeding** in battle wounds and has earned the folk names, soldier's woundwart, knight milfoil, staunchweed, and herbe militaris. It has also been used in civilian life to treat **internal and external bleeding** of all kinds: **wounds, sores, rashes and bleeding piles.**

Yarrow is native to Europe and western Asia, but has been naturalized in all temperate regions and is cultivated in cooler regions of Indo-China and Central America. The rich folklore of this plant in Europe has also become naturalized (with some modification), in North America and China.

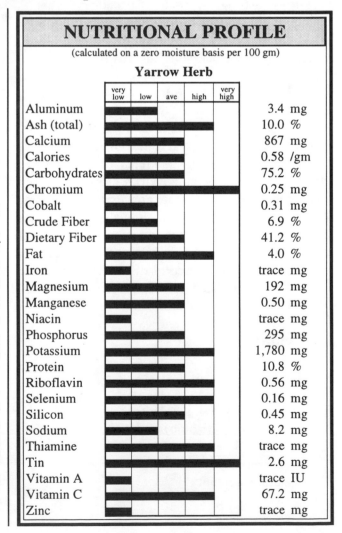

NUTRITIONAL PROFILE
(calculated on a zero moisture basis per 100 gm)

Yarrow Herb

Nutrient	very low	low	ave	high	very high	Value	Unit
Aluminum						3.4	mg
Ash (total)						10.0	%
Calcium						867	mg
Calories						0.58	/gm
Carbohydrates						75.2	%
Chromium						0.25	mg
Cobalt						0.31	mg
Crude Fiber						6.9	%
Dietary Fiber						41.2	%
Fat						4.0	%
Iron						trace	mg
Magnesium						192	mg
Manganese						0.50	mg
Niacin						trace	mg
Phosphorus						295	mg
Potassium						1,780	mg
Protein						10.8	%
Riboflavin						0.56	mg
Selenium						0.16	mg
Silicon						0.45	mg
Sodium						8.2	mg
Thiamine						trace	mg
Tin						2.6	mg
Vitamin A						trace	IU
Vitamin C						67.2	mg
Zinc						trace	mg

Yarrow has been used to brew beer, as tobacco and in salads and soups. It has been used in witchcraft to cast spells and in Christianity to ward off spells.

Medicinal Properties

Definite Action
    Antibacterial (volatile oil)
    Anti-inflammatory (volatile oil)
    Astringent (tannin)
    Hypotensive (alkaloids)
    Hypoglycemic (alkaloids)
    Antithrombotic (coumarins)
Probable Action
    Antipyretic (alkaloids)
    Diuretic (volatile oil)
    Expectorant (volatile oil)

The use of this herb in Western and Chinese folk medicine has been with respect to four activities: 1) astringency of the tannins, 2) irritant action of the volatile oils, 3) the antispasmodic effects of the flavonoids and 4) the hypotensive effects of the alkaloids. Yarrow is used as a **tonic, carminative, febrifuge, antispasmodic, astringent** and **hemostat.**

The volatile oils are responsible for the **carminative, febrifuge, expectorant, diuretic and antibiotic** properties of yarrow. The method of action being **stimulus of mucous membrane** and **bactericidal.**

The alkaloids have been shown to be **hypotensive** and **antipyretic.**

The flavonoids and coumarins are responsible for the **antispasmodic** action on smooth muscle and for the weak **antithrombotic** action.

Organic acids such as the tannins and salicylic acid are responsible for the **astringency** which is the major action of yarrow.

Typical Daily Usage

Fresh herb: 2-4 tablespoon
Dried herb: 3-6 gm
Extract: 4.5 gm dried flower, 22 ml alcohol, 23 ml
    water

Traditional Formulas

Golden Seal and Juniper combination
Alfalfa and Yucca combination
Pau D'Arco and Yellow Dock combination
Parthenium and Golden Seal combination
Parthenium and Myrrh combination
Chamomile and Rose Hips combination

Chemical Constituents

Aromatic compounds
    Volatile oil: 0.1-1.4%
        Terpenes
            Azulene, caryophyllene, cineole
    Fixed oil and Resin: 2-3%
        Fatty acids and waxes
Astringent compounds
    Tannins
    Salicylic acid
Bitter compounds
    Saponins
        Sitosterol and others
    Alkaloids
        Achilleine, trigonelline, betonicine,
            stachydrine

Nutrients of Note

Water when fresh: 82.3%
Water when air dried: 8.1%

Yellow Dock root
Rumex Crispus (Polygonaceae)

Properties: bitter , laxative, antimicrobial, hepatonic

Systems Affected: circulatory, digestive, glandular

Common Names: curled dock, narrow dock, sour dock, rumex, garden patience

Folk History and Use

Yellow dock is a common weed, found nearly world wide. Native to Europe and north Asia, this herb is now difficult to eradicate from gardens around the world. It quickly inhabits cultivated ground and grows along road sides and produces copious quantities of seed each fall.

The leaves of yellow dock can be gathered when young and used as a pot herb. They should be boiled once and the water discarded to take away the bitter taste, then boiled again. This is important because the leaves contain oxalate crystals, most likely potassium oxalate, which is quite toxic. The greens, as well as the root, contain much ascorbic acid and were formerly used as antiscorbutic agents.

The generic name for yellow dock, rumex, is derived from the Latin "rumex" meaning a lance in reference to the shape of its leaves. Its species name, crispus, is from the Latin "crisped" in reference to its leaves being crisped at the edges.

Yellow dock comes from a group of related docks and sorrels and is distinguished from related species by it yellow carrot-shaped root. The root possesses **astringent** qualities united with a **cathartic** principle and has been used as a substitute for rhubarb. It was used in Medieval times to cure **boils** and as a poultice to remedy **burns, scalds, blisters** and **syphylitic lesions**. It was also used to take the itch out of cutaneous eruptions like **psoriasis** and the rashes caused by stinging nettle.

The powdered root was formerly recommended as a **dentifrice** especially when the gums were spongy.

During the 19th century, it gained popularity as a remedy for **jaundice** and as a tonic for the **liver** and **gall bladder** and has since been included in nearly all herbal **liver remedies**. This belief apparently began during the Middle Ages with the Doctrine of Signatures when all yellow herbs were thought to represent bile and bilious diseases.

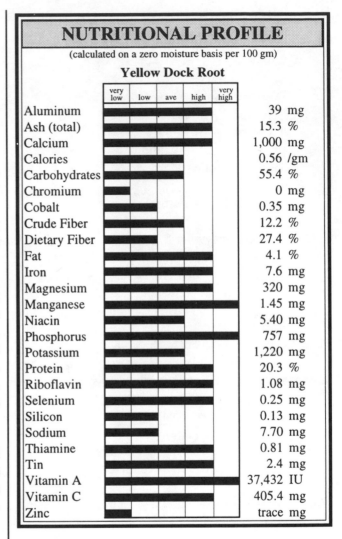

NUTRITIONAL PROFILE
(calculated on a zero moisture basis per 100 gm)

Yellow Dock Root

	very low	low	ave	high	very high		
Aluminum						39	mg
Ash (total)						15.3	%
Calcium						1,000	mg
Calories						0.56	/gm
Carbohydrates						55.4	%
Chromium						0	mg
Cobalt						0.35	mg
Crude Fiber						12.2	%
Dietary Fiber						27.4	%
Fat						4.1	%
Iron						7.6	mg
Magnesium						320	mg
Manganese						1.45	mg
Niacin						5.40	mg
Phosphorus						757	mg
Potassium						1,220	mg
Protein						20.3	%
Riboflavin						1.08	mg
Selenium						0.25	mg
Silicon						0.13	mg
Sodium						7.70	mg
Thiamine						0.81	mg
Tin						2.4	mg
Vitamin A						37,432	IU
Vitamin C						405.4	mg
Zinc						trace	mg

Medicinal Properties

Definite Action
  Astringent (tannin)
  Laxative (anthraquinones)
  Antiscorbutic (vitamin C content)
  Antimicrobial (anthraquinones)
Probable Action
  Nutrient source (iron)
Possible Action
  Hepatonic (?)

The action of yellow dock has been compared to that of various rhubarb species used as laxatives. The active principles in yellow dock are the **astringent** tannins and purgative anthraquinone glycosides based on emodin and chrysophenic acid. The primary use of this herb is in **purgative therapies.**

The tannins and the **antimicrobial** properties of the anthraquinones combine to make decoctions of the plant useful in scrofulous diseases of the skin, including psoriasis and eczema, and help explain the traditional use of yellow dock in treating **skin rashes** obtained from stinging nettles (Urtica spp.) and **syphylitic lesions.**

Its **astringent** and **antimicrobial** properties also explain its use as an **abrasive dentifrice**, especially in cases of spongy gums.

Many sorrels and dock species have a sour taste, apparently due to ascorbic and other organic acids. Our studies confirm that yellow dock has considerable amounts of ascorbic acid that accounts for its former success as an **antiscorbutic** agent.

Yellow dock has accumulated through the Doctrine of Signatures and from folk tradition the reputation of being a **liver tonic, gall bladder tonic** and the best organic source of iron available. One nutritional therapist recently claimed that yellow dock is 50 percent iron by weight.

Though yellow dock contains above average quantities of iron, it doesn't come close to its legendary esteem in this regard, but is useful as a nutritive tonic supplying many trace minerals. Its action on the liver and gall bladder may have some yet unproven efficacy, since most laxatives do stimulate bile production and the secretion of gastric fluids.

Typical Daily Usage

Fresh root: 2-4 tablespoon
Dried root: 3-6 gm
Extract: 4.5 gm dried root, 22 ml alcohol, 23 ml water

Traditional Formulas

Gentain and Cascara combination
Pau D' Arco combination
Red Beet and Yellow Dock combination
Pollen and Ginseng combination

Chemical Constituents

Aromatic compounds
  Volatile oil
  Fixed oil and resin: 3%
Astringent compounds
  Tannins
    Chrysophanic acid and others
Bitter compounds
  Anthraquinone glycosides
    Emodin and others

Nutrients of Note

Water when fresh: 74.3%
Water when air dried: 8.7%

Yerba Santa leaf
Eriodictyon californicum (Hydrophyllaceae)

Properties: bitter, aromatic, expectorant, antispasmodic, antiseptic, anti-inflammatory

Systems affected: respiratory, immune

Common Names: mountain balm, bear's weed, consumptive's weed, tarweed, gum bush

Folk History and Use

Yerba santa or holy herb was the name the Spanish priests gave to this aromatic shrub. It is an evergreen plant that grows in the desert mountains of Mexico and the southwest United States.

The Native American Indians used its thick resinous leaves to make a tea for the treatment of **colds, asthma, tuberculosis** and **rheumatism**. The Native Americans also applied yerba santa linaments to **reduce fever, treat bruises, relieve rheumatism** and **heal infected wounds**. It has a widespread use in treating **wounds and bruises on domestic animals.**

Yerba santa has a distinct odor and flavor that have been incorporated into many bitter pharmaceutical preparations both as an **expectorant** and to mask other bitter flavors, especially quinine.

Medicinal Properties

Definite action
  Expectorant (eriodictyol)
  Antiseptic (eriodictyol)
Probable action
  Antispasmodic (volatile oil)
  Anti-inflammatory (volatile oil)
  Antirheumatic (volatile oil)

Yerba santa contains a volatile oil that is responsible for its therapeutic actions. The leaves are very oily, containing up to 8% oil by weight. The oil consists of about 75% eriodictyonine, 10% eriodictyol and several other related compounds. No reports of toxicity either topically or internally have been reported in the scientific literature.

Typical Daily Usage

Fresh leaf: 1-2 teaspoon
Dried leaf: 1-2 gm.
Extract: 1 gm. dried leaf, 5 ml. alcohol, 5 ml. water

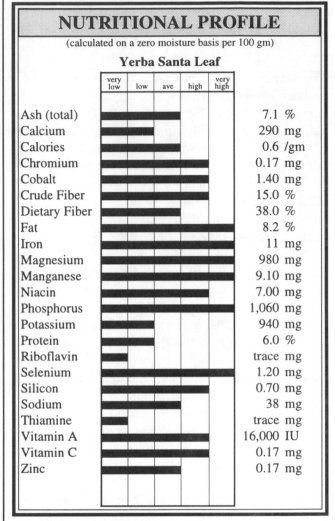

NUTRITIONAL PROFILE
(calculated on a zero moisture basis per 100 gm)

Yerba Santa Leaf

Nutrient	very low	low	ave	high	very high	Value	Unit
Ash (total)			■			7.1	%
Calcium			■			290	mg
Calories			■			0.6	/gm
Chromium				■		0.17	mg
Cobalt				■		1.40	mg
Crude Fiber				■		15.0	%
Dietary Fiber			■			38.0	%
Fat					■	8.2	%
Iron				■		11	mg
Magnesium					■	980	mg
Manganese					■	9.10	mg
Niacin				■		7.00	mg
Phosphorus					■	1,060	mg
Potassium		■				940	mg
Protein					■	6.0	%
Riboflavin	■					trace	mg
Selenium				■		1.20	mg
Silicon			■			0.70	mg
Sodium		■				38	mg
Thiamine	■					trace	mg
Vitamin A				■		16,000	IU
Vitamin C				■		0.17	mg
Zinc			■			0.17	mg

Traditional Formulas

Yerba Santa combination

Chemical Constituents

Aromatic compounds
  Volatile oil
  Resin: 4-8%
Astringent compounds
  Tannin
  Organic acids
    Formic and acetic
Bitter compounds
  Eriodictyol, eriodictyonine and others
Mucilaginous compounds
Gum:12%

Nutrients of Note

Water when fresh: 78%
Water when air dried: 7.6%
Sugars: 9% (galactose, rhamnose)

Yucca root
Yucca baccata (Liliaceae)

Properties: bitter, astringent, antibacterial, antifungal

Systems Affected: digestive

Common Names: soap root

Folk History and Use

This native of the Mojave Desert is a small shrub with a rosette of sword-shaped leaves 2-3 ft. long, rising from a very short stem. When soil and temperature conditions are proper, a spike shoots up from the rosette 5 or 6 feet above the ground and bears clusters of lily-like flowers. Several weeks later, the dried white fruit is ripe and provides a delicious snack to the initiated desert rat.

The most common folk name applied to this plant is soap root. Early settlers learned from the Indians that processed yucca root made a sudsy shampoo or general purpose soap, particularly for clothing.

The substances in the root which give it this property are steroidal saponins. Steroidal saponins are found in low concentrations in wild yam root, fenugreek and in some species of nightshade.

Yucca is also a constituent of some proprietary root beers where it is used as a foaming agent.

Yucca is most often included in formulas designed to **break up obstructions**, especially to reduce the inflammation in joints, which include the chronic degenerative diseases **arthritis** and **rheumatism**.

There has been some research in **antitumor** activity of yucca components. It has been found that there is a chemical in fresh flowers that affect one type of skin cancer in mice.

Medicinal Properties

Definite action
   Antibacterial (saponins)
   Antifungal (saponins)
Probable action
   Blood purifier (saponins)

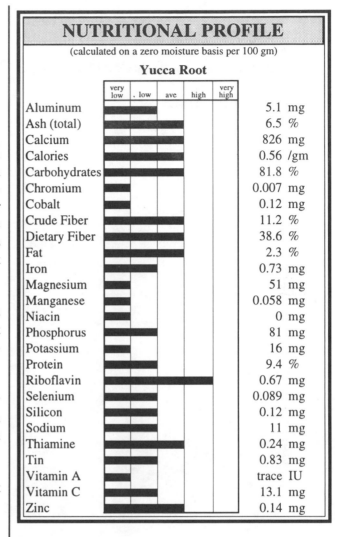

NUTRITIONAL PROFILE
(calculated on a zero moisture basis per 100 gm)

Yucca Root

	very low	low	ave	high	very high	
Aluminum						5.1 mg
Ash (total)						6.5 %
Calcium						826 mg
Calories						0.56 /gm
Carbohydrates						81.8 %
Chromium						0.007 mg
Cobalt						0.12 mg
Crude Fiber						11.2 %
Dietary Fiber						38.6 %
Fat						2.3 %
Iron						0.73 mg
Magnesium						51 mg
Manganese						0.058 mg
Niacin						0 mg
Phosphorus						81 mg
Potassium						16 mg
Protein						9.4 %
Riboflavin						0.67 mg
Selenium						0.089 mg
Silicon						0.12 mg
Sodium						11 mg
Thiamine						0.24 mg
Tin						0.83 mg
Vitamin A						trace IU
Vitamin C						13.1 mg
Zinc						0.14 mg

Recently, yucca root and extracts of yucca leaves and stems have been used to successfully treat **arthritis, rheumatism** and related disorders. The active ingredient in the treatment has been attributed to its steroidal saponins. It is now known that the saponin does not enter the bloodstream, but acts only on the intestinal flora to regulate the balance of the bacterial and yeast colonies in the colon. By stimulating friendly flora and inhibiting others, yucca saponins may indirectly stimulate the absorption of other nutritional factors and decrease the amount of toxins available for absorption from the digestive system.

The elimination systems of the body (kidneys, liver, lymph, and blood) are thus less taxed to remove poisons from the body. This lowers the build up of toxins in the joints and elsewhere which seem to be related to degenerative diseases like **arthritis.**

Typical Daily Usage

Fresh root: 1/4-1/2 cup
Dried root: 6-12 gm
Extract: 9 gm dried root, 45 ml alcohol, 45 ml water

Traditional Formulas

Alfalfa and Yucca combination

Chemical Constituents

Aromatic compounds
  Volatile oil: 0.1-0.2%
  Fixed oil and Resin
Astringent compounds
  Tannin
Bitter compounds
  Saponins
    Sarspogenin, tigogenin, and others

Nutrients of Note

Water when fresh: 79.2%
Water when air dried: 8.9%

Chapter 5

The Circulatory System

The circulatory system is made up of the heart, blood, blood vessels and lymphatic vessels. Its prime function is to transport blood throughout the body. Imbalances in the circulatory system can affect all other systems of the body but most often affect the nervous, respiratory and gastrointestinal systems. The names for the herbal combinations are chosen based on the properties of the key herbs in the formula.

Therapies for Relieving Excess Conditions

"Hardening of the arteries" or atherosclerosis is typical of an excess condition in the circulatory system resulting from toxin buildup in the blood. This condition is often associated with high blood pressure and herbalists use bitter and aromatic herbs to detoxify the blood and calm the nerves.

Excess conditions in the urinary system are often marked by patterns of minor aches, pains and ailments including: anxiety, nervousness, excitability, insecurity, inflammatory skin conditions, rapid speech, red eyes, insomnia, hypertension, hyperlipidemia, hypercholesterolemia, excessive perspiration, frequent urination, neurosis, fevers, stomatitis and painful urination. If left unchecked, these ailments may develop into illnesses including: atherosclerosis, cardiac arrhythmia, cardiac myopathy, cerebrovascular disease, vasculitis, stroke, thrombosis, embolism and heart murmur.

Early herbal therapies for these conditions consisted of single herbs like garlic which purify the blood. Garlic is not simply a blood purifier however, and with time and experience, herbalists recognized and recorded in their herbals the several properties of garlic. The British Herbal Pharmacopeia lists garlic as a diaphoretic, expectorant, spasmolytic, antiseptic, bacteriostatic, antiviral, immunostimulant, hypotensive and anthelmintic.

These lists of empirical properties of an herb are the key to understanding herbal combinations. Herbalists have found that they can enhance a particular property of a single herb by adding herbs that complement and support a given property. Conversely, the herbalist is able to minimize the effects of an unwanted property by adding herbs that counteract and balance that property.

Therapies for Supplementing Deficient Conditions

Weakness in the circulatory system is characterized by a lack of integrity in either the heart or blood vessels. This often results in capillary fragility, anemia and fluid accumulation.

Weakened conditions of the circulatory system are often associated with patterns of minor aches, pains and ailments including: iron deficiency, anemia, hemolytic anemia, vascular fragility, easy bruising, hypotension, edema, nervous exhaustion, forgetfulness, depression, leg pains, chest pains, insomnia, poor night vision, impotence, night sweats, frequent urination, amenorrhea and weak digestion. If left unchecked, these ailments may develop into one or more of the following illnesses: congestive heart failure, mitral valve prolapse, varicose veins, hemophilia diabetes, atherosclerosis and impotence.

Early herbal therapies for these conditions consisted of single herbs like hawthorn berries which are cardiotonic. Hawthorn is not simply a cardiotonic however, and with time and experience, herbalists recognized and recorded in their herbals the several properties of hawthorn. The British Herbal Pharmacopeia lists hawthorn as cardiotonic, coronary vasodilator and hypotensive.

These lists of empirical properties of an herb are the key to understanding herbal combinations. Herbalists have found that they can enhance a particular property of a single herb by adding herbs that complement and support a given property. Conversely, the herbalist is able to minimize an unwanted property by adding herbs that counteract and balance that property.

Therapies for Relieving Excess Conditions

Capsicum and Garlic Combination

Composition

Garlic
Capsicum
Parsley

Properties

Stimulant
Hypotensive
Diaphoretic
Carminative
Diuretic
Antiseptic

General Description

Capsicum and Garlic combination is a stimulant or sudorific formula. The herbs increase blood circulation and perspiration, reduce blood pressure, increase the production of digestive fluids and fight infections.

Chinese herbalists would describe this herbal combination as a fire reducing formula. It also reduces the wood element while enhancing the earth, water and metal elements.

Capsicum and Garlic combination has been used to treat **colds, coughs, hypertension, asthma, skin eruptions, impotence, hemorrhoids, rheumatism, indigestion, worms, parasites, chronic chills** and **poor circulation.**

Imbalances indicating the use of this formula are commonly noted in the heart acupressure point located directly over the heart area of the chest. Imbalances are often noted in the lymphatic rosary of both irises and in the 2:30 position of the left iris. Use caution in cases of acute inflammation of the kidneys and inflammatory conditions of the gastrointestinal tract.

This formula is commonly used in conjunction with the vitamin C family, vitamin A, hawthorn, ginger root, vitamin E, selenium, germanium, echinacea, goldenseal, spirulina, zinc and manganese.

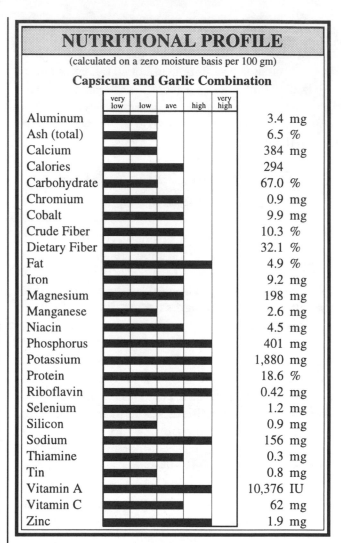

NUTRITIONAL PROFILE
(calculated on a zero moisture basis per 100 gm)

Capsicum and Garlic Combination

	very low	low	ave	high	very high		
Aluminum						3.4	mg
Ash (total)						6.5	%
Calcium						384	mg
Calories						294	
Carbohydrate						67.0	%
Chromium						0.9	mg
Cobalt						9.9	mg
Crude Fiber						10.3	%
Dietary Fiber						32.1	%
Fat						4.9	%
Iron						9.2	mg
Magnesium						198	mg
Manganese						2.6	mg
Niacin						4.5	mg
Phosphorus						401	mg
Potassium						1,880	mg
Protein						18.6	%
Riboflavin						0.42	mg
Selenium						1.2	mg
Silicon						0.9	mg
Sodium						156	mg
Thiamine						0.3	mg
Tin						0.8	mg
Vitamin A						10,376	IU
Vitamin C						62	mg
Zinc						1.9	mg

Individual Components

Garlic bulb contains aromatic compounds that lower blood pressure, heart rate and blood cholesterol while increasing coronary circulation. These compounds also fight infections, reduce muscle spasms, increase immune response, promote sweating, increase the production of digestive fluids and decrease the thickness while increasing the production of mucosal fluid. Garlic has been used to treat colds, coughs, asthma, coronary heart disease, hypertension, atherosclerosis, infections, inflammatory skin conditions and hemorrhoids.

Capsicum fruit contains aromatic resins that increase blood circulation, promote sweating, increase the production of digestive fluids and reduce muscle spasms. It has been used to treat flatulence, colic, ulcers, rheumatic arthritis, cold hands and feet and dropsy.

Parsley herb contains aromatic compounds that decrease the thickness and increase the production of mucosal fluids, increase the production of digestive fluids, increase menstrual and urine flow. It also contains bitter compounds that reduce muscle spasms and pains, reduce blood pressure and are antiseptic. Parsley is an excellent herbal source of trace minerals especially the electrolyte minerals including sodium, potassium, calcium and magnesium. It is also an excellent herbal source of vitamin A, vitamin C and chlorophyllins. Parsley has been used to treat urinary tract infections, amenorrhea, dysmenorrhea, dyspepsia, bronchitis, allergies, arthritis, asthma, flatulence, dysuria and nephritis.

Garlic Combination

Composition

Garlic	Ginger
Capsicum	Siberian Ginseng
Parsley	Goldenseal

Properties

Stimulant	Carminative
Hypotensive	Diaphoretic
Antiseptic	Diuretic

General Description

Garlic combination is a stimulant or sudorific formula that relieves stress in the circulatory system. The herbs work to promote efficient function in the eliminative organs particularly the liver and kidneys. This formula also increases blood circulation and perspiration. These actions result in lower blood pressure, increased coronary blood flow and elimination of toxins from the blood.

Chinese herbalists would describe this herbal combination as a fire reducing formula. It also enhances the water, earth and metal elements while reducing the wood elements.

Garlic Combination has traditionally been used to treat **atherosclerosis hypertension, hemorrhoids, rheumatism, chronic chills, poor circulation, colds, flu and indigestion.**

Imbalances indicating the use of this formula are commonly noted in the heart acupressure point located directly over the heart area of the chest. Imbalances are often noted at the 2:30 position of the left iris. Use caution in cases of acute inflammation of the kidneys, ulcers and colitis.

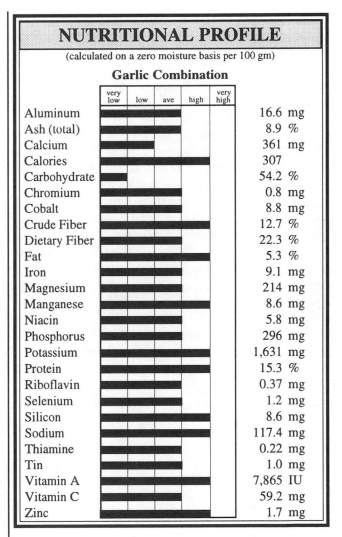

NUTRITIONAL PROFILE
(calculated on a zero moisture basis per 100 gm)

Garlic Combination

	very low	low	ave	high	very high	
Aluminum						16.6 mg
Ash (total)						8.9 %
Calcium						361 mg
Calories						307
Carbohydrate						54.2 %
Chromium						0.8 mg
Cobalt						8.8 mg
Crude Fiber						12.7 %
Dietary Fiber						22.3 %
Fat						5.3 %
Iron						9.1 mg
Magnesium						214 mg
Manganese						8.6 mg
Niacin						5.8 mg
Phosphorus						296 mg
Potassium						1,631 mg
Protein						15.3 %
Riboflavin						0.37 mg
Selenium						1.2 mg
Silicon						8.6 mg
Sodium						117.4 mg
Thiamine						0.22 mg
Tin						1.0 mg
Vitamin A						7,865 IU
Vitamin C						59.2 mg
Zinc						1.7 mg

This formula is commonly used in conjunction with hawthorn, yarrow, the vitamin C family, vitamin A, vitamin E, iron and copper.

Individual Components

Garlic bulb contains aromatic compounds that lower blood pressure, heart rate and blood cholesterol while increasing coronary circulation. These compounds also fight infections, reduce muscle spasms, increase immune response, promote sweating, increase the production of digestive fluids and decrease the thickness while increasing the production of mucosal fluid. Garlic has been used to treat colds, coughs, asthma, coronary heart disease, hypertension, atherosclerosis, infections, inflammatory skin conditions and hemorrhoids.

Capsicum fruit contains aromatic resins that increase blood circulation, promote sweating, increase the production of digestive fluids and reduce muscle spasms. It has been used to treat flatulence, colic, ulcers, rheumatic arthritis, cold hands and feet and dropsy.

Parsley herb contains aromatic compounds that decrease the thickness and increase the production of mucosal fluids, increase the production of digestive fluids, increase menstrual flow and increase urine flow. It also contains bitter compounds that reduce muscle spasms and pains, reduce blood pressure and are antiseptic. Parsley is an excellent herbal source of trace minerals especially the electrolyte minerals including sodium, potassium, calcium and magnesium. It is also an excellent herbal source of vitamin A, vitamin C and chlorophyllins. Parsley has been used to treat urinary tract infections, amenorrhea, dysmenorrhea, dyspepsia, bronchitis, allergies, arthritis, asthma, flatulence, dysuria and nephritis.

Ginger root contains aromatic compounds that increase the production of digestive fluids and enzymes, lower blood pressure, lower blood sugar and cholesterol. It also contains bitter compounds that reduce muscle spasms, increase blood circulation and dilate blood vessels. Ginger is an excellent herbal source of trace minerals, especially silicon, magnesium and manganese. It has been used to treat nausea, motion sickness, flatulence, colds, coughs, indigestion, fevers, vomiting, diarrhea, chronic bronchitis and cold hands and feet.

Siberian Ginseng root contains bitter compounds that help the body respond more quickly to stress. These compounds increase the production of DNA, RNA and proteins essential to all life processes. They also stimulate the adrenal, pancreas, and pituitary glands to lower blood sugar and reduce inflammation. Ginseng also increases the production of digestive fluids and is a mild sedative. It had been used to treat anemia, impotence, insomnia, diarrhea, fatigue debility, weak digestion and failing memory.

Goldenseal root is an excellent herbal source of trace minerals including cobalt, iron, magnesium, manganese, silicon and zinc. It is also an excellent herbal source of vitamin C. It has been used to treat hepatitis, gastritis, colitis, ulcers, menorrhagia, postpartum hemorrhage, dysmenorrhea, diabetes, infections, hemorrhoids, eczema, obesity and fevers.

Goldenseal root contains bitter astringent alkaloids that normalize liver and spleen functions by increasing the production of digestive fluids and enzymes, particularly bile. The compounds are antiseptic, constrict peripheral blood vessels, especially in the uterus, are laxative and relieve pain and inflammation in mucosal tissue. Goldenseal is an excellent herbal source of trace minerals including cobalt, iron, magnesium, manganese, silicon and zinc. It is also an excellent herbal source of vitamin C. It has been used to treat hepatitis, gastritis, colitis, ulcers, menorrhagia, postpartum hemorrhage, dysmenorrhea, diabetes, infections, hemorrhoids, eczema, obesity and fevers.

Therapies for Supplementing Deficient Conditions

Biota and Zizyphus Combination

Composition

Biota	Dong Quai
Zizyphus	Lycium Fruit
Cistanche	Polygala
Schizandra	Dioscorea
Succinum	Lotus Seed
Cuscuta	Siberian Ginseng
Acorus	Astragalus
Ophiopogon	Hoelen
Rehmannia	Polygonatum

Properties

Cardiotonic
Carminative
Diuretic
Adaptogen
Antidepressant

General Description

Biota and Zizyphus combination is a nerve tonic and a heart tonic. The herbs work to increase blood circulation, improve digestion, relieve depression, increase the flow of urine and allow the body to more quickly respond to stress. It is used to treat general weakness and debility resulting from chronic nervous disorders.

Chinese herbalists describe this herbal combination as a fire enhancing formula. It also enhances the earth and metal elements, reducing the wood and water elements.

Biota and Zizyphus combination has traditionally been used to treat **exhaustion, heart palpitations, angina, pains, insomnia, depression, anxiety, weak digestion, frequent urination, back pains, anemia** and **dry skin.**

Imbalances indicating the use of this formula are commonly noted in the stress acupressure point located on the forehead between the eyes. Imbalances are often noted at the 2:30 position of the left iris.

This formula is commonly used in conjunction with the vitamin C family, polyunsaturated fatty acids and hawthorn berries.

Individual Components

Biota seed contains aromatic compounds that have a sedative effect. These compounds also have a mild laxative effect. Biota has been used to treat heart palpitations, insomnia, debility and constipation.

Zizyphus seed contains bitter compounds that have a sedative effect, relieve pains, reduce fevers and lower blood pressure. It has been used to treat insomnia, heart palpitations, night sweats and nervous tension.

Cistanche herb contains bitter compounds that enhance the production of urine, rejuvenate renal function and have a mild laxative effect. It has been used to treat impotence, frequent urination and chronic constipation.

Schizandra fruit contains bitter compounds that allow the body to more quickly respond to stress. This increases the body's capacity for work and decreases fatigue. These compounds also increase blood circulation, blood sugar and bile production while lowering blood pressure. Schizandra also contains astringent compounds that increase the contraction of the heart muscle and the uterus and are antiseptic. The herb has been used to treat heart palpitations, dropsy, nervous exhaustion, asthma, diabetes, chronic diarrhea, night sweats, seminal emissions, insomnia, frequent urination and anxiety.

Succinum resin contains aromatic compounds that increase the flow of urine and increase blood circulation. These compounds also relieve pains, are antiseptic and have a sedative effect. Succinum has been used to treat insomnia, heart palpitations, epilepsy, urinary tract infections, kidney stones, amenorrhea and coronary heart disease.

Cuscuta seed contains bitter compounds that increase the flow of urine, detoxify the kidneys, lower blood pressure, enhance heart action and normalize liver functions. Cuscuta has been used to treat lumbago, impotence, frequent urination, kidney stones, poor eyesight and nocturnal emission.

Acorus root contains aromatic compounds that have a sedative effect, increase the production of digestive fluids, relieve muscle spasms, lower blood pressure, reduce fevers and are antiseptic. Acorus has been used to treat nervous tension, depression, epilepsy, poor appetite, gastritis and flatulence.

Ophiopogon root contains bitter compounds that have a sedative effect, promote the production of mucosal fluids, reduce muscle spasms and have an antiseptic effect. In addition, the herb lowers blood sugar and regenerates beta cells in the islets of langerhorn of the pancreas. Ophiopogon has been used to treat insomnia, coronary heart disease, heart palpitations, fear and dry coughs.

Rehmannia root contains astringent compounds that stop bleeding and reduce inflammation especially in the digestive system. The herb also contains bitter compounds that reduce capillary fragility. It has been used to treat ulcers, menorrhagia, thirst diabetes constipation, anemia and infertility.

Dong Quai root contains aromatic compounds that relieve smooth muscle spasms especially in the uterus, have a sedative effect and increase the production of digestive fluids. It also contains bitter compounds that regulate glycogen production in the liver pain and inflammation, increase blood flow especially to the heart, lower blood cholesterol, normalize uterine contractions and are antiseptic. Dong Quai is an excellent herbal source of iron, magnesium and niacin. It has been used to treat anemia, abdominal pains, dysmenorrhea, amenorrhea, arthritis, coronary heart disease, atherosclerosis, angina pectoris, indigestion and headaches.

Lycium fruit contains bitter compounds that lower blood sugar, promote the regeneration of liver cells and lower blood cholesterol. It has been used to treat atherosclerosis, backache,impotence, vertigo, poor eyesight and diabetes.

Polygala root contains bitter compounds that decrease the thickness and increase the production of mucosal fluids, have a sedative effect, and are antiseptic. These compounds also lower blood pressure and increase uterine tension. Polygala has been used to treat insomnia, heart palpitations, ulcers, inflammatory skin conditions, bronchitis and nervous tension.

Dioscorea root contains mucilaginous compounds that decrease the thickness and increase the production of mucosal fluids, enhance the efficiency of healing and increase the production of digestive fluids. It has been used to treat lack of appetite, diarrhea, asthma, dry coughs, nocturnal emissions, frequent urination, diabetes and inflammatory skin conditions.

Lotus seed contains mucilaginous compounds that absorb toxins from the digestive system and relieve smooth muscle spasms. It also contains astringent compounds that shrink inflamed tissue. Lotus seed has been used to treat chronic diarrhea, lack of appetite, insomnia and heart palpitations.

Siberian Ginseng root contains bitter compounds that help the body respond more quickly to stress. These compounds increase the production of DNA, RNA and proteins essential to all life processes. They also stimulate the adrenal, pancreas, and pituitary glands to lower blood sugar and reduce inflammation. Ginseng also increases the production of digestive fluids and is a mild sedative. It has been used to treat anemia, impotence, insomnia, diarrhea, fatigue, debility, weak digestion and failing memory.

Astragalus root contains bitter compounds that increase the flow of urine, are antiseptic, increase the production of digestive fluids including bile and relieve muscle spasms. Astragalus also contains mucilaginous compounds that enhance immune response, increasing the production of lymphocytes and macrophages. The herb also increases heart action and lowers blood pressure and blood sugar. It has been used to treat fatigue, debility, urinary tract infections, edema, nephritis, ulcers, prolapse of organs and night sweats.

Hoelen herb contains bitter compounds that increase the flow of urine, decrease blood sugar and have a sedative effect. It has been used to treat edema, dropsy, diarrhea, insomnia, frequent urination and heart palpitations.

Polygonatum root contains bitter compounds that have a cardiotonic effect that increases heart rate and lowers blood pressure. These compounds initially raise blood sugar then lower it. It is used to treat diabetes, coronary heart disease, tuberculosis and dry coughs.

Ginko and Hawthorn Combination

Composition

Ginkgo
Hawthorn

Properties

Cardiotonic
Stimulant

General Description

Ginkgo and Hawthorn combination is a circulatory stimulant. Its primary action is to increase vascular blood flow. This function improves alertness and one's sense of well being.

Chinese herbalists would describe this herbal combination as a fire enhancing formula. It also enhances the earth and metal elements while reducing the wood and water elements.

Ginkgo and Hawthorn combination has traditionally been used to treat **poor circulation, atherosclerosis, vertigo, headaches, tinnitus, deafness, diminished mental capacity, Alzheimer's disease, diabetes** and **skin disorders.**

Imbalances indicating the use of this formula are commonly noted in the heart acupressure point located approximately on the left side of the lower sternum. Imbalances are often noted at the 2:30 position of the iris.

This formula is commonly used in conjunction with butcher's broom, fish oil and the vitamin C family.

Individual Components

Ginkgo leaves contain bitter compounds (flavonoids) that decrease capillary permeability, thrombosis and platelet aggregation. These compounds increase peripheral blood flow and reduce inflammation. Ginkgo is an excellent herbal source of iron, calcium and

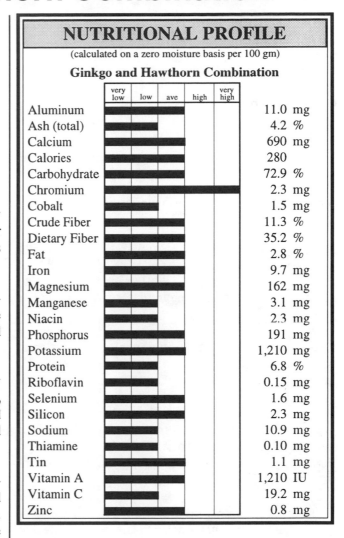

NUTRITIONAL PROFILE

(calculated on a zero moisture basis per 100 gm)

Ginkgo and Hawthorn Combination

	very low	low	ave	high	very high		
Aluminum						11.0	mg
Ash (total)						4.2	%
Calcium						690	mg
Calories						280	
Carbohydrate						72.9	%
Chromium						2.3	mg
Cobalt						1.5	mg
Crude Fiber						11.3	%
Dietary Fiber						35.2	%
Fat						2.8	%
Iron						9.7	mg
Magnesium						162	mg
Manganese						3.1	mg
Niacin						2.3	mg
Phosphorus						191	mg
Potassium						1,210	mg
Protein						6.8	%
Riboflavin						0.15	mg
Selenium						1.6	mg
Silicon						2.3	mg
Sodium						10.9	mg
Thiamine						0.10	mg
Tin						1.1	mg
Vitamin A						1,210	IU
Vitamin C						19.2	mg
Zinc						0.8	mg

vitamin C. It has been used to treat poor circulation, deafness, Alzheimer's disease and atherosclerosis.

Hawthorn berries contain bitter compounds that increase coronary blood flow and myocardial metabolism allowing the heart to function with less oxygen. These compounds also lower blood pressure by decreasing cardiac output and dilating peripheral blood vessels. It has been used to treat hypertension, coronary heart disease, atherosclerosis, blood clots and insomnia.

Hawthorn Combination

Composition

Hawthorn
Capsicum
Garlic

Properties

Cardiotonic
Stimulant

General Description

Hawthorn combination is a circulatory system stimulant. Its primary action is to increase coronary blood flow. This formula is particularly effective in treating chronic weaknesses of the circulatory system such as atherosclerosis.

Chinese herbalists would describe this combination as a fire enhancing formula. It also enhances the earth and metal elements while reducing the wood and water elements.

Hawthorn combination has traditionally been used to treat **dropsy, atherosclerosis, thrombosis, hyperlipidemia, hypercholesterolemia, edema, heart weakness** and **angina pains.**

Imbalances indicating the use of this formula are commonly noted in the heart acupressure point on the left side of the lower sternum. Imbalances are often noted at the 2:30 position of the left iris. Use caution in cases of inflammatory conditions of the gastrointestinal tract.

This formula is commonly used in conjunction with the vitamin C family, polyunsaturated fish oils, and a low sodium, low protein vegetarian diet.

Individual Components

Hawthorn berry contains bitter compounds that increase coronary blood flow and myocardial metabolism allowing the heart to function with less oxygen. These compounds also lower blood pressure by decreasing cardiac output and dilating peripheral blood vessels. It has been used to treat hypertension, coronary heart disease, atherosclerosis, blood clots and insomnia.

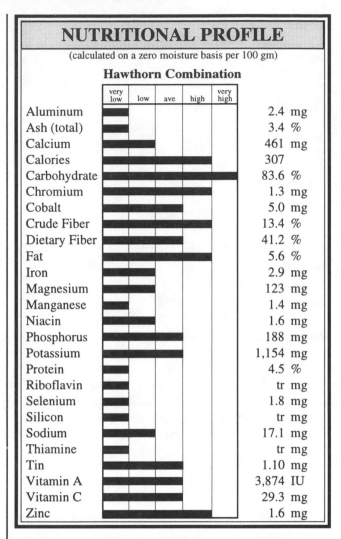

NUTRITIONAL PROFILE
(calculated on a zero moisture basis per 100 gm)
Hawthorn Combination

	very low	low	ave	high	very high	
Aluminum	■					2.4 mg
Ash (total)	■					3.4 %
Calcium		■				461 mg
Calories				■		307
Carbohydrate					■	83.6 %
Chromium					■	1.3 mg
Cobalt				■		5.0 mg
Crude Fiber				■		13.4 %
Dietary Fiber			■			41.2 %
Fat				■		5.6 %
Iron		■				2.9 mg
Magnesium			■			123 mg
Manganese		■				1.4 mg
Niacin	■					1.6 mg
Phosphorus		■				188 mg
Potassium					■	1,154 mg
Protein		■				4.5 %
Riboflavin	■					tr mg
Selenium		■				1.8 mg
Silicon	■					tr mg
Sodium			■			17.1 mg
Thiamine	■					tr mg
Tin				■		1.10 mg
Vitamin A				■		3,874 IU
Vitamin C		■				29.3 mg
Zinc					■	1.6 mg

Capsicum fruit contains aromatic resins that increase blood circulation, promote sweating, increase the production of digestive fluids and reduce muscle spasms. It has been used to treat flatulence, colic, ulcers, rheumatic arthritis, cold hands and feet and dropsy.

Garlic bulb contains aromatic compounds that lower blood pressure, heart rate and blood cholesterol while increasing coronary circulation. These compounds also fight infections, reduce muscle spasms, increase immune response, promote sweating, increase the production of digestive fluids and decrease the thickness while increasing the production of mucosal fluid. Garlic has been used to treat colds, coughs, asthma, coronary heart disease, hypertension, atherosclerosis, infections, inflammatory skin conditions and hemorrhoids.

Chapter 6

The Digestive System

The digestive system is made up of the alimentary canal and includes the mouth and salivary glands, the esophagus, stomach, liver, gall bladder, pancreas, small intestine and large intestine. Its prime function is to digest food, absorb nutrients and eliminate waste through the bowel. Imbalances in the digestive system often affect the circulatory system as unwanted toxins are absorbed and bowel elimination is slowed. The names for the herbal combinations are chosen based on the properties of the key herbs in the formula.

Therapies for Relieving Excess Conditions

Constipation is the most prevalent excess condition of the digestive system found in modern societies. The ingestion of large quantities of refined foods is the prime cause of this condition and results in unwanted toxins being absorbed into the circulatory system and elimination of waste being slowed.

Excess conditions in the digestive system are often marked by patterns of minor aches, pains and ailments including: flatulence, abdominal pains, anxiety, nervousness, selfishness, difficulty rising from bed, constipation, nausea, abdominal bloating, obesity, diarrhea, anemia, motion sickness, indigestion, headache and vomiting. If left unchecked, these ailments may develop into illnesses such as: diverticulosis, constipation, arthritis, gastric ulcers, obesity, anorexia, neuromuscular disorders and yeast infections.

Early herbal therapies for these conditions consisted of single herbs like cascara sagrada bark which is a laxative. Cascara is not simply a laxative however, and with time and experience, herbalists recognized and recorded in their herbals the several properties of cascara. The British Herbal Pharmacopoeia lists cascara as a laxative, cholagogue and mild purgative.

These lists of empirical properties of an herb are the key to understanding herbal combinations. Herbalists have found that they can enhance a particular property of a single herb by adding herbs that complement and support a given property. Conversely, the herbalist is also able to minimize an unwanted property by adding herbs that counteract to balance that property.

Therapies for Supplementing Deficient Conditions

Weakened conditions of the digestive system can result from poor blood circulation, inefficient function of the digestive organs, lifestyle or aging. Herbalists use aromatic herbs to stimulate blood flow and increase the production of digestive fluids and enzymes. Mucilaginous herbs are also employed to soothe inflamed tissues and provide bulk to the stool.

Weakened conditions of the digestive system are often associated with patterns of minor aches, pains and ailments including: diarrhea, hemorrhoids, hernia, joint pains, muscle cramps, cold hands and feet, lack of muscle tone, easy bruising, sinus congestion, vaginal discharge, indigestion, anemia and weight loss. If left unchecked, these ailments may develop into illnesses including: gastric ulcers, colitis, chronic enteritis, prolapse of organs, chronic diarrhea and Crohn's disease.

Early herbal therapies for these conditions consisted of single herbs like slippery elm bark which soothes inflamed tissues and absorbs toxins from the bowel. Slippery elm is not simply a demulcent however, and with time and experience, herbalists recognized and recorded in their herbals the several properties of slippery elm. The British Herbal Pharmacopoeia lists slippery elm as a demulcent, emollient, nutrient and antitussive.

These lists of empirical properties of an herb are the key to understanding herbal combinations. Herbalists have found that they can enhance a particular property of a single herb by adding herbs that complement and support that property. Conversely, the herbalist is also able to minimize an unwanted property by adding herbs that counteract or balance the property.

Therapies for Relieving Excess Conditions

Agastache and Shengu Combination

Composition

Agastache	Citrus
Shengu	Pinellia
Magnolia bark	Cardamon
Atractylodes	Crateagus
Saussurea	Ginger
Oryza	Licorice
Hoelen	Siberian Ginseng
Gastrodia	Platycodon

Properties

Anti-inflammatory
Carminative
Stimulant
Diuretic
Laxative

General Description

Agastache and Shengu combination enhances the digestive and detoxifying functions of the body. The herbs work to increase the production of digestive fluids. Enzymes soothe inflamed tissues, increase blood circulation, and increase the flow of urine and are mildly laxative.

Chinese herbalists describe this herbal combination as an earth reducing formula. It also reduces water and metal elements while enhancing the fire and wood elements.

Agastache and Shengu combination has traditionally been used to treat **nausea, bloating, food allergies, obesity, sluggish bowels, diarrhea, headaches, poor circulation, indigestion, flatulence, gastroenteritis, anxiety, difficulty rising from bed, sweet cravings, motion sickness and morning sickness.**

Imbalances indicating the use of this formula are commonly noted in the stomach acupressure point located approximately 2 inches below and 2 inches to the left of the sternum. Imbalances are often noted at the 4:30 position of the left iris and in the 7:30 position of the right iris. Use caution in cases of inflammatory skin conditions, high fevers and ulcers.

This formula is commonly used in conjunction with protein digestive (HCl) aids, food enzyme supplements, licorice, marshmallow, chamomile, vitamin A and zinc.

Individual Components

Agastache herb contains aromatic compounds that promote sweating, increase the production of digestive fluids, reduce muscle spasms and are antiseptic. It has been used to treat dyspepsia, indigestion, nausea, bloating, colds, fevers and flatulence.

Shengu is a combination of five herbs that contains digestive enzymes and nutrients that improve digestion. These herbs increase the production of digestive fluids and improve the nutritional value of other foods. It has been used to treat dyspepsia, indigestion and poor appetite.

Magnolia bark contains bitter compounds that relieve muscle cramps, are antiseptic and have sedative properties. It has been used to treat gastritis, coughs, asthma, diarrhea, vomiting and flatulence.

Atractylodes root contains aromatic compounds that are antiseptic, increase the production of digestive fluids and enzymes, increase blood pressure, are laxative, stimulate liver function and increase the flow of urine. It has been used to treat dyspepsia, flatulence, loss of appetite, nausea, indigestion, rheumatic arthritis and night blindness.

Saussurea root contains aromatic compounds that increase the production of digestive fluids, increase blood circulation and are antiseptic. It also contains bitter compounds that relieve smooth muscle spasms, lower blood pressure and relieve pains. Saussurea has been used to treat gastritis, chest pains, jaundice, gall stones and diarrhea.

Oryza seed contains mucilaginous compounds that absorb toxins and give bulk to the stool. In addition these compounds sooth inflamed tissues and make digestion more efficient. Oryza has been used to treat diarrhea, dyspepsia, frequent urination and indigestion.

Hoelen herb contains bitter compounds that increase the flow of urine, decrease blood sugar and have a sedative effect. It has been used to treat edema, dropsy, diarrhea, insomnia, frequent urination and heart palpitations.

Gastrodia root contains bitter compounds that are sedative, increase the secretion of bile and relieve pain and muscle spasms. It has been used to treat convulsions, arthritis, headaches, vertigo and hypertension.

Citrus peel contains aromatic compounds that are antiseptic, reduce muscle spasms and decrease the thickness while increasing the production of mucosal fluids. It also contains bitter compounds that are anti-inflammatory, reduce muscle spasms, increase the production of digestive fluid and increase blood circulation. Citrus peel has been used to treat coughs, colds, flu, fevers and bronchitis.

Pinellia root contains bitter compounds that decrease the thickness while increasing the production of mucosal fluids, relieve muscle spasms, increase the production of digestive fluids and absorb toxins. Pinellia root must by processed with alum or ginger root before ingestion since it is toxic. It has been used to treat morning sickness, nausea, vomiting, respiratory congestion, ulcers and blood poisoning.

Cardamon fruit contains aromatic compounds that promote sweating, increase the production of digestive fluids, and reduce smooth muscle spasms especially in the intestine and uterus. It has been used to treat diarrhea, to prevent miscarriage and to treat dyspepsia.

Crataegus fruit contains bitter compounds that increase coronary blood flow and myocardial metabolism allowing the heart to function with less oxygen. These compounds also lower blood pressure by decreasing cardiac output and dilating peripheral blood vessels. Crataegus has been used to treat hypertension, atherosclerosis, dyspepsia, postpartum depression and amenorrhea.

Ginger root contains aromatic compounds that increase the production of digestive fluids and enzymes, lower blood pressure, lower blood sugar and cholesterol. It also contains bitter compounds that reduce muscle spasms, increase blood circulation and dilate blood vessels. Ginger is an excellent herbal source of trace minerals especially silicon, magnesium and manganese. It has been used to treat nausea, motion sickness, flatulence, colds, coughs, indigestion, fevers, vomiting, diarrhea, chronic bronchitis and cold hands and feet.

Licorice root contains bitter compounds that reduce inflammation, decrease the thickness and increase the production of mucosal fluids and relieve muscle spasms. In addition, licorice stimulates adrenal functions, reduces the urge to cough, is mildly laxative and enhances immune response. It has been used to treat coughs, colds, arthritis, asthma, peptic ulcers, Addison's disease, dropsy and atherosclerosis.

Siberian Ginseng root contains bitter compounds that help the body respond more quickly to stress. These compounds increase the production of DNA, RNA and proteins essential to all life processes. They also stimulate the adrenal, pancreas, and pituitary glands to lower blood sugar and reduce inflammation. Ginseng also increases the production of digestive fluids and is a mild sedative. It had been used to treat anemia, impotence, insomnia, diarrhea, fatigue debility, weak digestion and failing memory.

Platycodon root contains bitter compounds that decrease the thickness while increasing the production of mucosal fluids, lower blood sugar, lower blood cholesterol, and are antiseptic. It is used to treat coughs, weak digestion, inflammatory skin conditions and respiratory tract infections.

Capsicum and Myrrh Combination

Composition

Capsicum
Goldenseal
Myrrh

Properties

Anti-inflammatory	Laxative
Antiseptic	Cholagogue
Analgesic	Vulnerary
Stimulant	

General Description

Capsicum and Myrrh combination is used to treat ulcers and other inflammations in the digestive system. The herbs reduce pain and inflammation, are antiseptic, increase blood circulation, are laxative and increase the production of digestive fluids and enzymes.

Chinese herbalists would describe this herbal combination as an earth reducing formula. It also reduces the water element while enhancing the wood and metal elements.

Capsicum and Myrrh combination has traditionally been used to treat **ulcers, indigestion, gastritis, worms, sinus congestion** and **chronic chills.**

Imbalances indicating the use of this formula are commonly noted in the stomach acupressure point located approximately two inches below the sternum. Imbalances are often noted in the autonomic nerve wreath surrounding both pupils. Use caution in cases of bloody stool, Crohn's disease and vomiting. Long term use can increase capillary permeability.

This formula is commonly used in conjunction with the vitamin A, chlorophyll, comfrey, the vitamin C family, vitamin E and cabbage.

Individual Components

Capsicum fruit contains aromatic resins that increase blood circulation, promote sweating, increase the production of digestive fluids and reduce muscle spasms.

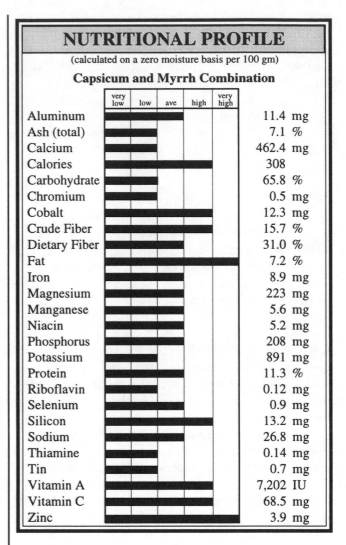

NUTRITIONAL PROFILE
(calculated on a zero moisture basis per 100 gm)

Capsicum and Myrrh Combination

	very low	low	ave	high	very high	
Aluminum						11.4 mg
Ash (total)						7.1 %
Calcium						462.4 mg
Calories						308
Carbohydrate						65.8 %
Chromium						0.5 mg
Cobalt						12.3 mg
Crude Fiber						15.7 %
Dietary Fiber						31.0 %
Fat						7.2 %
Iron						8.9 mg
Magnesium						223 mg
Manganese						5.6 mg
Niacin						5.2 mg
Phosphorus						208 mg
Potassium						891 mg
Protein						11.3 %
Riboflavin						0.12 mg
Selenium						0.9 mg
Silicon						13.2 mg
Sodium						26.8 mg
Thiamine						0.14 mg
Tin						0.7 mg
Vitamin A						7,202 IU
Vitamin C						68.5 mg
Zinc						3.9 mg

It has been used to treat flatulence, colic, ulcers, rheumatic arthritis, cold hands and feet and dropsy.

Goldenseal root contains bitter astringent alkaloids that normalize liver and spleen functions by increasing the production of digestive fluids and enzymes, particularly bile. The compounds are antiseptic, constrict peripheral blood vessels, especially in the uterus, are laxative and relieve pain and inflamation in mucosal tissue. Goldenseal is an excellent herbal source of trace minerals including cobalt, iron, magnesium, manganese, silicon and zinc. It is also an excellent herbal source of vitamin C. It has been used to treat hepatitis, gastritis, colitis, ulcers, menorrhagia, postpartum hemorrhage, dysmenorrhea, diabetes, infections, hemorrhoids, eczema, obesity, and fevers.

Myrrh gum contains astringent resins that promote the healing of sores. These compounds shrink inflamed tissue, are antiseptic and reduce pain in mucous membranes. Myrrh also decreases the thickness while increasing the production of mucosal fluids. It has been used to treat colds, coughs, bronchitis, asthma, dysmenorrhea, rheumatism and arthritis.

Cascara Combination

Composition

Cascara Sagrada	Ginger
Buckthorn	Couch Grass
Licorice	Red Clover
Barberry	Turkey Rhubarb
Capsicum	

Properties

Purgative
Carminative
Cholagogue
Antispasmodic

General Description

Cascara combination is a purgative formula. It is a colon stimulant that enhances elimination. The herbs are purgative, increase the production of digestive fluids and enzymes, especially bile, reduce smooth muscle cramps and promote the growth of friendly colonic bacteria.

Chinese herbalists would describe this herbal combination as an internal attacking or wood reducing formula. It also reduces the fire and metal elements while enhancing the earth and water elements.

Cascara combination has traditionally been used to treat **constipation, dry stool, obesity, fevers, skin inflammations, jaundice and liver dysfunction.**

Imbalances indicating the use of this formula are commonly noted in the colon acupressure point located halfway between the navel and the right hip bone. Imbalances are often noted just outside the nerve wreaths surrounding each pupil. Use caution in cases of pregnancy, diarrhea and a weakened constitution.

This formula is commonly used in conjunction with psyllium hulls, fruit juices, lactobacillus acidophilus, digestive enzyme supplements, the vitamin C family and the complex of B vitamins.

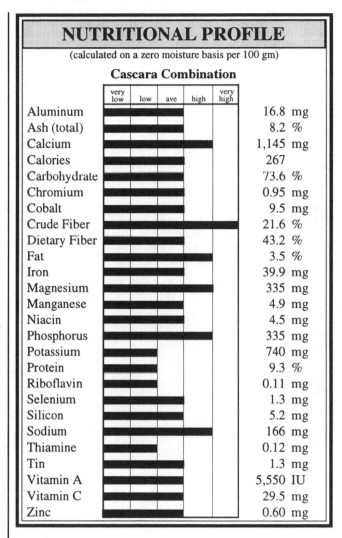

NUTRITIONAL PROFILE
(calculated on a zero moisture basis per 100 gm)

Cascara Combination

	very low	low	ave	high	very high		
Aluminum						16.8	mg
Ash (total)						8.2	%
Calcium						1,145	mg
Calories						267	
Carbohydrate						73.6	%
Chromium						0.95	mg
Cobalt						9.5	mg
Crude Fiber						21.6	%
Dietary Fiber						43.2	%
Fat						3.5	%
Iron						39.9	mg
Magnesium						335	mg
Manganese						4.9	mg
Niacin						4.5	mg
Phosphorus						335	mg
Potassium						740	mg
Protein						9.3	%
Riboflavin						0.11	mg
Selenium						1.3	mg
Silicon						5.2	mg
Sodium						166	mg
Thiamine						0.12	mg
Tin						1.3	mg
Vitamin A						5,550	IU
Vitamin C						29.5	mg
Zinc						0.60	mg

Individual Components

Cascara Sagrada bark is perhaps the most famous herbal laxative. It contains bitter compounds that increase peristalsis, are purgative, increase the release of bile and promote the growth of friendly colonic bacteria. Cascara is used to treat constipation, dyspepsia, liver congestion, gallstones, hemorrhoids, jaundice and intestinal parasites.

Buckthorn bark contains bitter compounds that increase peristalsis, are purgative and increase the release of bile. It has been used to treat constipation, fevers, inflammatory skin conditions, rheumatism, hemorrhoids and intestinal parasites.

Licorice root contains bitter compounds that reduce inflammation, decrease the thickness and increase the production of mucosal fluids and relieve muscle spasms. In addition, licorice stimulates adrenal functions, reduces the urge to cough, is mildly laxative and enhances immune response. It has been used to treat coughs, colds, arthritis, asthma, peptic ulcers, Addison's disease, dropsy and atherosclerosis.

Barberry contains bitter compounds that improve the efficiency of digestion, stimulate the production of bile, dilate blood vessels, and produce a mild laxative effect. It also contains astringent compounds that tighten inflamed tissues in the digestive system. Barberry has been used in cases of jaundice, dyspepsia, constipation and gallstones.

Capsicum fruit contains aromatic resins that increase blood circulation, promote sweating, increase the production of digestive fluids and reduce muscle spasms. It has been used to treat flatulence, colic, ulcers, rheumatic arthritis, cold hands and feet and dropsy.

Ginger root contains aromatic compounds that increase the production of digestive fluids and enzymes, lower blood pressure, lower blood sugar and cholesterol. It also contains bitter compounds that reduce muscle spasms, increase blood circulation and dilate blood vessels. Ginger is an excellent herbal source of trace minerals especially silicon, magnesium, and manganese. It has been used to treat nausea, motion sickness, flatulence, colds, coughs, indigestion, fevers, vomiting, diarrhea, chronic bronchitis and cold hands and feet.

Couch grass contains bitter compounds that increase the flow of urine and are antiseptic. It has been used to treat urinary tract infections, arthritis and rheumatism.

Red Clover flowers contain bitter compounds that increase the production of digestive fluids and enzymes, especially bile. These compounds also shrink inflammation and relieve pains. Red clover is an excellent herbal source of calcium, chromium, magnesium, phosphorus and potassium. It has been used to treat arthritis, jaundice, liver congestion, muscle cramps and inflammatory skin conditions.

Turkey Rhubarb stem contains bitter compounds that are purgative and increase the release of bile. It has been used to treat constipation, jaundice, and inflammatory skin conditions.

Cascara and Dong Quai Combination

Composition

Dong Quai	Ginger
Cascara sagrada	Barberry
Turkey rhubarb	Fennel
Goldenseal	Red Raspberry
Capsicum	

Properties

Purgative	Cholagogue
Carminative	Antispasmodic

General Description

Cascara and Dong Quai combination is a purgative formula. It enhances the eliminative and detoxifying functions of the body. The herbs are purgative, increase the production of digestive fluids and enzymes, especially bile, and reduce smooth muscle cramps.

Chinese herbalists would describe this herbal combination as a wood reducing formula. It also reduces the fire and metal elements while enhancing the earth and water elements.

Cascara and Dong Quai combination has traditionally been used to treat **constipation, jaundice, liver imbalances** and **weak digestion.**

Imbalances indicating the use of this formula are commonly noted in the colon acupressure point located halfway between the navel and the right hip bone. Imbalances are often noted just outside the nerve wreaths surrounding each pupil. Use caution in cases of diarrhea and pregnancy.

This formula is commonly used in conjunction with psyllium, dandelion, fruit juice, lactobacillus acidophilus, digestive enzymes supplements, the vitamin C family, the complex of B vitamins and vitamin A.

Individual Components

Dong Quai root contains aromatic compounds that relieve smooth muscle spasms especially in the uterus, have a sedative effect and increase the production of digestive fluids. It also contains bitter compounds that regulate glycogen production in the liver, reduce pain and inflammation, increase blood flow especially to the

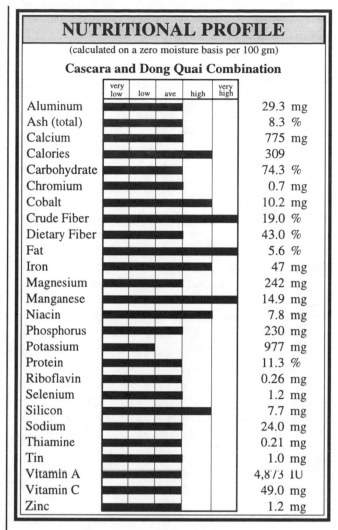

NUTRITIONAL PROFILE
(calculated on a zero moisture basis per 100 gm)

Cascara and Dong Quai Combination

	very low	low	ave	high	very high	
Aluminum						29.3 mg
Ash (total)						8.3 %
Calcium						775 mg
Calories						309
Carbohydrate						74.3 %
Chromium						0.7 mg
Cobalt						10.2 mg
Crude Fiber						19.0 %
Dietary Fiber						43.0 %
Fat						5.6 %
Iron						47 mg
Magnesium						242 mg
Manganese						14.9 mg
Niacin						7.8 mg
Phosphorus						230 mg
Potassium						977 mg
Protein						11.3 %
Riboflavin						0.26 mg
Selenium						1.2 mg
Silicon						7.7 mg
Sodium						24.0 mg
Thiamine						0.21 mg
Tin						1.0 mg
Vitamin A						4,873 IU
Vitamin C						49.0 mg
Zinc						1.2 mg

heart, lower blood cholesterol, normalize uterine contractions and are antiseptic. Dong Quai is an excellent herbal source of iron, magnesium and niacin. It has been used to treat anemia, abdominal pains, dysmenorrhea, amenorrhea, arthritis, coronary heart disease, atherosclerosis, angina pectoris, indigestion and headaches.

Cascara Sagrada bark is perhaps the most famous herbal laxative. It contains bitter compounds that increase peristalsis, are purgative, increase the release of bile and promote the growth of friendly colonic bacteria. Cascara is used to treat constipation, dyspepsia, liver congestion, gallstones, hemorrhoids, jaundice and intestinal parasites.

Turkey Rhubarb stem contains bitter compounds that are purgative, and increase the release of bile. It has been used to treat constipation, jaundice, and inflammatory skin conditions.

Goldenseal root contains bitter astringent alkaloids that normalize liver and spleen functions by increasing the production of digestive fluids and enzymes, particularly bile. The compounds are antiseptic, constrict peripheral blood vessels, especially in the uterus, are laxative and relieve pain and inflammation in mucosal tissue. Goldenseal is an excellent herbal source of trace minerals including cobalt, iron, magnesium, manganese, silicon and zinc. It is also an excellent herbal source of Vitamin C. It has been used to treat hepatitis, gastritis, colitis, ulcers, menorrhagia, postpartum hemorrhage, dysmenorrhea, diabetes, infections, hemorrhoids, eczema, obesity and fevers.

Capsicum fruit contains aromatic resins that increase blood circulation, promote sweating, increase the production of digestive fluids and reduce muscle spasms. It has been used to treat flatulence, colic, ulcers, rheumatic arthritis, cold hands and feet and dropsy.

Ginger root contains aromatic compounds that increase the production of digestive fluids and enzymes, lower blood pressure, lower blood sugar and cholesterol. It also contains bitter compounds that reduce muscle spasms, increase blood circulation and dilate blood vessels. Ginger is an excellent herbal source of trace minerals, especially silicon, magnesium and manganese. It has been used to treat nausea, motion sickness, flatulence, colds, coughs, indigestion, fevers, vomiting, diarrhea, chronic bronchitis and cold hands and feet.

Barberry contains bitter compounds that improve the efficiency of digestion, stimulate the production of bile, dilate blood vessels and produce a mild laxative effect. It also contains astringent compounds that tighten inflamed tissues in the digestive system. Barberry has been used in cases of jaundice, dyspepsia, constipation and gallstones.

Fennel seed contains aromatic compounds that stimulate the production of digestive fluids, relieve inflammation, are antiseptic, make one breathe deeply and more often, and increase the flow of urine. It has been used to treat indigestion, dyspepsia, anorexia, colic, flatulence, coughs and colds.

Red Raspberry leaf contains astringent compounds that relieve pain and shrink inflamed tissues, especially in the female reproductive system. It also contains bitter compounds that relieve smooth muscle spasms. Red Raspberry is an excellent herbal source of manganese. It has been used to treat morning sickness, nausea, dysmenorrhea, false labor, colds, flu and fevers.

Chickweed and Cascara Combination

Composition

Chickweed	Gotu Kola
Cascara Sagrada	Hawthorn
Licorice	Papaya
Safflower	Fennel
Parthenium	Dandelion
Black Walnut	

Properties

Laxative
Diuretic
Carminative
Cholagogue
Demulcent

General Description

Chickweed and Cascara combination is used to eliminate excess weight. The formula enhances the eliminative and detoxifying functions. The herbs are laxative, increase the flow of urine, increase the production of digestive fluids and enzymes and soothe inflamed tissues.

Chinese herbalists would describe this herbal combination as a wood reducing formula. It also reduces the metal and water elements while enhancing the earth and fire.

Chickweed and Cascara combination has traditionally been used to treat **obesity, constipation, arthritis** and **inflammatory skin conditions.**

Imbalances indicating the use of this formula are commonly noted in the colon acupressure point located approximately four inches to the right of the navel. Imbalances are often noted at the 7:30 position of the right iris. Use caution in cases of gastrointestinal weakness and impaired kidney function.

This formula is commonly used in conjunction with parsley, alfalfa, pumpkin seed, the complex of B vitamins, vitamin A and the vitamin C family.

Individual Components

Chickweed herb contains mucilaginous compounds that absorb toxins from the bowel, soothe inflamed

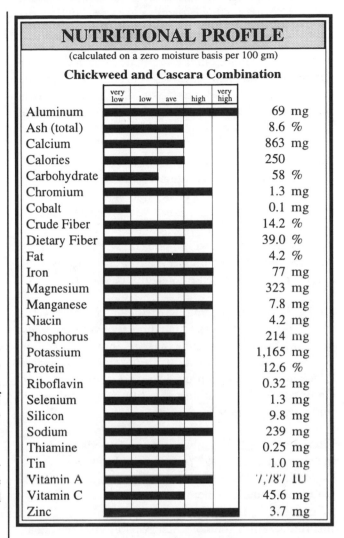

NUTRITIONAL PROFILE
(calculated on a zero moisture basis per 100 gm)

Chickweed and Cascara Combination

	very low	low	ave	high	very high		
Aluminum						69	mg
Ash (total)						8.6	%
Calcium						863	mg
Calories						250	
Carbohydrate						58	%
Chromium						1.3	mg
Cobalt						0.1	mg
Crude Fiber						14.2	%
Dietary Fiber						39.0	%
Fat						4.2	%
Iron						77	mg
Magnesium						323	mg
Manganese						7.8	mg
Niacin						4.2	mg
Phosphorus						214	mg
Potassium						1,165	mg
Protein						12.6	%
Riboflavin						0.32	mg
Selenium						1.3	mg
Silicon						9.8	mg
Sodium						239	mg
Thiamine						0.25	mg
Tin						1.0	mg
Vitamin A						7,787	IU
Vitamin C						45.6	mg
Zinc						3.7	mg

tissues, give bulk to the stool and increase the flow of urine. These compounds also decrease the thickness while increasing the production of mucosal fluids. Chickweed has been used to treat rheumatism, arthritis, inflammatory skin conditions and obesity.

Cascara Sagrada bark is perhaps the most famous herbal laxative. It contains bitter compounds that increase peristalsis, are purgative, increase the release of bile and promote the growth of friendly colonic bacteria. Cascara is used to treat constipation, dyspepsia, liver congestion, gallstones, hemorrhoids, jaundice and intestinal parasites.

Licorice root contains bitter compounds that reduce inflammation, decrease the thickness and increase the production of mucosal fluids and relieve muscle spasms. In addition, licorice stimulates adrenal functions, reduces the urge to cough, is mildly laxative and enhances immune response. It has been used to treat coughs, colds, arthritis, asthma, peptic ulcers, Addison's disease, dropsy and atherosclerosis.

Safflowers contain bitter compounds that increase the production and release of bile. It is an excellent herbal source of unsaturated fatty acids. Safflowers has been used to treat liver congestion, gallstones, gout, scarlet fevers, indigestion and amenorrhea.

Parthenium root contains mucilaginous compounds that increase immune response, sequester infection and sooth inflamed tissue. Parthenium also contains bitter compounds that increase immune response by increasing the production of T-lymphocytes, phagocytic macrophages, interferons and lymphokines. Parthenium has been used to treat wounds, infections, blood poisoning, inflammatory skin conditions and tonsillitis.

Black Walnut hull contains astringent compounds that shrink inflamed tissues of the digestive system. It also contains bitter compounds that are antifungal and decrease the secretion of fluids in the digestive system. Black walnut has been used to treat hemorrhoids, inflammatory skin conditions, colitis, intestinal worms and parasites and fevers.

Gotu Kola herb contains bitter compounds that have a sedative effect, dilate peripheral blood vessels and increase the flow of urine. It is an excellent herbal source of niacin, calcium, magnesium, manganese, silicon and sodium. Gotu kola has been used to treat insomnia, failing memory, schizophrenia, fevers, headache and inflammatory skin conditions.

Hawthorn berries contain bitter compounds that increase coronary blood flow and myocardial metabolism allowing the heart to function with less oxygen. These compounds also lower blood pressure by decreasing cardiac output and dilating peripheral blood vessels. Hawthorn has been used to treat hypertension, coronary heart disease, atherosclerosis, blood clots and insomnia.

Papaya fruit contains proteolytic enzymes that enhance protein digestion. It has been used to treat indigestion, flatulence, nausea and belching.

Fennel seed contains aromatic compounds that stimulate the production of digestive fluids, relieve inflammation, are antiseptic, make one breathe deeply and more often, and increase the flow of urine. It has been used to treat indigestion, dyspepsia, anorexia, colic, flatulence, coughs and colds.

Dandelion root contains bitter compounds that enhance the efficiency of the body's eliminative and detoxifying functions. These compounds help restore normal liver function, increase the production of digestive fluids and enzymes particularly bile, increase the flow of urine and have a laxative effect. Dandelion is an excellent herbal source of sodium, iron and vitamin A. It has been used to treat jaundice, gallstones, dyspepsia, constipation, inflammatory skin conditions, frequent urination, hepatitis, gout and rheumatism.

Gentain and Cascara Combination

Composition

Gentain	Safflower
Irish Moss	Yellow Dock
Cascara Sagrada	Barberry
Goldenseal	Dandelion
Fenugreek	Buchu
Comfrey	Chickweed
Black Walnut	Catnip
Parthenium	Cyani flower
Myrrh	

Properties

Laxative	Antiseptic
Diuretic	Immunostimulant
Carminative	Antispasmodic
Cholagogue	

General Description

Gentain and Cascara combination is used after a digestive system purge to eliminate residual toxins from the body. The formula enhances the detoxifying and eliminative functions of the liver, colon and kidneys. The herbs are laxative, increase the flow of urine, increase the production of digestive fluids and enzymes, especially bile, and relieve smooth muscle spasms. In addition, the herbs are antiseptic and enhance immune response.

Chinese herbalists would describe this herbal combination as a wood reducing formula. It also reduces the water and metal elements while enhancing the earth and fire elements.

Gentain and Cascara combination has traditionally been used to treat **infectious fevers, jaundice, hepatitis, diabetes, obesity, swollen glands, lymphatic inflammations, hemorrhoids, eczema** and **ulcers.**

Imbalances indicating the use of this formula are commonly noted in the colon acupressure point located approximately four inches to the right of the navel. Imbalances are often noted surrounding the nerve wreath of each pupil. Use caution in cases of anemia, emaciation, vertigo and chronic debility.

This formula is commonly used in conjunction with the vitamin C family.

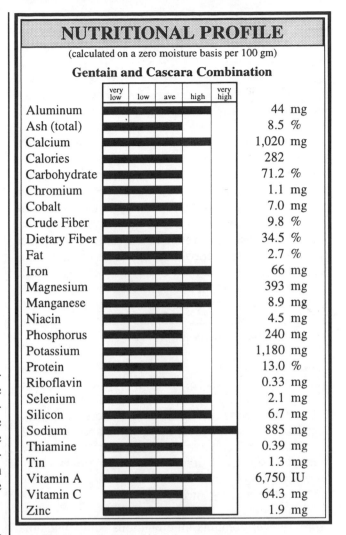

NUTRITIONAL PROFILE						
(calculated on a zero moisture basis per 100 gm)						
Gentain and Cascara Combination						
	very low	low	ave	high	very high	
Aluminum						44 mg
Ash (total)						8.5 %
Calcium						1,020 mg
Calories						282
Carbohydrate						71.2 %
Chromium						1.1 mg
Cobalt						7.0 mg
Crude Fiber						9.8 %
Dietary Fiber						34.5 %
Fat						2.7 %
Iron						66 mg
Magnesium						393 mg
Manganese						8.9 mg
Niacin						4.5 mg
Phosphorus						240 mg
Potassium						1,180 mg
Protein						13.0 %
Riboflavin						0.33 mg
Selenium						2.1 mg
Silicon						6.7 mg
Sodium						885 mg
Thiamine						0.39 mg
Tin						1.3 mg
Vitamin A						6,750 IU
Vitamin C						64.3 mg
Zinc						1.9 mg

Individual Components

Gentain root contains bitter compounds that increase appetite by enhancing the production of digestive fluids and enzymes, particularly bile. It is an excellent herbal source of vitamin B-1, niacin, magnesium, phosphorus, selenium and zinc. Gentain has been used to treat anorexia, dyspepsia, loss of appetite, indigestion and gallstones.

Irish Moss herb contains mucilaginous compounds that enhance the detoxifying and eliminative functions of the digestive system. These compounds absorb toxins from the bowel and provide bulk to the stool. Irish Moss is an excellent herbal source of the electrolyte minerals including calcium, magnesium, sodium and iodine. Iodine is essential to normal thyroid function. It is used to increase the metabolic rate and strengthen connective tissues including the hair, skin and nails. Irish moss has been used to treat enlarged glands, debility, fatigue, eczema, psoriasis, dry cough and nosebleeds.

Cascara Sagrada bark is perhaps the most famous herbal laxative. It contains bitter compounds that increase peristalsis, are purgative, increase the release of bile and promote the growth of friendly colonic bacteria. Cascara is used to treat constipation, dyspepsia, liver congestion, gallstones, hemorrhoids, jaundice and intestinal parasites.

Goldenseal root contains bitter astringent alkaloids that normalize liver and spleen functions by increasing the production of digestive fluids and enzymes, particularly bile. The compounds are antiseptic, constrict peripheral blood vessels, especially in the uterus, are laxative and relieve pain and inflammation in mucosal tissue. Goldenseal is an excellent herbal source of trace minerals including cobalt, iron, magnesium, manganese, silicon and zinc. It is also an excellent herbal source of vitamin C. It has been used to treat hepatitis, gastritis, colitis, ulcers, menorrhagia, postpartum hemorrhage, dysmenorrhea, diabetes, infections, hemorrhoids, eczema, obesity and fevers.

Fenugreek seed contains mucilaginous compounds that decrease the thickness while increasing the production of mucosal fluids and soothe inflamed tissue. It also contains bitter compounds that increase the production of digestive fluids and enzymes and have a mild laxative effect. Fenugreek is an excellent herbal source of iron and selenium. It has been used to treat bronchitis, dyspepsia, fevers, ulcers, respiratory tract infections, anorexia and gastritis.

Comfrey root contains mucilaginous compounds that decrease the thickness while increasing the production of mucosal fluid. These compounds increase the production of digestive fluids, decrease bowel transit time and absorb toxins from the bowel. Comfrey also contains astringent compounds that soothe inflamed tissue. It is an excellent source of allantoin, which promotes healing. Comfrey has been used to treat colitis, weak digestion, bronchitis, rheumatism, diarrhea and inflammatory skin conditions.

Black Walnut hull contains astringent compounds that shrink inflamed tissues of the digestive system. It also contains bitter compounds that are antifungal and decrease the secretion of fluids in the digestive system. Black walnut has been used to treat hemorrhoids, inflammatory skin conditions, colitis, intestinal worms and parasites and fevers.

Parthenium root contains mucilaginous compounds that increase immune response, sequester infection and soothe inflamed tissue. Parthenium also contains bitter compounds that increase immune response by increasing the production of T-lymphocytes, phagocytic macrophages, interferons and lymphokines. Parthenium has been used to treat wounds, infections, blood poisoning, inflammatory skin conditions and tonsillitis.

Myrrh gum contains astringent resins that promote the healing of sores. These compounds shrink inflamed tissue, are antiseptic and reduce pain in mucous membranes. Myrrh also decreases the thickness while increasing the production of mucosal fluids. It has been used to treat colds, coughs, bronchitis, asthma, dysmenorrhea, rheumatism and arthritis.

Safflower contains bitter compounds that increase the production and release of bile. It is an excellent herbal source of unsaturated fatty acids. Safflower has been used to treat liver congestion, gallstones, gout, scarlet fever, indigestion and amenorrhea.

Yellow dock contains bitter compounds that are laxative, increase the production of digestive fluids and enzymes, especially bile and increase the flow of urine. It also contains astringent compounds that shrink inflamed tissues. Yellow dock is an excellent herbal source of vitamin A, vitamin C, calcium, iron, magnesium, phosphorus and selenium. It has been used to treat liver congestion, constipation, arthritis, rheumatism, inflammatory bowel disorders and inflammatory skin conditions.

Barberry contains bitter compounds that improve the efficiency of digestion, stimulate the production of bile, dilate blood vessels and produce a mild laxative effect. It also contains astringent compounds that tighten inflamed tissues in the digestive system. Barberry has been used in cases of jaundice, dyspepsia, constipation and gallstones.

Dandelion root contains bitter compounds that enhance the efficiency of the body's eliminative and detoxifying functions. These compounds help restore normal liver function, increase the production of digestive fluids and enzymes particularly bile, increase the flow of urine and have a laxative effect. Dandelion is an excellent herbal source of sodium, iron, and vitamin A. It has been used to treat jaundice, gall stones, dyspepsia, constipation, inflammatory skin conditions, frequent urination, hepatitis, gout and rheumatism.

Buchu leaf contains aromatic compounds that increase the production of urine and are antiseptic. It also contains astringent compounds that shrink inflamed tissues. Buchu has been used to treat dysuria, urinary tract infections, gout, nephritis, arthritis and rheumatism.

Chickweed herb contains mucilaginous compounds that absorb toxins from the bowel, soothe inflamed tissues, give bulk to the stool and increase the flow of urine. These compounds also decrease the thickness while increasing the production of mucosal fluids. Chickweed has been used to treat rheumatism, arthritis, inflammatory skin conditions and obesity.

Catnip herb contains aromatic compounds that have a sedative effect, relieve smooth muscle spasms and induce sweating. It has been used to treat coughs, colds, anxiety, colic, fevers, influenza, lung congestion and nausea.

Cyani flower contains bitter compounds that increase the flow of urine, are sedative, relieve smooth muscle spasms, dilate peripheral blood vessels and are antiseptic. It has been used to treat fevers, inflammatory skin conditions, anxiety and urinary tract infections.

Ginger Combination

Composition

Ginger	Goldenseal
Capsicum	Licorice

Properties

Carminative	Antiseptic
Antispasmodic	Analgesic
Antiemetic	

General Description

Ginger combination is used to alleviate nausea and the urge to vomit, often associated with influenza. The herbs relieve muscle spasms, relieve pain associated with muscle aches, fight infections and promote the production of digestive fluids.

Chinese herbalists would describe this herbal combination as an earth reducing formula. It also reduces the water and wood element while enhancing the metal and fire elements.

Ginger combination has traditionally been used to treat **influenza, fevers, vomiting, motion sickness, chills, sore throats, headaches, swollen lymph glands, ear infections, belching, abdominal pains, hemorrhoids** and **dropsy.**

Imbalances indicating the use of this formula are commonly noted in the lymphatic rosary of both irises. This formula is used primarily for acute manifestations of influenza and is not designed for chronic debility or pains.

This formula is commonly used in conjunction with catnip, lobelia, scullcap, the vitamin C family, fruit juices and the complex of B vitamins.

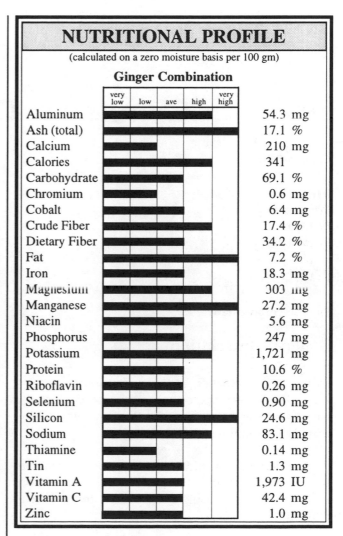

NUTRITIONAL PROFILE
(calculated on a zero moisture basis per 100 gm)

Ginger Combination

	very low	low	ave	high	very high	
Aluminum						54.3 mg
Ash (total)						17.1 %
Calcium						210 mg
Calories						341
Carbohydrate						69.1 %
Chromium						0.6 mg
Cobalt						6.4 mg
Crude Fiber						17.4 %
Dietary Fiber						34.2 %
Fat						7.2 %
Iron						18.3 mg
Magnesium						303 mg
Manganese						27.2 mg
Niacin						5.6 mg
Phosphorus						247 mg
Potassium						1,721 mg
Protein						10.6 %
Riboflavin						0.26 mg
Selenium						0.90 mg
Silicon						24.6 mg
Sodium						83.1 mg
Thiamine						0.14 mg
Tin						1.3 mg
Vitamin A						1,973 IU
Vitamin C						42.4 mg
Zinc						1.0 mg

Individual Components

Ginger root contains aromatic compounds that increase the production of digestive fluids and enzymes, lower blood pressure, lower blood sugar and cholesterol. It also contains bitter compounds that reduce muscle spasms, increase blood circulation and dilate blood vessels. Ginger is an excellent herbal source of trace minerals especially silicon, magnesium and manganese. It has been used to treat nausea, motion sickness, flatulence, colds, coughs, indigestion, fevers, vomiting, diarrhea, chronic bronchitis and cold hands and feet..

Capsicum fruit contains aromatic resins that increase blood circulation, promote sweating, increase the production of digestive fluids and reduce muscle spasms. It has been used to treat flatulence, colic, ulcers, rheumatic arthritis, cold hands and feet and dropsy.

Goldenseal root contains bitter astringent alkaloids that normalize liver and spleen functions by increasing the production of digestive fluids and enzymes, particularly bile. The compounds are antiseptic, constrict peripheral blood vessels, especially in the uterus, are laxative and relieve pain and inflammation in mucosal tissue. Goldenseal is an excellent herbal source of trace minerals including cobalt, iron, magnesium, manganese, silicon and zinc. It is also an excellent herbal source of vitamin C. It has been used to treat hepatitis, gastritis, colitis, ulcers, menorrhagia, postpartum hemorrhage, dysmenorrhea, diabetes, infections, hemorrhoids, eczema, obesity and fevers.

Licorice root contains bitter compounds that reduce inflammation, decrease the thickness and increase the production of mucosal fluids and relieve muscle spasms. In addition, licorice stimulates adrenal function, reduces the urge to cough, is mildly laxative and enhances immune response. It has been used to treat coughs, colds, arthritis, asthma, peptic ulcers, Addison's disease, dropsy and atherosclerosis.

Gymnema Combination

Composition

Gymnema
Brindleberry
Psyllium
Marshmallow

Properties

Appetite Suppressant

General Description

Gymnema combination is an appetite suppressant formula. The herbs work to reduce appetite, compete for carbohydrate absorption sites in the digestive tract and provide a sensation of fullness.

Chinese herbalists would describe this herbal combination as an earth reducing formula. It also reduces the fire element while enhancing the wood, water and metal elements.

Gymnema combination has traditionally been used to treat **obesity and diabetes.**

This formula is commonly used in conjunction with chickweed, yellow dock and goldenseal.

Individual Components

Gymnema leaf contains bitter compounds that compete for carbohydrate absorption sites in the digestive tract. This reduces the effective caloric value of ingested carbohydrates. Gymnema has been used to treat obesity and diabetes.

Brindleberry contains bitter compounds that reduce one's appetite for food. The method by which this is accomplished is as yet undetermined. Brindleberry is an excellent herbal source of vitamin C and beta carotene. It has been used to treat obesity, dysuria and diabetes.

Psyllium hulls contain mucilaginous compounds that give bulk to the stool, absorb toxins, soothe inflamed tissues and promote the growth of friendly colonic bacteria. It has been used to treat constipation, dysentery, chronic diarrhea and cystitis.

Marshmallow root contains mucilaginous compounds that decrease the thickness while increasing the production of mucosal fluids, soothe inflamed tissue, heat wounds and increase the flow of urine. It is an excellent herbal source of trace minerals, especially chromium, iron, magnesium, and selenium. Marshmallow has been used to treat allergies, gastritis, gastric ulcers, enteritis, coughs, cystitis and hay fevers.

Pumpkin and Cascara Combination

Composition

Pumpkin	Witch hazel
Culver's root	Mullein
Cascara Sagrada	Slippery Elm
Violet leaf	Marshmallow
Digenia	

Properties

Anthelmintic	Laxative
Antiseptic	Vulnerary

General Description

Pumpkin and Cascara combination is used to eliminate worms and parasites from the digestive tract. The herbs are anthelmintic, are purgative, shrink inflamed tissues and are antiseptic.

Chinese herbalists would describe this herbal combination as a metal enhancing formula. It also enhances the earth and fire elements while reducing the wood and water elements.

Pumpkin and Cascara combination has traditionally been used to treat **worms, parasites, irregular bowel movements, appetite disorders, stomachaches, swollen abdomens** and **food cravings.**

Imbalances indicating the use of this formula are commonly noted in the colon acupressure point located approximately four inches to the right of the navel. Imbalances are often noted surrounding the nerve wreaths surrounding each pupil. Use caution in cases of high fevers.

This formula is commonly used in conjunction with the vitamin C family, zinc, echinacea and germanium.

Individual Components

Pumpkin seeds contain bitter compounds that are anthelmintic and antiseptic. It is an excellent herbal source of zinc. Pumpkin has been used to treat intestinal worms, parasites and dysmenorrhea.

Culver's root contains bitter compounds that increase the production of digestive fluids and enzymes, espe-

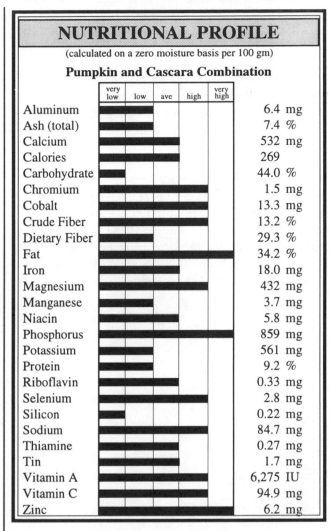

NUTRITIONAL PROFILE
(calculated on a zero moisture basis per 100 gm)

Pumpkin and Cascara Combination

	very low	low	ave	high	very high	
Aluminum						6.4 mg
Ash (total)						7.4 %
Calcium						532 mg
Calories						269
Carbohydrate						44.0 %
Chromium						1.5 mg
Cobalt						13.3 mg
Crude Fiber						13.2 %
Dietary Fiber						29.3 %
Fat						34.2 %
Iron						18.0 mg
Magnesium						432 mg
Manganese						3.7 mg
Niacin						5.8 mg
Phosphorus						859 mg
Potassium						561 mg
Protein						9.2 %
Riboflavin						0.33 mg
Selenium						2.8 mg
Silicon						0.22 mg
Sodium						84.7 mg
Thiamine						0.27 mg
Tin						1.7 mg
Vitamin A						6,275 IU
Vitamin C						94.9 mg
Zinc						6.2 mg

cially bile, are laxative and emetic. It has been used to treat indigestion, constipation, liver congestion and gallstones.

Cascara Sagrada bark is perhaps the most famous herbal laxative. It contains bitter compounds that increase peristalsis, are purgative, increase the release of bile and promote the growth of friendly colonic bacteria. Cascara is used to treat constipation, dyspepsia, liver congestion, gallstones, hemorrhoids, jaundice and intestinal parasites.

Violet leaf contains bitter compounds that increase the production and release of bile, decrease the thickness while increasing the production of mucosal fluids and increase the flow of urine. It has been used to treat jaundice, inflammatory skin conditions, gout and pleurisy.

Digenia herb contains mucilaginous compounds that are anthelmintic, soothe inflamed tissues, absorb toxins from the bowel and give bulk to the stool. It is an excellent source of sodium, calcium, magnesium and iodine. Digenia has been used to treat intestinal worms and parasites, colitis and ulcers.

Witch Hazel bark contains astringent compounds that shrink inflamed tissues, stop bleeding and are antiseptic. It has been used to treat varicose veins, hemorrhoids, burns and insect bites.

Mullein leaves contain mucilaginous compounds that decrease the thickness and increase the production of mucosal fluids. These compounds also soothe inflamed tissue. Mullein also contains aromatic compounds that increase the flow of urine. The herb has been used to treat bronchitis, coughs, colds, hayfevers, dysuria, nephritis and sinus congestion.

Slippery Elm bark contains mucilaginous compounds that decrease the thickness while increasing the production of mucosal fluids. These compounds soothe inflamed tissue, decrease bowel transit time and absorb toxins from the bowel. It also contains astringent compounds that shrink inflamed tissues. Slippery elm has been used to treat asthma, bronchitis, colitis, coughs, weak digestion and inflammatory bowel disease.

Marshmallow root contains mucilaginous compounds that decrease the thickness while increasing the production of mucosal fluids, soothe inflamed tissue, heal wounds and increase the flow of urine. It is an excellent herbal source of trace minerals, especially chromium iron, magnesium and selenium. Marshmallow has been used to treat allergies, gastritis, gastric ulcers, enteritis, coughs, cystitis and hay fevers.

Senna Combination

Composition

Ginger	Fennel
Catnip	Senna

Properties

Purgative	Antispasmodic
Stimulant	Carminative

General Description

Senna combination is a purgative formula. It is used as a colon stimulant to enhance elimination. The herbs are purgative, reduce smooth muscle spasms, increase the production of digestive fluids and enzymes, increase blood circulation and promote the growth of friendly colonic bacteria.

Chinese herbalists would describe this herbal combination as an internal attacking or wood reducing formula. It also reduces the fire and metal elements while enhancing the earth and water elements.

Senna combination has traditionally been used to treat **constipation, dry stool, obesity, fevers, skin inflammations, jaundice** and **liver dysfunction.**

Imbalances indicating the use of this formula are commonly noted in the colon acupressure point located halfway between the navel and the right hip bone. Imbalances are often noted just inside the nerve wreaths surrounding each pupil. Use caution in cases of pregnancy, diarrhea and a weakened constitution.

This formula is commonly used in conjunction with psyllium hulls, fruit juices, lactobacillus acidophilus, digestive enzyme supplements, the vitamin C family and the complex of B vitamins.

Individual Components

Ginger root contains aromatic compounds that increase the production of digestive fluids and enzymes, lower blood pressure, lower blood sugar and cholesterol. It also contains bitter compounds that reduce muscle spasms, increase blood circulation and dilate blood vessels. Ginger is an excellent herbal source of trace minerals, especially silicon, magnesium and manganese. It has been used to treat nausea, motion sickness, flatulence, colds, coughs, indigestion, fevers, vomiting, diarrhea, chronic bronchitis and cold hands and feet.

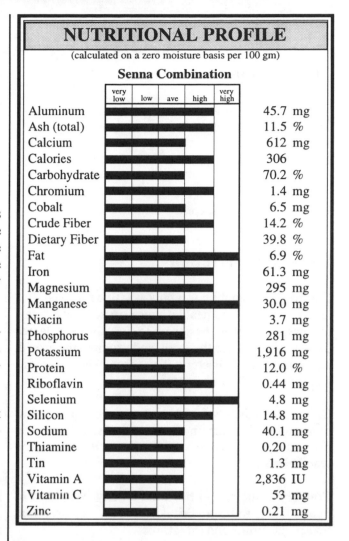

NUTRITIONAL PROFILE
(calculated on a zero moisture basis per 100 gm)

Senna Combination

	very low	low	ave	high	very high	Value	
Aluminum						45.7	mg
Ash (total)						11.5	%
Calcium						612	mg
Calories						306	
Carbohydrate						70.2	%
Chromium						1.4	mg
Cobalt						6.5	mg
Crude Fiber						14.2	%
Dietary Fiber						39.8	%
Fat						6.9	%
Iron						61.3	mg
Magnesium						295	mg
Manganese						30.0	mg
Niacin						3.7	mg
Phosphorus						281	mg
Potassium						1,916	mg
Protein						12.0	%
Riboflavin						0.44	mg
Selenium						4.8	mg
Silicon						14.8	mg
Sodium						40.1	mg
Thiamine						0.20	mg
Tin						1.3	mg
Vitamin A						2,836	IU
Vitamin C						53	mg
Zinc						0.21	mg

Catnip herb contains aromatic compounds that have a sedative effect, relieve smooth muscle spasms and induce sweating. It has been used to treat coughs, colds, anxiety, colic, fevers, influenza, lung congestion and nausea.

Fennel seed contains aromatic compounds that stimulate the production of digestive fluids, relieve inflammation, are antiseptic, make one breathe deeply and more often, and increase the flow of urine. It has been used to treat indigestion, dyspepsia, anorexia, colic, flatulence, coughs and colds.

Senna leaf contains bitter compounds that are purgative and increase the flow of bile. It is an excellent herbal source of vitamin B-1, vitamin B-2, vitamin C and niacin. Senna has been used to treat constipation, obesity, gout, jaundice and inflammatory skin conditions.

Therapies for Supplementing Deficient Conditions

Comfrey Combination

Composition

Comfrey	Slippery Elm
Goldenseal	Aloe Vera

Properties

Demulcent	Astringent
Vulnerary	Antiseptic
Bulk Laxative	

General Description

Comfrey combination is a bulk laxative formula. It is used to detoxify and heal inflamed tissues in the digestive system. The herbs absorb toxins, shrink inflamed tissues, give bulk to the stool, and promote the growth of friendly colonic bacteria. This formula is also used as a poultice.

Chinese herbalists would describe this herbal combination as an earth enhancing formula. It also enhances the fire and metal elements while reducing the water and wood elements.

Comfrey combination has traditionally been used to treat **ulcers, nausea, thirst, disurea, constipation, fevers, jaundice** and **infections.**

Imbalances indicating the use of this formula are commonly noted in the colon acupressure point located approximately four inches to the right of the naval. Imbalances are often noted surrounding each pupil. Use caution in cases of pregnancy or liver impairment.

This formula is commonly used in conjunction with zinc, echinacea, germanium, vitamin A and the vitamin C family.

Individual Components

Comfrey root contains mucilaginous compounds that decrease the thickness while increasing the production of mucosal fluid. These compounds also increase the production of digestive fluids, decrease bowel transit time and absorb toxins from the bowel. Comfrey also contains astringent compounds that soothe inflamed tissue. It is an excellent source of allantoin, which

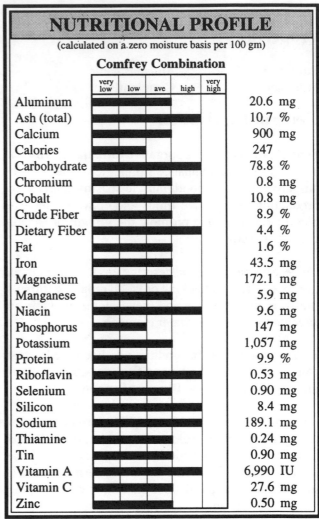

NUTRITIONAL PROFILE
(calculated on a zero moisture basis per 100 gm)

Comfrey Combination

	very low	low	ave	high	very high	
Aluminum						20.6 mg
Ash (total)						10.7 %
Calcium						900 mg
Calories						247
Carbohydrate						78.8 %
Chromium						0.8 mg
Cobalt						10.8 mg
Crude Fiber						8.9 %
Dietary Fiber						4.4 %
Fat						1.6 %
Iron						43.5 mg
Magnesium						172.1 mg
Manganese						5.9 mg
Niacin						9.6 mg
Phosphorus						147 mg
Potassium						1,057 mg
Protein						9.9 %
Riboflavin						0.53 mg
Selenium						0.90 mg
Silicon						8.4 mg
Sodium						189.1 mg
Thiamine						0.24 mg
Tin						0.90 mg
Vitamin A						6,990 IU
Vitamin C						27.6 mg
Zinc						0.50 mg

promotes healing. Comfrey has been used to treat colitis, weak digestion, bronchitis, rheumatism, diarrhea and inflammatory skin conditions.

Goldenseal root contains bitter astringent alkaloids that normalize liver and spleen functions by increasing the production of digestive fluids and enzymes, particularly bile. The compounds are antiseptic, constrict peripheral blood vessels, especially in the uterus, are laxative and relieve pain and inflammation in mucosal tissue. Goldenseal is an excellent herbal source of trace minerals including cobalt, iron, magnesium, manganese, silicon and zinc. It is also an excellent herbal source of vitamin C. It has been used to treat hepatitis, gastritis, colitis, ulcers, menorrhagia, postpartum hemorrhage, dysmenorrhea, diabetes, infections, hemorrhoids, eczema, obesity and fevers.

Slippery Elm bark contains mucilaginous compounds that decrease the thickness while increasing the production of mucosal fluids. These compounds also soothe inflamed tissue, decrease bowel transit time and absorb toxins from the bowel. It also contains astringent compounds that shrink inflamed tissues. Slippery elm has been used to treat asthma, bronchitis, colitis, coughs, weak digestion and inflammatory bowel disease.

Aloe Vera juice contains mucilaginous compounds that soothe inflamed tissues, absorb toxins, give bulk to the stool and promote the growth of friendly colonic bacteria. It also contains bitter compounds that are purgative. Aloe has been used to treat burns, ulcers, inflammatory skin conditions, hemorrhoids and constipation.

Ginger and Barberry Combination

Composition

Barberry	Peppermint
Ginger	Wild Yam
Cramp bark	Catnip
Fennel	

Properties

Antispasmodic	Bitter tonic
Carminative	Stimulant
Cholagogue	

General Description

Ginger and Barberry combination is a bitter tonic formula. It is used to improve the appetite and make digestion more efficient. The herbs increase the production of digestive fluids and enzymes especially bile. They also increase blood circulation, relieve smooth muscle spasms and soothe inflamed tissues.

Chinese herbalists would describe this herbal combination as a wood reducing formula. It also reduces the fire element while enhancing the water, metal, and earth elements.

Ginger and Barberry combination has traditionally been used to treat **bloating, flatulence, menstrual cramps, gall bladder congestion, chronic constipation, inflammatory skin conditions, jaundice, fevers and conjunctivitis.**

Imbalances indicating the use of this formula are commonly noted in the liver acupressure point located approximately four inches to the right of the sternum between the 7th and 8th ribs. Imbalances are often noted at the 7:45 position of the right iris. Use caution in cases of extreme pain in the gall bladder region, enlarged liver, gastritis, and dysentery.

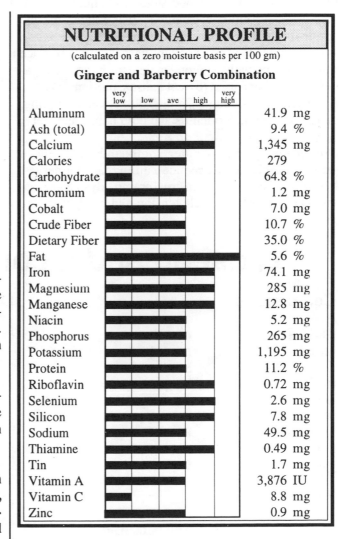

NUTRITIONAL PROFILE

(calculated on a zero moisture basis per 100 gm)

Ginger and Barberry Combination

	very low	low	ave	high	very high		
Aluminum						41.9	mg
Ash (total)						9.4	%
Calcium						1,345	mg
Calories						279	
Carbohydrate						64.8	%
Chromium						1.2	mg
Cobalt						7.0	mg
Crude Fiber						10.7	%
Dietary Fiber						35.0	%
Fat						5.6	%
Iron						74.1	mg
Magnesium						285	mg
Manganese						12.8	mg
Niacin						5.2	mg
Phosphorus						265	mg
Potassium						1,195	mg
Protein						11.2	%
Riboflavin						0.72	mg
Selenium						2.6	mg
Silicon						7.8	mg
Sodium						49.5	mg
Thiamine						0.49	mg
Tin						1.7	mg
Vitamin A						3,876	IU
Vitamin C						8.8	mg
Zinc						0.9	mg

This formula is commonly used in conjunction with lecithin, dandelion, methionine, the complex of B vitamins, choline, vitamin A, iron, the vitamin C family, vitamin D and vitamin E.

Individual Components

Barberry contains bitter compounds that improve the efficiency of digestion, stimulate the production of bile, dilate blood vessels and produce a mild laxative effect. It also contains astringent compounds that tighten inflamed tissues in the digestive system. Barberry has been used in cases of jaundice, dyspepsia, constipation and gallstones.

Ginger root contains aromatic compounds that increase the production of digestive fluids and enzymes, lower blood pressure, lower blood sugar and cholesterol. It also contains bitter compounds that reduce muscle spasms, increase blood circulation and dilate blood vessels. Ginger is an excellent herbal source of trace minerals especially silicon, magnesium, and manganese. It has been used to treat nausea, motion sickness, flatulence, colds, coughs, indigestion, fevers, vomiting, diarrhea, chronic bronchitis and cold hands and feet.

Cramp bark contains bitter compounds that relieve smooth muscle spasms, reduce pain and calm the nerves. It has been used to treat menstrual cramps, dysmenorrhea, rheumatism, colic, muscle tension and headaches.

Fennel seed contains aromatic compounds that stimulate the production of digestive fluids, relieve inflammation, are antiseptic, make one breathe deeply and more often, and increase the flow of urine. It has been used to treat indigestion, dyspepsia, anorexia, colic, flatulence, coughs and colds.

Peppermint leaf contains aromatic compounds that increase the production of digestive fluids, relieve muscle spasms, increase blood circulation, reduce pains, promote sweating and are antiseptic. It also contains astringent compounds which shrink inflamed tissues. Peppermint has been used to treat indigestion, flatulence, mouth sores, loss of appetite, muscle cramps, nausea, morning sickness and dysmenorrhea.

Wild Yam root contains bitter compounds that promote sweating, relieve muscle cramps and reduce inflammation. It has been used to treat arthritis, menstrual cramps, rheumatism and gastritis.

Catnip herb contains aromatic compounds that have a sedative effect, relieve smooth muscle spasms and induce sweating. It has been used to treat coughs, colds, anxiety, colic, fevers, influenza, lung congestion and nausea.

Ginseng and Licorice Combination

Composition

Siberian Ginseng	Citrus
Licorice	Dong Quai
Atractylodes	Saussurea
Hoelen	Magnolia bark
Ginger	Chaenomeles
Dioscorea	Zanthoxylum
Lotus seed	Pinellia
Dolichos	Galanga
Astragalus	Cardamon

Properties

Carminative	Anti-inflammatory
Stimulant	Demulcent
Immunostimulant	Adaptogen
Antiseptic	

General Description

Ginseng and Licorice combination is a general tonic formula. The formula works to rejuvenate and enhance the digestive, circulatory and immune functions. The herbs increase the production of digestive fluids and enzymes, increase blood circulation, enhance immune response, are antiseptic and reduce inflammation.

Chinese herbalists would describe this herbal combination as an earth enhancing formula. It also enhances the metal and fire elements while reducing the water and wood elements.

Ginseng and Licorice combination has traditionally been used to treat **hemorrhoids, diarrhea, menstrual cramps, poor appetite, ulcers, colitis, indigestion, fatigue, chills, flu, leg cramps, poor circulation, hernia, depression** and **arthritis.**

Imbalances indicating the use of this formula are commonly noted in the stomach acupressure point located one inch below and one inch to the left of the sternum. Imbalances are often noted at the 7 o'clock position of the left iris.

Ginseng and Licorice combination is commonly used in conjunction with the complex of B vitamins and the vitamin C family.

Individual Components

Siberian Ginseng root contains bitter compounds that help the body respond more quickly to stress. These compounds increase the production of DNA, RNA and proteins essential to all life processes. They stimulate the adrenal, pancreas, and pituitary glands to lower blood sugar and reduce inflammation. Ginseng also increases the production of digestive fluids and is a mild sedative. It has been used to treat anemia, impotence, insomnia, diarrhea, fatigue, debility, weak digestion and failing memory.

Licorice root contains bitter compounds that reduce inflammation, decrease the thickness and increase the production of mucosal fluids and relieve muscle spasms. In addition, licorice stimulates adrenal function, reduces the urge to coughs, is mildly laxative and enhances immune response. It has been used to treat coughs, colds, arthritis, asthma, peptic ulcers, Addison's disease, dropsy and atherosclerosis.

Atractylodes root contains aromatic compounds that are antiseptic, increase the production of digestive fluids and enzymes, increase blood pressure, are laxative, stimulate liver function and increase the flow of urine. It has been used to treat dyspepsia, flatulence, loss of appetite, nausea, indigestion, rheumatic arthritis and night blindness.

Hoelen herb contains bitter compounds that increase the flow of urine, decrease blood sugar and has a sedative effect. It has been used to treat edema, dropsy, diarrhea, insomnia, frequent urination and heart palpitations.

Ginger root contains aromatic compounds that increase the production of digestive fluids and enzymes, lower blood pressure, lower blood sugar and cholesterol. It also contains bitter compounds that reduce muscle spasms, increase blood circulation and dilate blood vessels. Ginger is an excellent herbal source of trace minerals especially silicon, magnesium, and manganese. It has been used to treat nausea, motion sickness, flatulence, colds, coughs, indigestion, fevers, vomiting, diarrhea, chronic bronchitis and cold hands and feet.

Dioscorea root contains mucilaginous compounds that decrease the thickness and increase the production of mucosal fluids, enhance the efficiency of healing and increase the production of digestive fluids. It has been used to treat lack of appetite, diarrhea, asthma, dry coughs, nocturnal emissions, frequent urination, diabetes and inflammatory skin conditions.

Lotus seed contains mucilaginous compounds that absorb toxins from the digestive system and relieve smooth muscle spasms. It also contains astringent compounds that shrink inflamed tissue. Lotus seed has been used to treat chronic diarrhea, lack of appetite, insomnia and heart palpitations.

Dolichos seed contains mucilaginous compounds that absorb toxins from the bowel and soothe inflamed tissues. These compounds also lower blood sugar and blood cholesterol and give bulk to the stool. Dolichos has been used to treat fevers, chills, diarrhea, nausea, food poisoning, intoxication and sunstroke.

Astragalus root contains bitter compounds that increase the flow of urine, are antiseptic, increase the production of digestive fluids including bile and relieve muscle spasms. Astragalus also contains mucilaginous compounds that enhance immune response, increasing the production of lymphocytes and macrophages. The herb also increases heart action and lowers blood pressure and blood sugar. It has been used to treat fatigue, debility, urinary tract infections, edema, nephritis, ulcers, prolapse of organs and night sweats.

Citrus peel contains aromatic compounds that are antiseptic, reduce muscle spasms and decrease the thickness while increasing the production of mucosal fluids. It also contains bitter compounds that are antiinflammatory, reduce muscle spasms, increase the production of digestive fluid and increase blood circulation. Citrus peel has been used to treat coughs, colds, flu, fevers and bronchitis.

Dong Quai root contains aromatic compounds that relieve smooth muscle spasms especially in the uterus, have a sedative effect and increase the production of digestive fluids. It also contains bitter compounds that regulate glycogen production in the liver, reduce pain and inflammation, increase blood flow especially to the heart, lower blood cholesterol, normalize uterine contractions and are antiseptic. Dong quai is an excellent herbal source of iron, magnesium and niacin. It has been used to treat anemia, abdominal pains, dysmenorrhea, amenorrhea, arthritis, coronary heart disease, atherosclerosis, angina pectoris, indigestion and headaches.

Saussurea root contains aromatic compounds that increase the production of digestive fluids, increase blood circulation and are antiseptic. It also contains bitter compounds that relieve smooth muscle spasms, lower blood pressure and relieve pains. Saussurea has been used to treat gastritis, chest pains, jaundice, gall stones and diarrhea.

Magnolia bark contains bitter compounds that relieve muscle cramps, are antiseptic, and have sedative properties. It has been used to treat gastritis, coughs, asthma, diarrhea, vomiting and flatulence.

Chaenomeles fruit contains bitter compounds that relieve muscle spasms and increase the production of digestive fluids. It has been used to treat rheumatism, rheumatic arthritis, leg cramps, vomiting, diarrhea and dyspepsia.

Zanthoxylum bark contains bitter compounds that are antiseptic, increase the flow of urine, are laxative and relieve pains. It has been used to treat dyspepsia, abdominal pains, intestinal worms, inflammatory skin conditions and dysentery.

Pinellia root contains bitter compounds that decrease the thickness while increasing the production of mucosal fluids, relieve muscle spasms, increase the production of digestive fluids and absorb toxins. Pinellia root must by processed with alum or ginger root before ingestion since it is toxic. It has been used to treat morning sickness, nausea, vomiting, respiratory congestion, ulcers and blood poisoning.

Galanga root contains aromatic compounds that are antiseptic, increase the production of digestive fluids and increase blood circulation. It also contains bitter compounds that relieve smooth muscle spasms. Galanga has been used to treat dyspepsia, gastritis, flatulence, chronic enteritis, poor circulation and vomiting.

Cardamon fruit contains aromatic compounds that promote sweating, increase the production of digestive fluids and reduce smooth muscle spasms especially in the intestine and uterus. It has been used to treat diarrhea, to prevent miscarriage and to treat dyspepsia.

Papaya and Peppermint Combination

Composition

Papaya	Wild Yam
Ginger	Dong Quai
Peppermint	Catnip
Fennel	Spearmint

Properties

Carminative
Stimulant
Antispasmodic
Diaphoretic

General Description

Papaya and Peppermint combination is a carminative formula. It is used to enhance the digestive function. The herbs increase the production of digestive fluids and enzymes, increase blood circulation, relieve muscle spasms and promote sweating.

Chinese herbalists would describe this herbal combination as an earth enhancing formula. It also enhances the fire and metal elements while reducing the water and wood elements.

Papaya and Peppermint combination has traditionally been used to treat **indigestion, belching, abdominal pains, nausea, cramps, flatulence and difficult urination.**

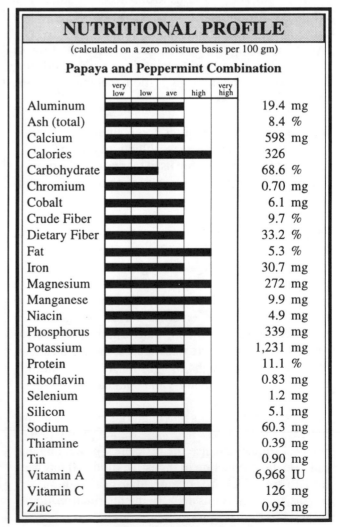

NUTRITIONAL PROFILE
(calculated on a zero moisture basis per 100 gm)
Papaya and Peppermint Combination

	value
Aluminum	19.4 mg
Ash (total)	8.4 %
Calcium	598 mg
Calories	326
Carbohydrate	68.6 %
Chromium	0.70 mg
Cobalt	6.1 mg
Crude Fiber	9.7 %
Dietary Fiber	33.2 %
Fat	5.3 %
Iron	30.7 mg
Magnesium	272 mg
Manganese	9.9 mg
Niacin	4.9 mg
Phosphorus	339 mg
Potassium	1,231 mg
Protein	11.1 %
Riboflavin	0.83 mg
Selenium	1.2 mg
Silicon	5.1 mg
Sodium	60.3 mg
Thiamine	0.39 mg
Tin	0.90 mg
Vitamin A	6,968 IU
Vitamin C	126 mg
Zinc	0.95 mg

Imbalances indicating the use of this formula are commonly noted in the stomach acupressure point located approximately two inches below and two inches to the left of the sternum. Imbalances are often noted at the 4:30 position of the left iris and the 7:30 position of the right iris. Use caution in cases of inflammatory skin conditions, high fevers and ulcers.

This formula is commonly used in conjunction with protein digestive (HCl) acids, food enzyme supplements, licorice, marshmallow, chamomile, vitamin A and zinc.

Individual Components

Papaya fruit contains proteolytic enzymes that enhance protein digestion. It has been used to treat indigestion, flatulence, nausea and belching.

Ginger root contains aromatic compounds that increase the production of digestive fluids and enzymes, lower blood pressure, lower blood sugar and cholesterol. It also contains bitter compounds that reduce muscle spasms, increase blood circulation and dilate blood vessels. Ginger is an excellent herbal source of trace minerals especially silicon, magnesium and manganese. It has been used to treat nausea, motion sickness, flatulence, colds, coughs, indigestion, fevers, vomiting, diarrhea, chronic bronchitis and cold hands and feet.

Peppermint leaf contains aromatic compounds that increase the production of digestive fluids, relieve muscle spasms, increase blood circulation, reduce pains, promote sweating and are antiseptic. It also contains astringent compounds which shrink inflamed tissues. Peppermint has been used to treat indigestion, flatulence, mouth sores, loss of appetite, muscle cramps, nausea, morning sickness and dysmenorrhea.

Fennel seed contains aromatic compounds that stimulate the production of digestive fluids, relieve inflammation, are antiseptic, make one breath deeply and more often, and increase the flow of urine. It has been used to treat indigestion, dyspepsia, anorexia, colic, flatulence, coughs and colds.

Wild Yam root contains bitter compounds that promote sweating, relieve muscle cramps and reduce inflammation. It has been used to treat arthritis, menstrual cramps, rheumatism and gastritis.

Dong Quai root contains aromatic compounds that relieve smooth muscle spasms especially in the uterus, have a sedative effect and increase the production of digestive fluids. It also contains bitter compounds that regulate glycogen production in the liver, reduce pain and inflammation, increase blood flow especially to the heart, lower blood cholesterol, normalize uterine contractions and are antiseptic. Dong quai is an excellent herbal source of iron, magnesium and niacin. It has been used to treat anemia, abdominal pains, dysmenorrhea, amenorrhea, arthritis, coronary heart disease, atherosclerosis, angina pectoris, indigestion and headaches.

Catnip herb contains aromatic compounds that have a sedative effect, relieve smooth muscle spasms and induce sweating. It has been used to treat coughs, colds, anxiety, colic, fevers, influenza, lung congestion and nausea.

Spearmint leaf contains aromatic compounds that increase the production of digestive fluids and enzymes, relieve smooth muscle spasms, increase blood circulation, promote sweating, relieve pain and are antiseptic. It also contains astringent compounds that shrink inflamed tissues. Spearmint has been used to treat indigestion, morning sickness, nausea, menstrual cramps, flatulence, muscle aches, flu and vomiting.

Plantain Combination

Composition

Plantain	Rose hips
Marshmallow	Chamomile
Slippery Elm	Bugleweed

Properties

Demulcent
Vulnerary
Antispasmodic
Anti-inflammatory

General Description

Plantain combination is used to relieve inflammatory conditions in the digestive system. The herbs absorb toxins, reduce inflammation, promote healing, soothe the bowel, give bulk to the stool and promote the growth of friendly colonic bacteria.

Chinese herbalists would describe this herbal combination as an earth enhancing or moistening formula. It also enhances the water and wood elements while reducing the fire and metal elements.

Plantain combination has traditionally been used to treat **ulcers, colitis, Crohn's disease, celiac disease** and **other inflammatory conditions of the gastrointestinal tract.**

Imbalances indicating the use of this formula are commonly noted in the colon acupressure point located halfway between the navel and right hip bone. Imbalances are often noted just inside the nerve wreaths surrounding each pupil.

This formula is commonly used in conjunction with lobelia, comfrey, licorice, goldenseal, barberry, the vitamin C family, pantothenic acid, germanium and zinc.

Individual Components

Plantain seed contains mucilaginous compounds that absorb toxins from the bowel, soothe inflamed tissues and promote normal bowel function. Plantain has been used to treat chronic constipation, colitis, dysentery, coughs, ulcers and diarrhea.

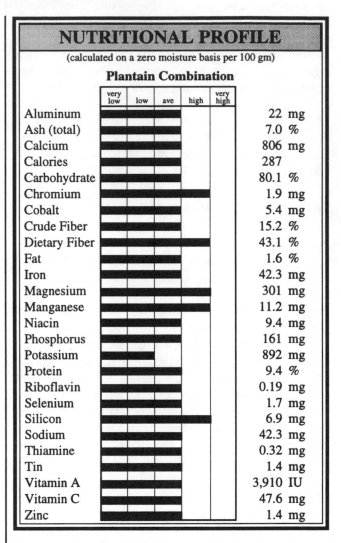

NUTRITIONAL PROFILE
(calculated on a zero moisture basis per 100 gm)

Plantain Combination

Nutrient	Amount
Aluminum	22 mg
Ash (total)	7.0 %
Calcium	806 mg
Calories	287
Carbohydrate	80.1 %
Chromium	1.9 mg
Cobalt	5.4 mg
Crude Fiber	15.2 %
Dietary Fiber	43.1 %
Fat	1.6 %
Iron	42.3 mg
Magnesium	301 mg
Manganese	11.2 mg
Niacin	9.4 mg
Phosphorus	161 mg
Potassium	892 mg
Protein	9.4 %
Riboflavin	0.19 mg
Selenium	1.7 mg
Silicon	6.9 mg
Sodium	42.3 mg
Thiamine	0.32 mg
Tin	1.4 mg
Vitamin A	3,910 IU
Vitamin C	47.6 mg
Zinc	1.4 mg

Marshmallow root contains mucilaginous compounds that decrease the thickness while increasing the production of mucosal fluids, soothe inflamed tissue, heat wounds and increase the flow of urine. It is an excellent herbal source of trace minerals, especially chromium, iron, magnesium and selenium. Marshmallow has been used to treat allergies, gastritis, gastric ulcers, enteritis, coughs, cystitis and hay fevers.

Slippery Elm bark contains mucilaginous compounds that decrease the thickness while increasing the production of mucosal fluids. These compounds also soothe inflamed tissue, decrease bowel transit time and absorb toxins from the bowel. It also contains astringent compounds that shrink inflamed tissues. Slippery Elm has been used to treat asthma, bronchitis, colitis, coughs, weak digestion and inflammatory bowel disease.

Rose hips contains bitter compounds called bioflavonoids which enhance the absorption of vitamin C and strengthen connective tissue. This results in decreased capillary fragility. It also contains astringent compounds which shrink inflamed tissue and reduce the secretion of mucosal fluid. Rose hips is an excellent herbal source of vitamin C. It has been used to treat the common cold, influenza, fevers, infections, inflammatory skin conditions, easy bruising, varicose veins, debility, capillary fragility and hemorrhoids.

Chamomile flowers contain aromatic compounds that increase the production of digestive fluids, reduce muscle spasms and pains, reduce inflammation and are antiseptic. In addition, these compounds have a sedative effect.

Chamomile is one of the best herbal sources of niacin, magnesium and essential fatty acids. It has been used to treat dyspepsia, flatulence, nausea, vomiting, dysmenorrhea, bronchitis, urinary tract infections, insomnia, headaches and menstrual cramps.

Bugleweed herb contains astringent compounds that stop bleeding and shrink inflamed tissues. It also contains aromatic compounds that relieve pain and are mildly sedative. These compounds also lower heart rate while increasing cardiac output. Bugleweed has been used to treat arrhythmia, hemorrhage, angina pains, colitis and ulcers.

Psyllium Combination

Composition

Psyllium
Hibiscus
Licorice

Properties

Bulk laxative
Demulcent

General Description

Psyllium combination is a bulk laxative formula. The herbs give bulk to the stool, soothe inflamed tissues, absorb toxins and promote the growth of friendly colonic bacteria.

Chinese herbalists would describe this herbal combination as an earth enhancing formula. It also enhances the fire and metal elements while reducing the water and wood elements.

Psyllium combination has traditionally been used to treat **constipation, hemorrhoids, indigestion, ulcers** and **arthritis.**

Imbalances indicating the use of this formula are commonly noted in colon acupressure point located over the navel. Imbalances are often noted just outside the nerve wreath of each iris. Use caution in cases of hypertension.

This formula is commonly used in conjunction with chlorophyllins, vitamin A, the vitamin C family and cascara sagrada.

Individual Components

Psyllium hulls contain mucilaginous compounds that give bulk to the stool, absorb toxins, soothe inflamed tissues and promote the growth of friendly colonic bacteria. It has been used to treat constipation, dysentery, chronic diarrhea and cystitis.

Hibiscus flower contains bitter compounds that increase blood circulation, soothe inflamed tissues and relieve smooth muscle spasms. It has been used to treat menstrual cramps and poor circulation.

Licorice root contains bitter compounds that reduce inflammation, decrease the thickness and increase the production of mucosal fluids and relieve muscle spasms. In addition, licorice stimulates adrenal function, reduces the urge to coughs, is mildly laxative and enhances immune response. It has been used to treat coughs, colds, arthritis, asthma, peptic ulcers, Addison's disease, dropsy and atherosclerosis.

Slippery Elm Combination

Composition

Slippery Elm
Wild Yam
Marshmallow
Dong Quai
Ginger

Properties

Demulcent
Carminative
Vulnerary
Stimulant
Diuretic
Anti-inflammatory

General Description

Slippery Elm combination is a poultice formula. It is used to absorb toxins and reduce inflammation in the colon. The herbs absorb toxins, shrink inflamed tissues, give bulk to the stool and promote the growth of friendly colonic bacteria. They also increase blood circulation and the flow of urine.

Chinese herbalists would describe this combination as an earth enhancing or moistening formula. It also enhances the water and wood elements while reducing the fire and metal elements.

Slippery Elm combination has traditionally been used to treat **ulcers, colitis, malnutrition, debility, convalescence, constitutional weakness,** and **inflammatory conditions of the gastrointestinal tract.**

Imbalances indicating the use of this formula are commonly noted in the colon acupressure point located halfway between the navel and right hipbone. Imbalances are often noted just inside the nerve wreaths surrounding each pupil. Use caution in cases of constipation or gallstones.

Imbalances indicating the use of this formula are commonly noted in the colon acupressure point located halfway between the navel and right hipbone. Imbalances are often noted just inside the nerve wreaths surrounding each pupil. Use caution in cases of constipation or gallstones.

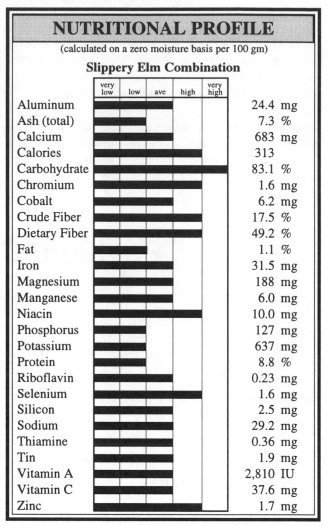

NUTRITIONAL PROFILE
(calculated on a zero moisture basis per 100 gm)

Slippery Elm Combination

	very low	low	ave	high	very high	
Aluminum						24.4 mg
Ash (total)						7.3 %
Calcium						683 mg
Calories						313
Carbohydrate						83.1 %
Chromium						1.6 mg
Cobalt						6.2 mg
Crude Fiber						17.5 %
Dietary Fiber						49.2 %
Fat						1.1 %
Iron						31.5 mg
Magnesium						188 mg
Manganese						6.0 mg
Niacin						10.0 mg
Phosphorus						127 mg
Potassium						637 mg
Protein						8.8 %
Riboflavin						0.23 mg
Selenium						1.6 mg
Silicon						2.5 mg
Sodium						29.2 mg
Thiamine						0.36 mg
Tin						1.9 mg
Vitamin A						2,810 IU
Vitamin C						37.6 mg
Zinc						1.7 mg

This formula is commonly used in conjunction with lobelia, comfrey, licorice, chamomile, goldenseal, zinc and vitamin C.

Individual Components

Slippery Elm bark contains mucilaginous compounds that decrease the thickness while increasing the production of mucosal fluids. These compounds also soothe inflamed tissue, decrease bowel transit time and absorb toxins from the bowel. It also contains astringent compounds that shrink inflamed tissues. Slippery elm has been used to treat asthma, bronchitis, colitis, coughs, weak digestion and inflammatory bowel disease.

Wild Yam root contains bitter compounds that promote sweating, relieve muscle cramps and reduce inflammation. It has been used to treat arthritis, menstrual cramps, rheumatism and gastritis.

Marshmallow root contains mucilaginous compounds that decrease the thickness while increasing the production of mucosal fluids, soothe inflamed tissue, heal wounds and increase the flow of urine. It is an excellent herbal source of trace minerals especially chromium, iron, magnesium and selenium. Marshmallow has been used to treat allergies, gastritis, gastric ulcers, enteritis, coughs, cystitis and hay fevers.

Dong Quai root contains aromatic compounds that relieve smooth muscle spasms especially in the uterus, have a sedative effect and increase the production of digestive fluids. It also contains bitter compounds that regulate glycogen production in the liver, reduce pain and inflammation, increase blood flow especially to the heart, lower blood cholesterol, normalize uterine contractions and are antiseptic. Dong quai is an excellent

herbal source of iron, magnesium and niacin. It has been used to treat anemia, abdominal pains, dysmenorrhea, amenorrhea, arthritis, coronary heart disease, atherosclerosis, angina pectoris, indigestion and headaches.

Ginger root contains aromatic compounds that increase the production of digestive fluids and enzymes, lower blood pressure, lower blood sugar and cholesterol. It also contains bitter compounds that reduce muscle spasms, increase blood circulation and dilate blood vessels. Ginger is an excellent herbal source of trace minerals especially silicon, magnesium and manganese. It has been used to treat nausea, motion sickness, flatulence, colds, coughs, indigestion, fevers, vomiting, diarrhea, chronic bronchitis and cold hands and feet.

Chapter 7

The Glandular System

The glandular system is made up of the hormone producing organs of the body, including the pituitary, thyroid, parathyroid, thymus, adrenal and pancreas. These glands perform a myriad of regulatory functions in the body, including temperature control and metabolic rate. Herbalists use herbs rich in trace minerals to supplement the production of hormones and enhance the efficiency of the glandular system. The names for the herbal combinations are chosen based on the properties of the key herbs in the formula.

Therapies for Relieving Excess Conditions

Blood sugar swings and metabolic fluctuations are examples of excess conditions of the glandular system. The hormone imbalances that disrupt the body's thermostat are also expressed as skin disorders.

Excess conditions in the glandular system are often marked by patterns of minor aches, pains and ailments including: backache, abdominal cramps, an inability to gain weight, sore throats, itching skin, burning skin, burning urination, fear, anxiety, hyperactivity, fatigue, agitation, hot hands and feet, vertigo, fevers, thirst, dry skin, mouth sores, tinnitis, dry coughs and vertigo. If left unchecked, these ailments may develop into illnesses including: hypoglycemia, hypothyroidism, hypertension, deafness, arthritis, autoimmune diseases, constipation, respiratory tract infections, dysmenorrhea, amenorrhea and menorrhagia.

Early herbal therapies for these conditions consisted of single herbs like black cohosh that is employed whenever anxiety and muscular spasms are encountered. Black cohosh is not simply an antispasmodic however, and with time and experience, herbalists recognized and recorded in their herbals the several properties of black cohosh. The British Herbal Pharmacopoeia lists black cohosh as an antirheumatic, antitussive, sedative and emmenagogue.

These lists of empirical properties of an herb are the key to understanding herbal combinations. Herbalists have found that they can enhance a particular property of a single herb by adding herbs that complement and support a given property. Conversely, the herbalist is also able to minimize an unwanted property by adding herbs that counteract or balance that property.

Therapies for Supplementing Deficient Conditions

Weakness in the glandular system is marked by serious conditions such as diabetes and Addison's disease as well as less serious and more common expressions of glandular deficiency such as hypothyroidism and obesity.

Deficient conditions of the glandular system are often associated with patterns of minor aches, pains, and ailments including: dry eyes, anemia, scanty menstruation, nail problems, muscle inflammation, frustration, depression, anger, fatigue, poor appetite, muscle spasms, obesity, inflammatory skin conditions, dry hair and insomnia. If left unchecked, these ailments may develop into illnesses including: diabetes, Addison's disease, hypothyroidism, hepatitis, shingles, tumors, hemorrhoids, gallstones, deafness, dysmenorrhea, prostatitis, painful urination, premenstrual syndrome and menopausal distress.

Early herbal therapies for these conditions consisted of single herbs like ginseng that is noted for its tonic and regenerative powers. Ginseng is not simply a tonic however, and with time and experience, herbalists recognized and recorded in their herbals the several properties of ginseng. The British Herbal Pharmacopoeia lists ginseng as a thymoleptic, sedative, demulcent, stomachic and aphrodisiac.

These empirical lists of properties of an herb are the key to understanding herbal combinations. Herbalists have found that they can enhance a particular property of a single herb by adding herbs that complemented and supported that property. Conversely, the herbalist is also able to minimize an unwanted property by adding herbs that counteract or balance the property.

Black Cohosh Combination

Composition

Black Cohosh	Capsicum
Licorice	Goldenseal
Kelp	Ginger
Gotu Kola	Dong Quai

Properties

Antispasmodic	Antiseptic
Anti-inflammatory	Stimulant
Demulcent	Analgesic

General Description

Black Cohosh combination is a prostatitis formula. It is used to reduce inflammation, swelling and muscle spasms in the urinary system especially the prostate. The herbs relieve smooth muscle spasms, shrink and sooth inflamed tissues, are antiseptic, increase blood circulation and relieve pains.

Chinese herbalists would describe this herbal combination as a water reducing formula. It also reduces the earth and wood elements while enhancing the fire and metal elements.

Black Cohosh combination has traditionally been used to treat **prostatitis, lumbago, painful urination** and **urinary tract infections.**

Imbalances indicating the use of this formula are commonly noted in the prostate acupressure point located at the top of the right hip bone along the inside of the inguinal ligament. Imbalances are often noted at the 5 o'clock position of each iris.

This formula is commonly used in conjunction with vitamin A, saw palmetto, pumpkin, almond, vitamin C, zinc and bee pollen.

Individual Components

Black Cohosh root contains bitter compounds that relieve smooth muscle spasms, reduce blood pressure

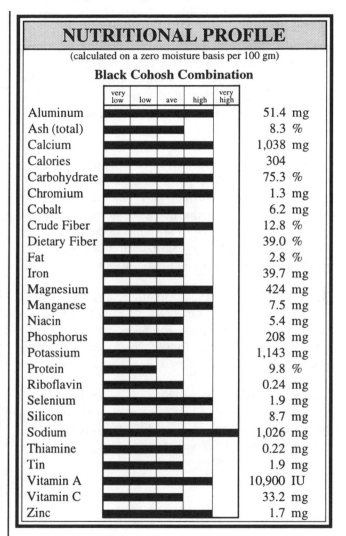

NUTRITIONAL PROFILE
(calculated on a zero moisture basis per 100 gm)

Black Cohosh Combination

	very low	low	ave	high	very high	
Aluminum						51.4 mg
Ash (total)						8.3 %
Calcium						1,038 mg
Calories						304
Carbohydrate						75.3 %
Chromium						1.3 mg
Cobalt						6.2 mg
Crude Fiber						12.8 %
Dietary Fiber						39.0 %
Fat						2.8 %
Iron						39.7 mg
Magnesium						424 mg
Manganese						7.5 mg
Niacin						5.4 mg
Phosphorus						208 mg
Potassium						1,143 mg
Protein						9.8 %
Riboflavin						0.24 mg
Selenium						1.9 mg
Silicon						8.7 mg
Sodium						1,026 mg
Thiamine						0.22 mg
Tin						1.9 mg
Vitamin A						10,900 IU
Vitamin C						33.2 mg
Zinc						1.7 mg

and dilate peripheral blood vessels. It also contains astringent compounds that shrink inflamed tissue. Black cohosh has been employed in most inflammatory conditions associated with spasms or tension. It is an excellent herbal source of iron and vitamin A. Black cohosh has been used to treat menstrual cramps, nervous tension, anxiety, dysmenorrhea, hysteria, menopause, fevers and headaches.

Licorice root contains bitter compounds that reduce inflammation, decrease the thickness and increase the production of mucosal fluids and relieve muscle spasms. In addition, licorice stimulates adrenal function, reduces the urge to coughs, is mildly laxative and enhances immune response. It has been used to treat coughs, colds, arthritis, asthma, peptic ulcers, Addison's disease, dropsy and atherosclerosis.

Kelp herb contains mucilaginous compounds that enhance the detoxifying and eliminative functions of the digestive system. These compounds absorb toxins from the bowel and provide bulk to the stool. Kelp is an excellent herbal source of calcium, magnesium, sodium and iodine. Iodine is essential to normal thyroid function. It is used to increase the metabolic rate and strengthen connective tissues including the hair, skin and nails. Kelp has been used to treat hypothyroidism, enlarged glands, debility, fatigue, eczema, psoriasis, arthritis and obesity.

Gotu Kola herb contains bitter compounds that have a sedative effect, dilate peripheral blood vessels and increase the flow of urine. It is an excellent herbal source of niacin, calcium, magnesium, manganese, silicon and sodium. Gotu kola has been used to treat insomnia, failing memory, schizophrenia, fevers, headaches and inflammatory skin conditions.

Capsicum fruit contains aromatic resins that increase blood circulation, promote sweating, increase the production of digestive fluids and reduce muscle spasms. It has been used to treat flatulence, colic, ulcers, rheumatic arthritis, cold hands and feet and dropsy.

Goldenseal root contains bitter, astringent alkaloids that normalize liver and spleen function by increasing the production of digestive fluids and enzymes, particularly bile. These compounds are antiseptic, constrict peripheral blood vessels especially in the uterus, are laxative, and relieve pain and inflammation in mucosal tissue. Goldenseal is an excellent herbal source of trace minerals including cobalt, iron, magnesium, manganese, silicon and zinc. It is also an excellent herbal source of vitamin C. It has been used to treat hepatitis, gastritis, colitis, ulcers, menorrhagia, postpartum hemorrhages, dysmenorrhea, diabetes, infections, hemorrhoids, eczema, obesity and fevers.

Ginger root contains aromatic compounds that increase the production of digestive fluids and enzymes, lower blood pressure, lower blood sugar and cholesterol. It also contains bitter compounds that reduce muscle spasms, increase blood circulation and dilate blood vessels. Ginger is an excellent herbal source of trace minerals especially silicon, magnesium and manganese. It has been used to treat nausea, motion sickness, flatulence, colds, coughs, indigestion, fevers, vomiting, diarrhea, chronic bronchitis and cold hands and feet.

Dong Quai root contains aromatic compounds that relieve smooth muscle spasms especially in the uterus, have a sedative effect and increase the production of digestive fluids. It also contains bitter compounds that regulate glycogen production in the liver, reduce pain and inflammation, increase blood flow especially to the heart, lower blood cholesterol, normalize uterine contractions and are antiseptic. Dong quai is an excellent herbal source of iron, magnesium and niacin. It has been used to treat anemia, abdominal pains, dysmenorrhea, amenorrhea, arthritis, coronary heart disease, atherosclerosis, angina pectoris, indigestion and headaches.

Black Cohosh and Blessed Thistle Combination

Composition

Black Cohosh	Sarsaparilla
Licorice	Blessed Thistle
False Unicorn	Squawvine
Siberian Ginseng	

Properties

Antispasmodic	Anti-inflammatory
Analgesic	Adaptogen
Nervine	

General Description

Black Cohosh and Blessed Thistle combination is used during menopause to enhance the female body's response to and recovery from the cessation of menstrual activity. The herbs relieve smooth muscle spasms, relieve pains, calm the nerves, reduce inflammation, increase adrenal activity, improve the body's response to stress and normalize metabolism.

Chinese herbalists would describe this herbal combination as a water enhancing formula. It also enhances the earth and metal elements while reducing the wood and fire elements.

Black Cohosh and Blessed Thistle combination has traditionally been used to treat **hot flashes, insomnia, menopause, nervous irritability, hormonal imbalances** and **sexual disinterest.**

Imbalances indicating the use of this formula are commonly noted in the uterus acupressure point located just above the pubic bone. Imbalances are often noted at the 7 o'clock position of the left iris and at the 5 o'clock position of the right iris. Use caution in cases of constipation and hypertension.

This formula is commonly used in conjunction with vitamin E, evening primrose oil, the complex of B vitamins and the vitamin C family.

Individual Components

Black Cohosh root contains bitter compounds that relieve smooth muscle spasms, reduce blood pressure

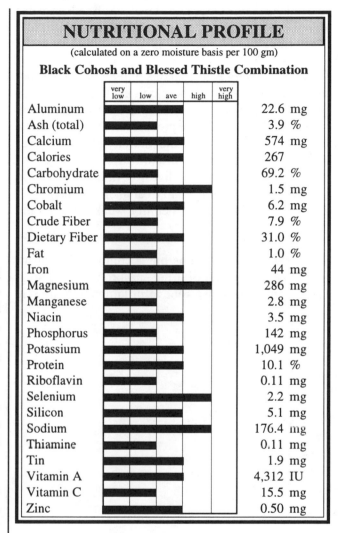

NUTRITIONAL PROFILE
(calculated on a zero moisture basis per 100 gm)
Black Cohosh and Blessed Thistle Combination

	very low	low	ave	high	very high	
Aluminum						22.6 mg
Ash (total)						3.9 %
Calcium						574 mg
Calories						267
Carbohydrate						69.2 %
Chromium						1.5 mg
Cobalt						6.2 mg
Crude Fiber						7.9 %
Dietary Fiber						31.0 %
Fat						1.0 %
Iron						44 mg
Magnesium						286 mg
Manganese						2.8 mg
Niacin						3.5 mg
Phosphorus						142 mg
Potassium						1,049 mg
Protein						10.1 %
Riboflavin						0.11 mg
Selenium						2.2 mg
Silicon						5.1 mg
Sodium						176.4 mg
Thiamine						0.11 mg
Tin						1.9 mg
Vitamin A						4,312 IU
Vitamin C						15.5 mg
Zinc						0.50 mg

and dilate peripheral blood vessels. It also contains astringent compounds that shrink inflamed tissue. Black cohosh has been employed in most inflammatory conditions associated with spasms or tension. It is an excellent herbal source of iron and vitamin A. Black cohosh has been used to treat menstrual cramps, nervous tension, anxiety, dysmenorrhea, hysteria, menopause, fevers and headaches.

Licorice root contains bitter compounds that reduce inflammation, decrease the thickness and increase the production of mucosal fluids and relieve muscle spasms. In addition, licorice stimulates adrenal function, reduces the urge to cough, is mildly laxative and enhances immune response. It has been used to treat coughs, colds, arthritis, asthma, peptic ulcers, Addison's disease, dropsy and atherosclerosis.

False Unicorn herb contains bitter compounds that enhance the function of the uterus and ovaries. These compounds relieve congestive dysmenorrhea, increase the flow of urine, reduce swelling and inflammation and help balance female hormone levels. False unicorn has been used to treat dysmenorrhea, edema, nephritis and amenorrhea.

Siberian Ginseng root contains bitter compounds that helps the body respond more quickly to stress. These compounds increase the production of DNA, RNA and proteins essential to all life processes. They also stimulate the adrenal, pancreas, and pituitary glands to lower blood sugar and reduce inflammation. Ginseng also increases the production of digestive fluids and is a mild sedative. It has been used to treat anemia, impotence, insomnia, diarrhea, fatigue debility, weak digestion and failing memory.

Sarsaparilla root contains bitter compounds that increase the production of urine and promote sweating. These compounds also relieve inflammation, muscle spasms and are antiseptic. Sarsaparilla is an excellent herbal source of chromium, cobalt, iron, and selenium. It has been used to treat rheumatism, gout, fevers, inflammatory skin conditions, prostatitis and impotence.

Blessed Thistle contains bitter compounds that decrease the thickness while increasing the production of mucosal fluids particularly in the digestive and respiratory systems. It also contains astringent compounds that are antiseptic, dilate peripheral blood vessels and shrink inflamed tissue. Blessed thistle is an excellent herbal source of potassium and sodium. The herb has been used to treat dysmenorrhea, amenorrhea, arthritis, dysuria, jaundice, fevers and respiratory allergies.

Squawvine herb contains astringent compounds that relieve erratic muscle spasms, shrink inflamed tissues and stop bleeding. It also contains bitter compounds that relieve anxiety and pains. Squawvine has been used to treat dysmenorrhea, menorrhagia, edema, varicose veins and postpartum depression.

Black Cohosh and Goldenseal Combination

Composition

Goldenseal	Queen of the Meadow
Red Raspberry	Marshmallow
Black Cohosh	Ginger
Dong Quai	Capsicum
Blessed Thistle	

Properties

Astringent	Nervine
Antispasmodic	Antiseptic
Vasoconstrictor	

General Description

Black Cohosh and Goldenseal combination is used to relieve excessive uterine bleeding. The herbs are noted for their ability to shrink the uterus and restrict peripheral blood flow. They also balance female hormone levels, reduce anxiety and are antiseptic.

Chinese herbalists would describe this herbal combination as a water reducing formula. It also reduces the earth and wood elements, while enhancing the fire and metal elements.

Black cohosh and Goldenseal combination has traditionally been used to treat **uterine hemorrhages, nephritis, edema, postpartum weakness, hemorrhoids** and **anemia.**

Imbalances indicating the use of this formula are commonly noted in the uterus acupressure point located just above the pubic bone. Imbalances are often noted at the 7 o'clock position of the left iris. Use caution in cases of constipation and hypertension.

This formula is commonly used in conjunction with vitamin E, evening primrose oil, the complex of B vitamins and the vitamin C family.

Individual Components

Goldenseal root contains bitter, astringent alkaloids that normalize liver and spleen function by increasing the production of digestive fluids and enzymes, particularly bile. These compounds are antiseptic, constrict peripheral blood vessels especially in the uterus, are laxative, and relieve pain and inflammation in mucosal tissue. Goldenseal is an excellent herbal source of trace minerals including cobalt, iron, magnesium, manganese, silicon and zinc. It is also an excellent herbal source of vitamin C. It has been used to treat hepatitis, gastritis, colitis, ulcers, menorrhagia, postpartum hemorrhages, dysmenorrhea, diabetes, infections, hemorrhoids, eczema, obesity and fevers.

Red Raspberry leaf contains astringent compounds that relieve pain and shrink inflamed tissues, especially in the female reproductive system. It also contains bitter compounds that relieve smooth muscle spasms. Red raspberry is an excellent herbal source of manganese. It has been used to treat morning sickness, nausea, dysmenorrhea, false labor, colds, flu and fevers.

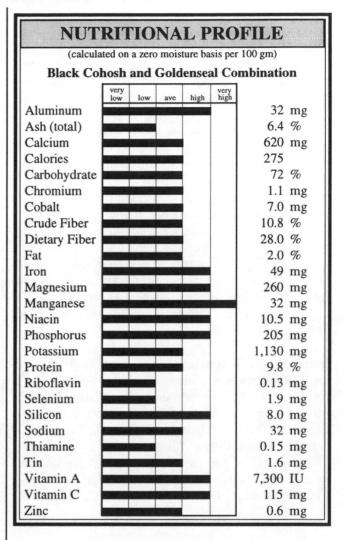

NUTRITIONAL PROFILE
(calculated on a zero moisture basis per 100 gm)

Black Cohosh and Goldenseal Combination

	very low	low	ave	high	very high	Value
Aluminum				■		32 mg
Ash (total)		■				6.4 %
Calcium			■			620 mg
Calories			■			275
Carbohydrate			■			72 %
Chromium			■			1.1 mg
Cobalt				■		7.0 mg
Crude Fiber			■			10.8 %
Dietary Fiber			■			28.0 %
Fat		■				2.0 %
Iron				■		49 mg
Magnesium			■			260 mg
Manganese					■	32 mg
Niacin			■			10.5 mg
Phosphorus			■			205 mg
Potassium				■		1,130 mg
Protein			■			9.8 %
Riboflavin			■			0.13 mg
Selenium		■				1.9 mg
Silicon				■		8.0 mg
Sodium		■				32 mg
Thiamine			■			0.15 mg
Tin			■			1.6 mg
Vitamin A				■		7,300 IU
Vitamin C				■		115 mg
Zinc			■			0.6 mg

Black Cohosh root contains bitter compounds that relieve smooth muscle spasms, reduce blood pressure and dilate peripheral blood vessels. It also contains astringent compounds that shrink inflamed tissue. Black cohosh has been employed in most inflammatory conditions associated with spasms or tension. It is an excellent herbal source of iron and vitamin A. Black cohosh has been used to treat menstrual cramps, nervous tension, anxiety, dysmenorrhea, hysteria, menopause, fevers and headaches.

Dong Quai root contains aromatic compounds that relieve smooth muscle spasms, especially in the uterus, have a sedative effect and increase the production of digestive fluids. It also contains bitter compounds that regulate glycogen production in the liver, reduce pain and inflammation, increase blood flow especially to the heart, lower blood cholesterol, normalize uterine contractions and are antiseptic. Dong quai is an excellent herbal source of iron, magnesium and niacin. It has been used to treat anemia, abdominal pains, dysmenorrhea, amenorrhea, arthritis, coronary heart disease, atherosclerosis, angina pectoris, indigestion and headaches.

Blessed Thistle contains bitter compounds that decrease the thickness while increasing the production of mucosal fluids particularly in the digestive and respiratory systems. It also contains astringent compounds that are antiseptic, dilate peripheral blood vessels and shrink inflamed tissue. Blessed thistle is an excellent herbal source of potassium and sodium. The herb has been used to treat dysmenorrhea, amenorrhea, arthritis, dysuria, jaundice, fevers and respiratory allergies.

Queen of the Meadow contains bitter compounds that increase the flow of urine and provide an antiseptic action on the urinary sytem. Queen of the Meadow has been used to treat urinary tract infections, gout, edema, lumbago, rheumatism and kidney stones.

Marshmallow root contains mucilaginous compounds that decrease the thickness while increasing the production of mucosal fluids, soothe inflamed tissue, heat wounds and increase the flow of urine. It is an excellent herbal source of trace minerals, especially chromium, iron, magnesium and selenium. Marshmallow has been used to treat allergies, gastritis, gastric ulcers, enteritis, coughs, cystis and hay fevers.

Ginger root contains aromatic compounds that increase the production of digestive fluids and enzymes, lower blood pressure, lower blood sugar and cholesterol. It also contains bitter compounds that reduce muscle spasms, increase blood circulation and dilate blood vessels. Ginger is an excellent herbal source of trace minerals, especially silicon, magnesium and manganese. It has been used to treat nausea, motion sickness, flatulence, colds, coughs, indigestion, fevers, vomiting, diarrhea, chronic bronchitis and cold hands and feet.

Capsicum fruit contains aromatic resins that increase blood circulation, promote sweating, increase the production of digestive fluids and reduce muscle spasms. It has been used to treat flatulence, colic, ulcers, rheumatic arthritis, cold hands and feet and dropsy.

Black Cohosh and Raspberry Combination

Composition

Black Cohosh
Squawvine
Dong Quai
Butcher's Broom
Red Raspberry

Properties

Antispasmodic
Nervine
Analgesic
Astringent

General Description

Black Cohosh and Raspberry combination is used to assist pregnant women to an easier pregnancy and childbirth. The combined action of the herbs in this formula are particularly directed to the smooth muscle of the uterus. It is used during the third trimester of pregnancy to tone the uterus and coordinate uterine contractions during childbirth. The formula relieves irritability, calms muscle spasms and relieves pain and anxiety associated with pregnancy and childbirth.

Chinese herbalists would describe this herbal combination as a water enhancing formula. It also enhances the earth and wood elements while enhancing the fire and metal elements.

Black Cohosh and Raspberry combination has traditionally been used to treat **dysmenorrhea, menstrual disorders, morning sickness, miscarriage, hot flashes** and **in preparation for childbirth.**

Imbalances indicating the use of this formula are commonly noted in the uterus acupressure point located just above the pubic bone. Imbalances are often noted at the 7 o'clock position of the left iris and at the 5 o'clock position of the right iris. Use caution in cases of constipation and hypertension.

This formula is commonly used in conjunction with vitamin E, evening primrose oil, the complex of B vitamins and the vitamin C family.

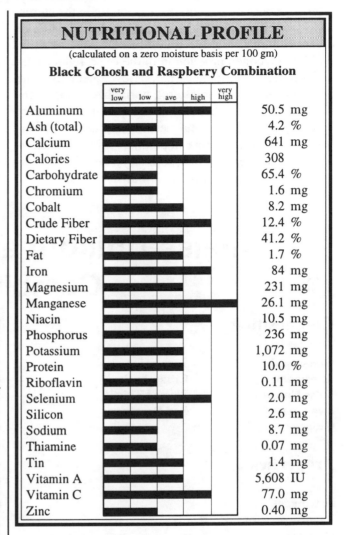

NUTRITIONAL PROFILE
(calculated on a zero moisture basis per 100 gm)
Black Cohosh and Raspberry Combination

	very low	low	ave	high	very high	
Aluminum				■		50.5 mg
Ash (total)	■					4.2 %
Calcium			■			641 mg
Calories				■		308
Carbohydrate			■			65.4 %
Chromium		■				1.6 mg
Cobalt			■			8.2 mg
Crude Fiber			■			12.4 %
Dietary Fiber				■		41.2 %
Fat			■			1.7 %
Iron				■		84 mg
Magnesium			■			231 mg
Manganese					■	26.1 mg
Niacin			■			10.5 mg
Phosphorus		■				236 mg
Potassium		■				1,072 mg
Protein		■				10.0 %
Riboflavin		■				0.11 mg
Selenium			■			2.0 mg
Silicon		■				2.6 mg
Sodium	■					8.7 mg
Thiamine		■				0.07 mg
Tin		■				1.4 mg
Vitamin A			■			5,608 IU
Vitamin C		■				77.0 mg
Zinc	■					0.40 mg

Individual Components

Black Cohosh root contains bitter compounds that relieve smooth muscle spasms, reduce blood pressure and dilate peripheral blood vessels. It also contains astringent compounds that shrink inflamed tissue. Black cohosh has been employed in most inflammatory conditions associated with spasms or tension. It is an excellent herbal source of iron and vitamin A. Black cohosh has been used to treat menstrual cramps, nervous tension, anxiety, dysmenorrhea, hysteria, menopause, fevers and headaches.

Squawvine herb contains astringent compounds that relieve erratic muscle spasms, shrink inflamed tissues and stop bleeding. It also contains bitter compounds that relieve anxiety and pains. Squawvine has been used to treat dysmenorrhea, menorrhagia, edema, varicose veins, and postpartum depression.

Dong Quai root contains aromatic compounds that relieve smooth muscle spasms especially in the uterus, have a sedative effect and increase the production of digestive fluids. It also contains bitter compounds that regulate glycogen production in the liver, reduce pain and inflammation, increase blood flow especially to the heart, lower blood cholesterol, normalize uterine contractions and are antiseptic. Dong quai is an excellent herbal source of iron, magnesium and niacin. It has been used to treat anemia, abdominal pains, dysmenorrhea, amenorrhea, arthritis, coronary heart disease, atherosclerosis, angina pectoris, indigestion and headaches.

Butcher's Broom herb contains bitter compounds that decrease capillary permeability and thrombosis. These compounds also relieve inflammation, increase the flow of urine and constrict peripheral blood vessels without increasing blood pressure. Butcher's broom is an excellent herbal source of iron and silicon. It has been used to treat post operative thrombosis, phlebitis, varicose veins, hemorrhoids, edema and dysmenorrhea.

Red Raspberry leaf contains astringent compounds that relieve pain and shrink inflamed tissues, especially in the female reproductive system. It also contains bitter compounds that relieve smooth muscle spasms. Red Raspberry is an excellent herbal source of manganese. It has been used to treat morning sickness, nausea, dysmenorrhea, false labor, colds, flu and fevers.

False Unicorn and Goldenseal Combination

Composition

Goldenseal	**Squawvine**
Capsicum	**Crampbark**
False Unicorn	**Blessed Thistle**
Uva Ursi	**Red Raspberry**
Ginger	

Properties

Astringent
Vasoconstrictor
Diuretic
Antiseptic
Antispasmodic

General Description

False Unicorn and Goldenseal combination is used to relieve excessive uterine bleeding. The herbs are noted for their ability to shrink the uterus and restrict peripheral blood flow. They also balance female hormone levels, increase the flow of urine and are antiseptic.

Chinese herbalists would describe this herbal combination as a water reducing formula. It also reduces the earth and wood elements while enhancing the fire and metal elements.

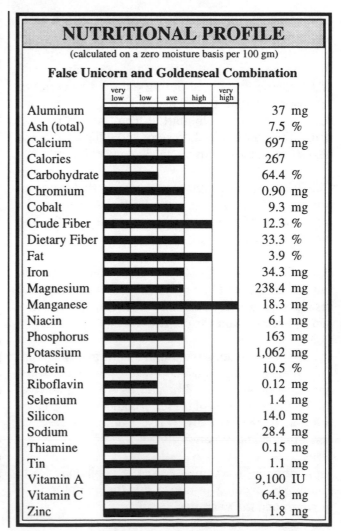

NUTRITIONAL PROFILE
(calculated on a zero moisture basis per 100 gm)

False Unicorn and Goldenseal Combination

	very low	low	ave	high	very high	
Aluminum						37 mg
Ash (total)						7.5 %
Calcium						697 mg
Calories						267
Carbohydrate						64.4 %
Chromium						0.90 mg
Cobalt						9.3 mg
Crude Fiber						12.3 %
Dietary Fiber						33.3 %
Fat						3.9 %
Iron						34.3 mg
Magnesium						238.4 mg
Manganese						18.3 mg
Niacin						6.1 mg
Phosphorus						163 mg
Potassium						1,062 mg
Protein						10.5 %
Riboflavin						0.12 mg
Selenium						1.4 mg
Silicon						14.0 mg
Sodium						28.4 mg
Thiamine						0.15 mg
Tin						1.1 mg
Vitamin A						9,100 IU
Vitamin C						64.8 mg
Zinc						1.8 mg

False Unicorn and Goldenseal combination has traditionally been used to treat **uterine hemorrhage, nephritis, edema, postpartum weakness, hemorrhoids, anemia** and **female hormonal balance.**

Imbalances indicating the use of this formula are commonly noted in the uterus acupressure point located just above the pubic bone. Imbalances are often noted at the 7 o'clock position of the left iris and the 5 o'clock position of the right iris. Use caution in cases of constipation and hypertension.

This formula is commonly used in conjunction with vitamin E, evening primrose oil, the complex of B vitamins and the vitamin C family.

Individual Components

Goldenseal is an excellent herbal source of trace minerals including cobalt, iron, magnesium, manganese, silicon and zinc. It is also an excellent herbal source of vitamin C. It has been used to treat hepatitis, gastritis, colitis, ulcers, menorrhagia, postpartum hemorrhage, dysmenorrhea, diabetes, infections, hemorrhoids, eczema, obesity and fevers.

Capsicum fruit contains aromatic resins that increase blood circulation, promote sweating, increase the production of digestive fluids and reduce muscle spasms. It has been used to treat flatulence, colic, ulcers, rheumatic arthritis, cold hands and feet and dropsy.

False Unicorn herb contains bitter compounds that enhance the function of the uterus and ovaries. These compounds relieve congestive dysmenorrhea, increase the flow of urine, reduce swelling and inflammation and help balance female hormone levels. False unicorn has been used to treat dysmenorrhea, edema, nephritis and amenorrhea.

Uva Ursi fruit contains bitter compounds that are antiseptic and increase the flow of urine. It also contains astringent compounds that shrink inflamed tissue.

It has been used to treat urinary tract infections, kidney stones, cystitis, nephritis, hemorrhoids and diarrhea.

Ginger root contains aromatic compounds that increase the production of digestive fluids and enzymes, lower blood pressure, lower blood sugar and cholesterol. It also contains bitter compounds that reduce muscle spasms, increase blood circulation and dilate blood vessels. Ginger is an excellent herbal source of trace minerals especially silicon, magnesium and manganese. It has been used to treat nausea, motion sickness, flatulence, colds, coughs, indigestion, fevers, vomiting, diarrhea, chronic bronchitis and cold hands and feet.

Squawvine herb contains astringent compounds that relieve erratic muscle spasms, shrink inflamed tissues and stop bleeding. It also contains bitter compounds that relieve anxiety and pains. Squawvine has been used to treat dysmenorrhea, menorrhagia, edema, varicose veins and postpartum depression.

Cramp bark contains bitter compounds that relieve smooth muscle spasms, reduce pain and calm the nerves. It has been used to treat menstrual cramps, dysmenorrhea, rheumatism, colic, muscle tension and headaches.

Blessed Thistle contains bitter compounds that decrease the thickness while increasing the production of mucosal fluids particularly in the digestive and respiratory systems. It also contains astringent compounds that are antiseptic, dilate peripheral blood vessels and shrink inflamed tissue. Blessed thistle is an excellent herbal source of potassium and sodium. The herb has been used to treat dysmenorrhea, amenorrhea, arthritis, dysuria, jaundice, fevers, and respiratory allergies.

Red Raspberry leaf contains astringent compounds that relieve pain and shrink inflamed tissues especially in the female reproductive system. It also contains bitter compounds that relieve smooth muscle spasms. Red raspberry is an excellent herbal source of manganese. It has been used to treat morning sickness, nausea, dysmenorrhea, false labor, colds, flu and fevers.

Licorice Combination

Composition

Licorice	Dandelion
Safflower	Horseradish

Properties

Anti-inflammatory	Stimulant
Carminative	Stomachic

General Description

Licorice combination is a hypoglycemic formula. It is used to balance the metabolic rate and minimize blood sugar changes by enhancing the function of the adrenal glands, pancreas, liver and digestive system. The herbs reduce inflammation, especially in the pancreas, increase the production of digestive fluids and enzymes, enhance adrenal activity and increase blood circulation.

Chinese herbalists would describe this herbal combination as a wood reducing formula. It also reduces the fire element while enhancing the metal earth and water elements.

Licorice combination has traditionally been used to treat **hypoglycemia, anemia, fatigue** and **restlessness.**

Imbalances indicating the use of this formula are commonly noted in the pancreas acupressure point located approximately four inches below and three inches to the left of the sternum. Imbalances are often noted at the 7 o'clock position of the right iris. Use caution in cases of hypertension, obesity and edema.

This formula is commonly used in conjunction with pantothenic acid.

Individual Components

Licorice root contains bitter compounds that reduce inflammation, decrease the thickness and increase the production of mucosal fluids and relieve muscle spasms. In addition, licorice stimulates adrenal function, reduces the urge to cough, is mildly laxative and enhances immune response. It has been used to treat coughs, colds, arthritis, asthma, peptic ulcers, Addison's disease, dropsy and atherosclerosis.

Safflowers contain bitter compounds that increase the production and release of bile. It is an excellent herbal source of unsaturated fatty acids. Safflowers has been used to treat liver congestion, gallstones, gout, scarlet fever, indigestion and amenorrhea.

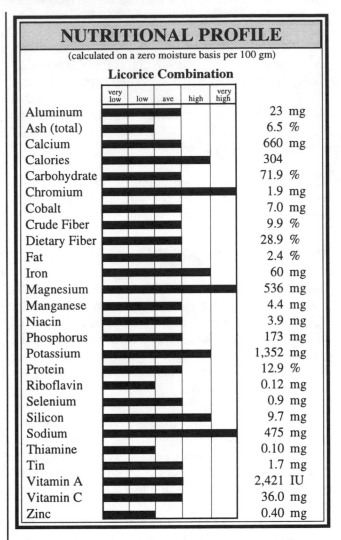

NUTRITIONAL PROFILE
(calculated on a zero moisture basis per 100 gm)

Licorice Combination

	very low	low	ave	high	very high	Value	Unit
Aluminum						23	mg
Ash (total)						6.5	%
Calcium						660	mg
Calories						304	
Carbohydrate						71.9	%
Chromium						1.9	mg
Cobalt						7.0	mg
Crude Fiber						9.9	%
Dietary Fiber						28.9	%
Fat						2.4	%
Iron						60	mg
Magnesium						536	mg
Manganese						4.4	mg
Niacin						3.9	mg
Phosphorus						173	mg
Potassium						1,352	mg
Protein						12.9	%
Riboflavin						0.12	mg
Selenium						0.9	mg
Silicon						9.7	mg
Sodium						475	mg
Thiamine						0.10	mg
Tin						1.7	mg
Vitamin A						2,421	IU
Vitamin C						36.0	mg
Zinc						0.40	mg

Dandelion root contains bitter compounds that enhance the efficiency of the body's eliminative and detoxifying functions. These compounds help restore normal liver function, increase the production of digestive fluids and enzymes particularly bile, increase the flow of urine and have a laxative effect. Dandelion is an excellent herbal source of sodium, iron and vitamin A. It has been used to treat jaundice, gallstones, dyspepsia, constipation, inflammatory skin conditions, frequent urination, hepatitis, gout and rheumatism.

Horseradish root contains aromatic compounds that increase circulation, are antiseptic and promote sweating. These compounds also decrease the thickness while increasing the production of mucosal fluid. Horseradish has been used to treat asthma, bronchitis, coughs, colds, fevers and rheumatism.

Raspberry and Dong Quai Combination

Composition

Red Raspberry	Black Cohosh
Dong Quai	Blessed Thistle
Ginger	Queen of the Meadow
Licorice	Marshmallow

Properties

Nervine
Antispasmodic
Analgesic
Diuretic
Stimulant

General Description

Raspberry and Dong Quai combination is used to relieve dysmenorrhea. It effectively relieves congestive dysmenorrhea which tends to be associated with premenstrual tension and the symptoms of water retention and pelvic inflammation. It also works to dispel cramping or spasmodic dysmenorrhea which follows the onset of menses. The herbs in this formula calm the nerves, relieve muscle spasms and relieve pain and anxiety associated with muscular spasms and tensions.

Chinese herbalists would describe this herbal combination as a water enhancing formula. It also enhances the earth and wood elements while enhancing the fire and metal elements.

Raspberry and Dong Quai combination has traditionally been used to treat **dysmenorrhea, menstrual disorders, morning sickness, muscle cramps** and **hot flashes.**

Imbalances indicating the use of this formula are commonly noted in the uterus acupressure point located just above the pubic bone. Imbalances are often noted at the 7 o'clock position of the left iris and at the 5 o'clock position of the right iris. Use caution in cases of edema and hypertension.

This formula is commonly used in conjunction with vitamin E, evening primrose oil, the complex of B vitamins and the vitamin C family.

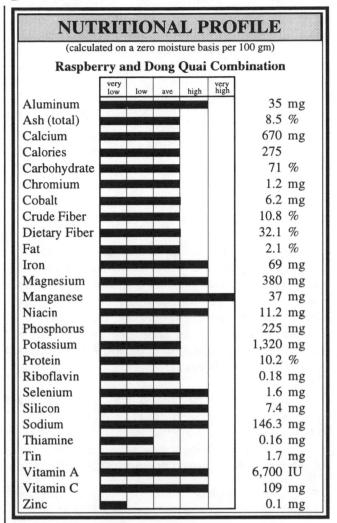

NUTRITIONAL PROFILE
(calculated on a zero moisture basis per 100 gm)
Raspberry and Dong Quai Combination

	very low	low	ave	high	very high	
Aluminum						35 mg
Ash (total)						8.5 %
Calcium						670 mg
Calories						275
Carbohydrate						71 %
Chromium						1.2 mg
Cobalt						6.2 mg
Crude Fiber						10.8 %
Dietary Fiber						32.1 %
Fat						2.1 %
Iron						69 mg
Magnesium						380 mg
Manganese						37 mg
Niacin						11.2 mg
Phosphorus						225 mg
Potassium						1,320 mg
Protein						10.2 %
Riboflavin						0.18 mg
Selenium						1.6 mg
Silicon						7.4 mg
Sodium						146.3 mg
Thiamine						0.16 mg
Tin						1.7 mg
Vitamin A						6,700 IU
Vitamin C						109 mg
Zinc						0.1 mg

Individual Components

Red Raspberry leaf contains astringent compounds that relieve pain and shrink inflamed tissues, especially in the female reproductive system. It also contains bitter compounds that relieve smooth muscle spasms. Red Raspberry is an excellent herbal source of manganese. It has been used to treat morning sickness, nausea, dysmenorrhea, false labor, colds, flu and fevers.

Dong Quai root contains aromatic compounds that relieve smooth muscle spasms especially in the uterus, have a sedative effect and increase the production of digestive fluids. It also contains bitter compounds that regulate glycogen production in the liver, reduce pain and inflammation, increase blood flow, especially to the heart, lower blood cholesterol, normalize uterine contractions and are antiseptic. Dong quai is an excellent herbal source of iron, magnesium and niacin. It has been used to treat anemia, abdominal pains, dysmenorrhea, amenorrhea, arthritis, coronary heart disease, atherosclerosis, angina pectoris, indigestion and headaches.

Ginger root contains aromatic compounds that increase the production of digestive fluids and enzymes, lower blood pressure, lower blood sugar and cholesterol. It also contains bitter compounds that reduce muscle spasms, increase blood circulation and dilate blood vessels. Ginger is an excellent herbal source of trace minerals especially silicon, magnesium and manganese. It has been used to treat nausea, motion sickness, flatulence, colds, coughs, indigestion, fevers, vomiting, diarrhea, chronic bronchitis and cold hands and feet.

Licorice root contains bitter compounds that reduce inflammation, decrease the thickness and increase the production of mucosal fluids and relieve muscle spasms. In addition, licorice stimulates adrenal function, reduces the urge to cough, is mildly laxative and enhances immune response. It has been used to treat coughs, colds, arthritis, asthma, peptic ulcers, Addison's disease, dropsy and atherosclerosis.

Black Cohosh root contains bitter compounds that relieve smooth muscle spasms, reduce blood pressure and dilate peripheral blood vessels. It also contains astringent compounds that shrink inflamed tissue. Black cohosh has been employed in most inflammatory conditions associated with spasms or tension. It is an excellent herbal source of iron and vitamin A. Black cohosh has been used to treat menstrual cramps, nervous tension, anxiety, dysmenorrhea, hysteria, menopause, fevers and headaches.

Blessed Thistle contains bitter compounds that decrease the thickness while increasing the production of mucosal fluids particularly in the digestive and respiratory systems. It also contains astringent compounds that are antiseptic, dilate peripheral blood vessels and shrink inflamed tissue. Blessed thistle is an excellent herbal source of potassium and sodium. The herb has been used to treat dysmenorrhea, amenorrhea, arthritis, dysuria, jaundice, fevers and respiratory allergies.

Queen of the Meadow contains bitter compounds that increase the flow of urine and provide an antiseptic action on the urinary system. Queen of the Meadow has been used to treat urinary tract infections, gout, edema, lumbago, rheumatism and kidney stones.

Marshmallow root contains mucilaginous compounds that decrease the thickness while increasing the production of mucosal fluids, soothe inflamed tissue, heal wounds and increase the flow of urine. It is an excellent herbal source of trace minerals especially chromium, iron, magnesium and selenium. Marshmallow has been used to treat allergies, gastritis, gastric ulcers, enteritis, coughs, cystitis and hay fevers.

Rehmannia and Ophiopogon Combination

Composition

Rehmannia	Moutan	Achyranthes
Dendrobium	Alisma orientale	Eucommia
Schizandra	Ophiopogon	Cornus
Phellodendron	Trichosanthes	Anemarrhena
Asphodeloides	Hoelen	Pueraria
Licorice		Asparagus

Properties

Expectorant	Diuretic
Stimulant	Carminative
Demulcent	Bulk Laxative

General Description

Rehmannia and Ophiopogon combination is used to normalize hormone imbalances often associated with metabolic processes, such as sugar metabolism, menopause, and dryness of the skin, throat or bowel. The herbs soothe inflamed tissues, decrease the thickness while increasing the production of mucosal fluids, increase the production of digestive fluids and enzymes, increase blood circulation, stimulate adrenal activity, increase the flow of urine and absorb toxins from the bowel.

Chinese herbalists would describe this herbal combination as a water enhancing formula. It also enhances the wood element while reducing the earth, fire and metal elements.

Rehmannia and Ophiopogon combination has traditionally been used to treat **hypoglycemia, menopause, dry coughs, thirst, night sweats, constipation, insomnia, diabetes, dry skin, hypertension, dysuria** and **sore throat.**

Imbalances indicating the use of this formula are commonly noted in the thymus acupressure point located in the center of the sternum. Imbalances are often noted at the 6 o'clock position of the right iris. Use caution in cases of hypertension.

This formula is commonly used in conjunction with the vitamin C family, goldenseal, the complex of B vitamins, calcium, chromium and manganese.

Individual Components

Rehmennia root contains astringent compounds that stop bleeding and reduce inflammation, especially in the digestive system. The herb also contains bitter compounds that reduce capillary fragility. It has been used to treat ulcers, menorrhagia, thirst, diabetes, constipation, anemia and infertility.

Dendrobium herb contains bitter compounds that increase the production of digestive fluids and enzymes, reduce fevers and pains, raise blood sugar and lower blood pressure. It has been used to treat hypoglycemia, thirst, dry mouth and dry coughs.

Schizandra fruit contains bitter compounds that allow the body to more quickly respond to stress. This increases the body's capacity for work and decreases fatigue. These compounds also increase blood circulation, blood sugar and bile production while lowering blood pressure. Schizandra also contains astringent compounds that increase the contraction of the heart muscle and the uterus and are antiseptic. The herb has been used to treat heart palpitations, dropsy, nervous exhaustion, asthma, diabetes, chronic diarrhea, night sweats, seminal emissions, insomnia, frequent urination and anxiety.

Phellodendron bark contains bitter compounds that increase the production of digestive fluids and enzymes, particularly bile. These compounds are also antiseptic and laxative, relieve pain and inflammation in mucosal tissue and constrict peripheral blood vessels. Phellodendron has been used to treat diarrhea, jaundice, urinary tract infections, eczema, boils, fevers and night sweats.

Hoelen herb contains bitter compounds that increase the flow of urine, decrease blood sugar and have a sedative effect. It has been used to treat edema, dropsy, diarrhea, insomnia, frequent urination and heart palpitations.

Asparagus root contains bitter compounds that decrease the thickness while increasing the production of mucosal fluids, relieve muscle spasms, are antiseptic and enhance immune response. It has been used to treat bronchitis, asthma, dry coughs, colds, flu, night sweats and dry stool.

Moutan root contains bitter compounds that are antiseptic, lower blood pressure, relieve inflammation, are sedative, decrease capillary permeability and increase blood circulation. It has been used to treat arthritis, gastric pains, dry skin, inflammatory skin conditions, amenorrhea, dysmenorrhea and fevers.

Alisma orientale root contains bitter compounds that increase the flow of urine, reduce blood pressure, lower blood sugar and cholesterol and are antiseptic. It has been used to treat edema, nephritis, diarrhea, cholesterolemia and urinary tract infections.

Ophiopogon root contains bitter compounds that have a sedative effect, promote the production of mucosal fluids, reduce muscle spasms and have an antiseptic effect. In addition, the herb lowers blood sugar and regenerates beta cells in the islets of langerhorn of the pancreas. Ophiopogon has been used to treat insomnia, coronary heart disease, heart palpitations, fear and dry coughs.

Trichosanthes root contains bitter compounds that raise blood sugar, induce labor, relieve inflammation and decrease the thickness while increasing the production of mucosal fluid. It has been used to treat hypoglycemia, dry coughs, abscesses and fevers.

Pueraria root contains bitter compounds that promote sweating, lower blood pressure, relieve pains, relieve muscle spasms, lower blood sugar, increase blood circulation and increase coronary blood flow. It has been used to treat hypertension, atherosclerosis, headaches, measles and inflammatory skin conditions.

Achyranthes root contains bitter compounds that increase the production of urine, relieve pains, lower blood pressure and decrease peristalsis. These compounds increase the contraction of the uterus and promote menstruation. It also contains mucilaginous compounds that sooth inflamed tissue and increase the production of mucosal fluids. Achyranthes has been used to treat amenorrhea, backache, hypertension, muscle aches and dysuria.

Eucommia bark contains bitter compounds that reduce blood pressure, relieve muscle spasms especially in the uterus and calm the mind. It also contains mucilaginous compounds that absorb toxins from the bowel, lower cholesterol absorption and enhance the production of mucosal fluids especially in the urinary system. Eucommia has been used to treat backache, dysuria, impotence, muscular weakness, osteoporosis, and to prevent miscarriage.

Cornus fruit contains astringent compounds that shrink inflamed tissue, reduce menstrual flow and are antiseptic. It also contains bitter compounds that increase the flow of urine, lower blood pressure and increase immune response. Cornus has been used to treat backaches, dysuria, impotence, uterine bleeding, menorrhagia and vertigo.

Anemarrhena asphodeloides root contains bitter compounds that reduce fevers, lower blood sugar, are antiseptic and increase the production of urine. These compounds also decrease the thickness while increasing the production of mucosal fluids. It has been used to treat fevers, thirst, respiratory tract infections, bronchitis, lumbago, constipation and dysuria.

Licorice root contains bitter compounds that reduce inflammation, decrease the thickness and increase the production of mucosal fluids and relieve muscle spasms. In addition, licorice stimulates adrenal function, reduces the urge to cough, is mildly laxative and enhances immune response. It has been used to treat coughs, colds, arthritis, asthma, peptic ulcers, Addison's disease, dropsy and atherosclerosis.

Therapies for Supplementing Deficient Conditions

Dong Quai and Peony Combination

Composition

Dong Quai	Alisma	Siberian Ginseng
Peony	Lycium fruit	Ligustrum
Rehmannia	Cornus	Achyranthes
Ligusticum	Salvia	Atractylodes
Bupleurum	Ganoderma	Ho Shou Wu
Astragalus	Curcuma	Cyperus

Properties

Blood Tonic	Stimulant
Immunostimulant	Emmenagogue
Adaptogen	Antispasmodic
Hepatic tonic	Diuretic

General Description

Dong Quai and Peony combination is a traditional blood tonic. It is used to overcome blood deficiencies and hormone imbalances associated with chronic liver dysfunction. The herbs work to enhance immune response, are antioxidant, improve blood circulation, calm the nerves, relieve muscle spasms, increase the flow of urine and increase menstrual flow.

Chinese herbalists describe this herbal combination as a wood enhancing formula. It also enhances the fire and metal element while reducing the water and earth elements.

Dong Quai and Peony combination has traditionally been used to treat **dysmenorrhea, hepatitis, cirrhosis, alcoholism, infertility, immune deficiency, fatigue, loss of appetite, anemia, postpartum depression, deafness** and **loss of eye sight.**

Imbalances indicating the use of this formula are commonly noted in the liver acupressure point located approximately four inches to the right of the sternum between the 7th and 8th ribs. Imbalances are often noted at the 7:30 position of the left iris.

This formula is commonly used in conjunction with black cohosh, vitamin E, vitamin B-6, iron, manganese, iodine, the complex of B vitamins and the vitamin C family.

Individual Components

Dong Quai root contains aromatic compounds that relieve smooth muscle spasms especially in the uterus, have a sedative effect and increase the production of digestive fluids. It also contains bitter compounds that regulate glycogen production in the liver, reduce pain and inflammation, increase blood flow, especially to the heart, lower blood cholesterol, normalize uterine contractions and are antiseptic. Dong quai is an excellent herbal source of iron, magnesium and niacin. It has been used to treat anemia, abdominal pains, dysmenorrhea, amenorrhea, arthritis, coronary heart disease, atherosclerosis, angina pectoris, indigestion and headaches.

Peony root contains bitter compounds that are sedative, antiseptic and relieve pains. These compounds also lower blood pressure and decrease capillary permeability. It has been used to treat arthralgia, gastric pains, inflammatory skin conditions and dysmenorrhea.

Rehmannia root contains astringent compounds that stop bleeding and reduce inflammation especially in the digestive system. The herb also contains bitter compounds that reduce capillary fragility. It has been used to treat ulcers, menorrhagia, thirst, diabetes, constipation, anemia and infertility.

Ligusticum root contains aromatic compounds that promote sweating, increase blood circulation, relieve pain and inflammation and relieve muscle spasms. It has been used to treat headaches, migraine headaches, arthritis, rheumatism, dysmenorrhea, flu, colds, inflammatory skin conditions and anemia.

Bupleurum root contains bitter compounds that have an anti-depressant effect, relieve pain and inflammation, reduce fevers and have an antiseptic effect. In addition, these compounds reduce blood cholesterol and triglyceride levels and reduce fat cell production and inflammation in the liver. Bupleurum has been used to treat premenstrual syndrome, dysmenorrhea, lung congestion, malaria, muscle cramps, tumors, inflammatory skin conditions, angina pains, epilepsy and depression.

Astragalus root contains bitter compounds that increase the flow of urine, are antiseptic, increase the production of digestive fluids including bile, and relieve muscle spasms. Astragalus also contains mucilaginous compounds that enhance immune response, increasing the production of lymphocytes and macrophages. The herb also increases heart action and lowers blood pressure and blood sugar. It has been used to treat fatigue, debility, urinary tract infections, edema, nephritis, ulcers, prolapse of organs and night sweats.

Alisma root contains bitter compounds that increase the flow of urine, reduce blood pressure, lower blood sugar and cholesterol and are antiseptic. It has been used to treat edema, nephritis, diarrhea, cholesterolemia and urinary tract infections.

Lycium fruit contains bitter compounds that lower blood sugar, promote the regeneration of liver cells and lower blood cholesterol. It has been used to treat atherosclerosis, backaches, impotence, vertigo, poor eyesight and diabetes.

Cornus fruit contains astringent compounds that shrink inflamed tissue, reduce menstrual flow and are antiseptic. It also contains bitter compounds that increase the flow of urine, lower blood pressure and increase immune response. Cornus has been used to treat backache, dysuria, impotence, uterine bleeding, menorrhagia and vertigo.

Salvia root contains bitter compounds that increase coronary blood flow, dilate peripheral blood vessels, lower blood pressure, lower blood sugar, lower blood cholesterol and allow the heart to function more efficiently with less oxygen. These compounds also calm the nerves, enhance immune response and are antiseptic. Salvia has been used to treat atherosclerosis, hypertension, insomnia, angina pains, dysmenorrhea and amenorrhea.

Ganoderma herb contains bitter compounds that increase coronary blood flow, lower blood pressure, lower blood cholesterol and allow the heart to function more efficiently on less oxygen. These compounds also calm the nerves, relieve pain and are antiseptic. Ganoderma also contains mucilaginous compounds that improve immune response and decrease the thickness while increasing the production of mucosal fluids. The herb has been used to treat insomnia, atherosclerosis, asthma, bronchitis, angina pains, hypertension and immune deficiency.

Curcuma root contains bitter compounds that relieve pain and inflammation in mucosal tissue and increase the production of bile. It also contains aromatic compounds that increase the production of digestive fluids and are antiseptic. It has been used to treat angina pains, anxiety, hepatitis, gall stones and dysmenorrhea.

Siberian Ginseng root contains bitter compounds that help the body respond more quickly to stress. These compounds increase the production of DNA, RNA and proteins essential to all life processes. They stimulate the adrenal, pancreas, and pituitary glands to lower blood sugar and reduce inflammation. Ginseng also increases the production of digestive fluids and is a mild sedative. It had been used to treat anemia, impotence, insomnia, diarrhea, fatigue debility, weak digestion and failing memory.

Ligustrum fruit contains bitter compounds that are cardiotonic, relieve pains, increase the flow of urine and are laxative. In addition, these compounds are antiseptic, increase immune response by stimulating the production of white blood cells and reduce inflammation in the eye. Ligustrum has been used to treat lumbago, constipation, cataracts, retinitis, pneumonia, bronchitis, urinary tract infections, gastroenteritis, colds, flu and dysmenorrhea.

Achyranthes root contains bitter compounds that increase the production of urine, relieve pains, lower blood pressure and decrease peristalsis. These compounds also increase the contraction of the uterus and promote menstruation. It also contains mucilaginous compounds that sooth inflamed tissue and increase the production of mucosal fluids. Achyranthes has been used to treat amenorrhea, backaches, hypertension, muscle aches and dysuria.

Atractylodes root contains aromatic compounds that are antiseptic, increase the production of digestive fluids and enzymes, increase blood pressure, are laxative, stimulate liver function and increase the flow of urine. It has been used to treat dyspepsia, flatulence, loss of appetite, nausea, indigestion, rheumatic arthritis and night blindness.

Ho Shou Wu root contains bitter compounds that have a laxative effect, lower blood cholesterol and are antiseptic. These compounds also increase the flow of urine, relieve smooth muscle spasms and are cardiotonic. Ho shou wu is an excellent herbal source of lecithin. It has been used to treat constipation, hypertension, inflammatory skin conditions, hypercholesterolemia and lumbago.

Cyperus root contains aromatic compounds that relieve smooth muscle spasms especially in the uterus, increase the production of digestive fluids and relieve pains. It has been used to treat dyspepsia, dysmenorrhea, nausea, flatulence, abdominal pain and menorrhagia.

Ginger and Dong Quai Combination

Composition

Dong Quai	Parsley
Uva Ursi	Ginger
Juniper Berry	Marshmallow
Goldenseal	

Properties

Carminative	Diuretic
Anti-inflammatory	Stimulant
Antiseptic	Male tonic

General Description

Ginger and Dong Quai Combination is a male tonic formula. It is used to restore sexual function, improve digestion and enhance the body's detoxifying function. The herbs increase the flow of urine, shrink inflamed tissues, are antiseptic, increase the production of digestive fluids and enzymes and increase blood circulation.

Chinese herbalists would describe this herbal combination as an earth reducing formula. It also reduces the water and wood elements while enhancing the fire and metal elements.

Ginger and Dong Quai combination has traditionally been used to treat **indigestion, bloating, nausea, food allergies, diarrhea, scanty urine, difficult urination** and **sleepiness after eating.**

Imbalances indicating the use of this formula are commonly noted in the pancreas acupressure point located just above the navel. Imbalances are often noted at the 6:30 position of the left iris and at the 7 o'clock position of the right iris. Use caution in cases of nephritis.

This formula is commonly used in conjunction with the vitamin C family, raw or slightly cooked foods, digestive enzymes, potassium, manganese and magnesium.

Individual Components

Dong Quai root contains aromatic compounds that relieve smooth muscle spasms especially in the uterus, have a sedative effect and increase the production of digestive fluids. It also contains bitter compounds that regulate glycogen production in the liver, reduce pain and inflammation, increase blood flow, especially to the heart, lower blood cholesterol, normalize uterine

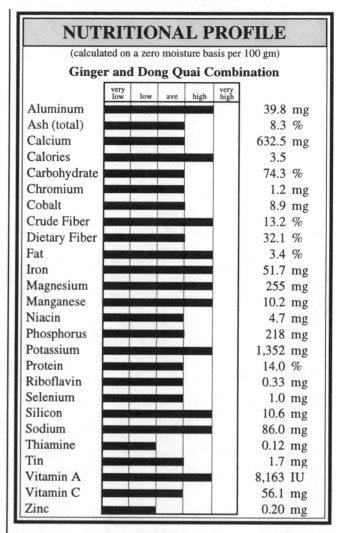

NUTRITIONAL PROFILE
(calculated on a zero moisture basis per 100 gm)

Ginger and Dong Quai Combination

	very low	low	ave	high	very high	
Aluminum						39.8 mg
Ash (total)						8.3 %
Calcium						632.5 mg
Calories						3.5
Carbohydrate						74.3 %
Chromium						1.2 mg
Cobalt						8.9 mg
Crude Fiber						13.2 %
Dietary Fiber						32.1 %
Fat						3.4 %
Iron						51.7 mg
Magnesium						255 mg
Manganese						10.2 mg
Niacin						4.7 mg
Phosphorus						218 mg
Potassium						1,352 mg
Protein						14.0 %
Riboflavin						0.33 mg
Selenium						1.0 mg
Silicon						10.6 mg
Sodium						86.0 mg
Thiamine						0.12 mg
Tin						1.7 mg
Vitamin A						8,163 IU
Vitamin C						56.1 mg
Zinc						0.20 mg

contractions and are antiseptic. Dong quai is an excellent herbal source of iron, magnesium and niacin. It has been used to treat anemia, abdominal pains, dysmenorrhea, amenorrhea, arthritis, coronary heart disease, atherosclerosis, angina pectoris, indigestion and headaches.

Uva ursi fruit contains bitter compounds that are antiseptic and increase the flow of urine. It also contains astringent compounds that shrink inflamed tissue. It has been used to treat urinary tract infections, kidney stones, cystitis, nephritis, hemorrhoids and diarrhea.

Juniper berry contains aromatic compounds that increase the flow of urine, increase the production of digestive fluids, relieve pain and are antiseptic. The herb has been used to treat cystitis, flatulence, burning urination, dysuria, urinary tract infections, kidney stones, rheumatism, gout and edema.

Goldenseal root is an excellent herbal source of trace minerals including cobalt, iron, magnesium, manganese, silicon and zinc. It is also an excellent herbal source of vitamin C. It has been used to treat hepatitis, gastritis, colitis, ulcers, menorrhagia, postpartum hemorrhage, dysmenorrhea, diabetes, infections, hemorrhoids, eczema, obesity and fevers.

Parsley herb contains aromatic compounds that decrease the thickness and increase the production of mucosal fluids, increase the production of digestive fluids, increase menstrual and urine flow. It contains bitter compounds that reduce muscle spasms and pains, reduce blood pressure and are antiseptic. Parsley is an excellent herbal source of trace minerals especially the electrolyte minerals including sodium, potassium, calcium and magnesium. It is also an excellent herbal source of vitamin A, vitamin C and chlorophyllins. Parsley has been used to treat urinary tract infections, amenorrhea, dysmenorrhea, dyspepsia, bronchitis, allergies, arthritis, asthma, flatulence, dysuria and nephritis.

Ginger root contains aromatic compounds that increase the production of digestive fluids and enzymes, lower blood pressure, lower blood sugar and cholesterol. It also contains bitter compounds that reduce muscle spasms, increase blood circulation and dilate blood vessels. Ginger is an excellent herbal source of trace minerals especially silicon, magnesium and manganese. It has been used to treat nausea, motion sickness, flatulence, colds, coughs, indigestion, fevers, vomiting, diarrhea, chronic bronchitis and cold hands and feet.

Marshmallow root contains mucilaginous compounds that decrease the thickness while increasing the production of mucosal fluids, soothe inflamed tissue, heal wounds and increase the flow of urine. It is an excellent herbal source of trace minerals especially chromium, iron, magnesium, and selenium. Marshmallow has been used to treat allergies, gastritis, gastric ulcers, enteritis, coughs, cystitis and hay fever.

Ginseng Combination

Composition

Siberian Ginseng	Pollen	Peppermint
Ho Shou Wu	Bayberry	Capsicum
Licorice	Fennel	Eucalyptus
Gentain	Slippery Elm	Lemongrass
Black Walnut	Myrrh	Safflower

Properties

Carminative	Adaptogen
Stimulant	Nutritive

General Description

Ginseng combination is a stress relieving formula. It is used where unusual stress increases the demand for nutrients such as athletic competition or periods of convalescence. The herbs increase the production of digestive fluids, increase circulation, enhance the absorption of nutrients and improve the body's response to stress.

Chinese herbalists would describe this herbal combination as an earth enhancing formula. It also enhances the fire and metal element while reducing the water and wood elements.

Ginseng combination has traditionally been used to treat **anorexia, dyspepsia, athletic training, fevers**

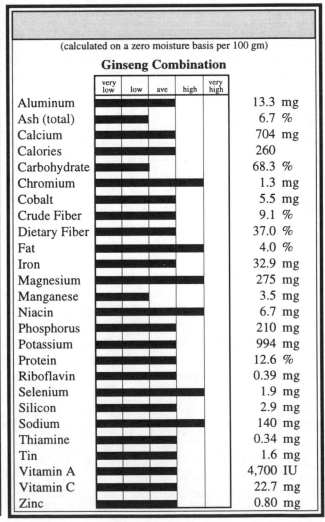

(calculated on a zero moisture basis per 100 gm)

Ginseng Combination

	very low	low	ave	high	very high		
Aluminum						13.3	mg
Ash (total)						6.7	%
Calcium						704	mg
Calories						260	
Carbohydrate						68.3	%
Chromium						1.3	mg
Cobalt						5.5	mg
Crude Fiber						9.1	%
Dietary Fiber						37.0	%
Fat						4.0	%
Iron						32.9	mg
Magnesium						275	mg
Manganese						3.5	mg
Niacin						6.7	mg
Phosphorus						210	mg
Potassium						994	mg
Protein						12.6	%
Riboflavin						0.39	mg
Selenium						1.9	mg
Silicon						2.9	mg
Sodium						140	mg
Thiamine						0.34	mg
Tin						1.6	mg
Vitamin A						4,700	IU
Vitamin C						22.7	mg
Zinc						0.80	mg

with chills, headaches, jet lag, muscle spasms, parasites and geriatric patients who lack appetite.

Imbalances indicating the use of this formula are commonly noted in the stomach acupressure point located approximately one inch below and one inch to the left of the sternum. Imbalances are often noted in the nerve wreath surrounding each pupil.

This formula is commonly used in conjunction with the vitamin C family, the complex of B vitamins, calcium and zinc.

Individual Components

Siberian Ginseng root contains bitter compounds that help the body respond more quickly to stress. These compounds increase the production of DNA, RNA and proteins essential to all life processes. They also stimulate the adrenal, pancreas, and pituitary glands to lower blood sugar and reduce inflammation. Ginseng also increases the production of digestive fluids and is a mild sedative. It had been used to treat anemia, impotence, insomnia, diarrhea, fatigue debility, weak digestion and failing memory.

Ho Shou Wu root contains bitter compounds that have a laxative effect, lower blood cholesterol, and are antiseptic. These compounds also increase the flow of urine, relieve smooth muscle spasms and are cardiotonic. Ho shou wu is an excellent herbal source of lecithin. It has been used to treat constipation, hyper tension, inflammatory skin conditions, hypercholesterolemia and lumbago.

Licorice root contains bitter compounds that reduce inflammation, decrease the thickness and increase the production of mucosal fluids and relieve muscle spasms. In addition, licorice stimulates adrenal function, reduces the urge to cough, is mildly laxative and enhances immune response. It has been used to treat coughs, colds, arthritis, asthma, peptic ulcers, Addison's disease, dropsy and atherosclerosis.

Gentain root contains bitter compounds that increase appetite by enhancing the production of digestive fluids and enzymes, particularly bile. It is an excellent herbal source of vitamin B-1, niacin, magnesium, phosphorus, selenium and zinc. Gentain has been used to treat anorexia, dyspepsia, loss of appetite, indigestion and gallstones.

Black Walnut hull contains astringent compounds that shrink inflamed tissues of the digestive system. It also contains bitter compounds that are antifungal and decrease the secretion of fluids in the digestive system. Black walnut has been used to treat hemorrhoids, inflammatory skin conditions, colitis, intestinal worms and parasites and fevers.

Pollen is gathered by bees from a variety of flowers. It is an excellent source of carbohydrates which may in part account for its reputation as an energy booster. Pollen has been used to treat fatigue, sexual dysfunction, poor memory and convalescence.

Bayberry bark contains astringent compounds that reduce the secretion of fluids, reduce pain and shrink inflamed tissues. These compounds also promote sweating, increase blood circulation and dilate peripheral blood vessels. It has been used to treat diarrhea, colds, intestinal flu, inflammatory conditions of the gastrointestinal tract, asthma, bronchitis, fevers and sinus congestion.

Fennel seed contains aromatic compounds that stimulate the production of digestive fluids, relieve inflammation, are antiseptic, make one breath deeply and more often and increase the flow of urine. It has been used to treat indigestion, dyspepsia, anorexia, colic, flatulence, coughs and colds.

Slippery Elm bark contains mucilaginous compounds that decrease the thickness while increasing the production of mucosal fluids. These compounds soothe inflamed tissue, decrease bowel transit time and absorb toxins from the bowel. It also contains astringent compounds that shrink inflamed tissues. Slippery elm has been used to treat asthma, bronchitis, colitis, coughs, weak digestion and inflammatory bowel diseases.

Myrrh gum contains astringent resins that promote the healing of sores. These compounds shrink inflamed tissue, are antiseptic and reduce pain in mucous membranes. Myrrh also decreases the thickness while increasing the production of mucosal fluids. It has been used to treat colds, coughs, bronchitis, asthma, dysmenorrhea, rheumatism and arthritis.

Peppermint leaf contains aromatic compounds that increase the production of digestive fluids, relieve muscle spasms, increase blood circulation, reduce pains, promote sweating and are antiseptic. It also contains astringent compounds which shrink inflamed tissues. Peppermint has been used to treat indigestion, flatulence, mouth sores, loss of appetite, muscle cramps, nausea, morning sickness and dysmenorrhea.

Capsicum fruit contains aromatic resins that increase blood circulation, promote sweating, increase the production of digestive fluids and reduce muscle spasms. It has been used to treat flatulence, colic, ulcers, rheumatic arthritis, cold hands and feet and dropsy.

Eucalyptus leaf contains aromatic compounds that decrease the thickness while increasing the production of mucosal fluids, are antiseptic, relieve smooth muscle spasms, promote sweating and relieve pains. It has been used to treat bronchitis, asthma, backaches, inflammatory skin conditions, fevers, colds, flu and respiratory tract infections.

Lemongrass herb contains aromatic compounds that have a sedative effect, decrease the secretion of fluids and are antiseptic. It has been used to treat colds, flu, nausea, indigestion and anxiety.

Safflowers contain bitter compounds that increase the production and release of bile. It is an excellent herbal source of unsaturated fatty acids. Safflowers has been used to treat liver congestion, gallstones, gout, scarlet fever, indigestion and amenorrhea.

Ginseng and Saw Palmetto Combination

Composition

Siberian Ginseng	Damiana	Garlic
Saw Palmetto	Sarsaparilla	Capsicum
Parthenium	Horsetail	Chickweed
Gotu Kola		

Properties

Stimulant	Antiseptic
Anti-inflammatory	Astringent
Diuretic	Adaptogen
Carminative	Nervine

General Description

Ginseng and Saw Palmetto combination is a male corrective formula. It is used to reduce inflammation in the reproductive and urinary systems particularly the prostate and kidneys. The herbs increase the flow of urine, shrink inflamed tissue, are antiseptic, increase blood circulation, enhance the body's response to stress, increase the production of digestive fluids and calm the nerves.

Chinese herbalists would describe this herbal combination as an earth enhancing formula. It also enhances the fire and metal elements while reducing the water and wood elements.

Ginseng and Saw Palmetto combination has traditionally been used to treat **decreased libido, insomnia, chronic weakness, debility, impotence, night sweats, nocturnal emissions, prostatitis, diarrhea, turbid urine** and **anorexia.**

Imbalances indicating the use of this formula are commonly noted in the prostate acupressure point located just above the pubic bone. Imbalances are often noted at the 7 o'clock position of the left iris and the 5 o'clock position of the right iris. Use caution in cases of gallstones.

This formula is commonly used in conjunction with the vitamin C family, zinc, parsley, pumpkin, bee pollen, calcium and magnesium.

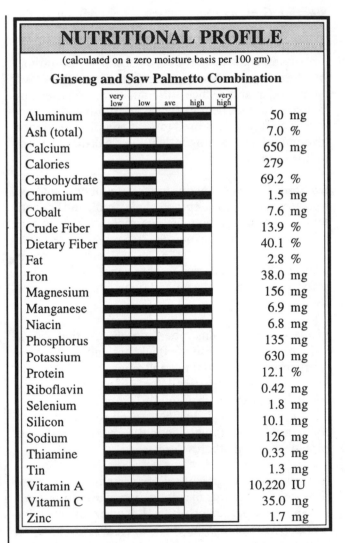

NUTRITIONAL PROFILE

(calculated on a zero moisture basis per 100 gm)

Ginseng and Saw Palmetto Combination

Nutrient	Amount
Aluminum	50 mg
Ash (total)	7.0 %
Calcium	650 mg
Calories	279
Carbohydrate	69.2 %
Chromium	1.5 mg
Cobalt	7.6 mg
Crude Fiber	13.9 %
Dietary Fiber	40.1 %
Fat	2.8 %
Iron	38.0 mg
Magnesium	156 mg
Manganese	6.9 mg
Niacin	6.8 mg
Phosphorus	135 mg
Potassium	630 mg
Protein	12.1 %
Riboflavin	0.42 mg
Selenium	1.8 mg
Silicon	10.1 mg
Sodium	126 mg
Thiamine	0.33 mg
Tin	1.3 mg
Vitamin A	10,220 IU
Vitamin C	35.0 mg
Zinc	1.7 mg

Individual Components

Siberian Ginseng root contains bitter compounds that help the body respond more quickly to stress. These compounds increase the production of DNA, RNA and proteins essential to all life processes. They stimulate the adrenal, pancreas, and pituitary glands to lower blood sugar and reduce inflammation. Ginseng also increases the production of digestive fluids and is a mild sedative. It has been used to treat anemia, impotence, insomnia, diarrhea, fatigue, debility, weak digestion and failing memory.

Saw Palmetto berry contains aromatic compounds that increase the flow of urine, are antiseptic and shrink inflamed tissues in the urinary system. It has been used to treat prostatitis, impotence and urinary tract infections.

Parthenium root contains mucilaginous compounds that increase immune response, sequester infection and soothe inflamed tissue. Parthenium also contains bitter compounds that increase immune response by increasing the production of T-lymphocytes, phagocytic macrophages, interferons and lymphokines. Parthenium has been used to treat wounds, infections, blood poisoning, inflammatory skin conditions and tonsilitis.

Gotu Kola herb contains bitter compounds that have a sedative effect, dilate peripheral blood vessels and increase the flow of urine. It is an excellent herbal source of niacin, calcium, magnesium, manganese, silicon and sodium. Gotu kola has been used to treat insomnia, failing memory, schizophrenia, fevers, headache and inflammatory skin conditions.

Damiana herb contains aromatic compounds that increase blood circulation, calm the nerves and relieve smooth muscle spasms. It is an excellent herbal source of vitamin A, vitamin C and niacin. Damiana has been used to treat anxiety, prostatitis, impotence, hot flashes and fatigue.

Sarsaparilla root contains bitter compounds that increase the production of urine and promote sweating. These compounds also relieve inflammation, muscle spasms and are antiseptic. Sarsaparilla is an excellent herbal source of chromium, cobalt, iron, and selenium. It has been used to treat rheumatism, gout, fevers, inflammatory skin conditions, prostatitis and impotence.

Horsetail herb contains bitter compounds that increase the production of urine and shrink inflamed mucosal tissue, particularly the prostate. Horsetail is most noted for its trace mineral profile since it is an excellent herbal source of bioavailable silicon, calcium, magnesium, chromium, iron, manganese and potassium. It has been used to treat prostatitis, osteoporosis, enuresis, urinary tract infections and muscle cramps.

Garlic bulb contains aromatic compounds that lower blood pressure, heart rate and blood cholesterol while increasing coronary circulation. These compounds also fight infections, reduce muscle spasms, increase immune response, promote sweating, increase the production of digestive fluids and decrease the thickness while increasing the production of mucosal fluid. Garlic has been used to treat colds, coughs, asthma, coronary heart disease, hypertension, atherosclerosis, infections, inflammatory skin conditions and hemorrhoids.

Capsicum fruit contains aromatic resins that increase blood circulation, promote sweating, increase the production of digestive fluids and reduce muscle spasms. It has been used to treat flatulence, colic, ulcers, rheumatic arthritis, cold hands and feet and dropsy.

Chickweed herb contains mucilaginous compounds that absorb toxins from the bowel, soothe inflamed tissues, give bulk to the stool and increase the flow of urine. These compounds also decrease the thickness while increasing the production of mucosal fluids. Chickweed has been used to treat rheumatism, arthritis, inflammatory skin conditions and obesity.

Goldenseal and Juniper Combination

Composition

Goldenseal	Garlic	Marshmallow
Juniper berry	Yarrow	Buchu
Uva Ursi	Capsicum	White Oak
Huckleberry	Dandelion	Licorice
Mullein		

Properties

Carminative	Male tonic
Diuretic	Expectorant
Cholagogue	Demucent
Anti-inflammatory	

General Description

Goldenseal and Juniper combination relieves inflammation in the glandular system especially the prostate and pancreas. The herbs increase the flow of urine, increase the flow of digestive fluids and enzymes particularly pancreatin and bile. They also soothe inflamed tissues and increase the production of mucosal fluids.

Chinese herbalists would describe this herbal combination as an earth enhancing formula. It also enhances the fire element while reducing the wood, water, and metal elements.

Goldenseal and Juniper combination has traditionally been used to treat **pancreatitis, acid indigestion, nausea, flatulence** and **abdominal flu.**

Imbalances indicating the use of this formula are commonly noted in the pancreas acupressure point located approximately four inches below and three inches to the left of the sternum. Imbalances are often noted at the 7 o'clock position of the right iris. Use caution in cases of chronic debility and convalescence.

This formula is commonly used in conjunction with chromium, vitamin C family, complex of B vitamins, vitamin A and vitamin E.

Individual Components

Goldenseal root contains bitter astringent alkaloids that normalize liver and spleen functions by increasing the production of digestive fluids and enzymes, particularly bile. The compounds are antiseptic, constrict peripheral blood vessels, especially in the uterus, are laxative and relieve pain and inflammation in mucosal tissue. Goldenseal is an excellent herbal source of trace minerals including cobalt, iron, magnesium, manganese, silicon and zinc. It is also an excellent herbal source of vitamin C. It has been used to treat hepatitis, gastritis, colitis, ulcers, menorrhagia, postpartum hemorrhages, dysmenorrhea, diabetes, infections, hemorrhoids, eczema, obesity and fevers.

Juniper berry contains aromatic compounds that increase the flow of urine, increase the production of digestive fluids, relieve pain and are antiseptic. The herb has been used to treat cystitis, flatulence, burning urination, dysuria, urinary tract infections, kidney stones, rheumatism, gout and edema.

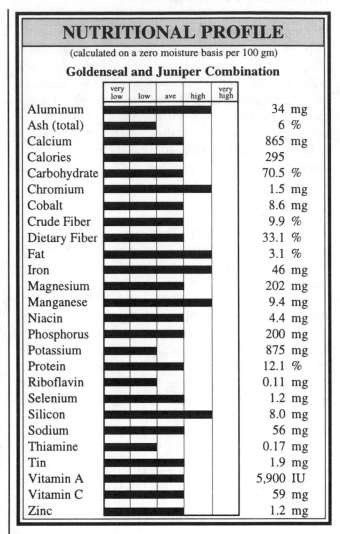

NUTRITIONAL PROFILE
(calculated on a zero moisture basis per 100 gm)

Goldenseal and Juniper Combination

	very low	low	ave	high	very high		
Aluminum						34	mg
Ash (total)						6	%
Calcium						865	mg
Calories						295	
Carbohydrate						70.5	%
Chromium						1.5	mg
Cobalt						8.6	mg
Crude Fiber						9.9	%
Dietary Fiber						33.1	%
Fat						3.1	%
Iron						46	mg
Magnesium						202	mg
Manganese						9.4	mg
Niacin						4.4	mg
Phosphorus						200	mg
Potassium						875	mg
Protein						12.1	%
Riboflavin						0.11	mg
Selenium						1.2	mg
Silicon						8.0	mg
Sodium						56	mg
Thiamine						0.17	mg
Tin						1.9	mg
Vitamin A						5,900	IU
Vitamin C						59	mg
Zinc						1.2	mg

Uva ursi fruit contains bitter compounds that are antiseptic and increase the flow of urine. It also contains astringent compounds that shrink inflamed tissue. It has been used to treat urinary tract infections, kidney stones, cystitis, nephritis, hemorrhoids and diarrhea.

Huckleberry contains bitter compounds that increase the flow of urine and raise blood sugar. It also contains astringent compounds that are antiseptic and shrink inflamed tissues. Huckleberry has been used to treat diabetes, dysuria and pancreatitis.

Mullein leaves contain mucilaginous compounds that decrease the thickness and increase the production of mucosal fluids. These compounds also soothe inflamed tissue. Mullein also contains aromatic compounds that increase the flow of urine. The herb has been used to treat bronchitis, coughs, colds, hay fever, dysuria, nephritis and sinus congestion.

Garlic bulb contains aromatic compounds that lower blood pressure, heart rate and blood cholesterol while increasing coronary circulation. These compounds also fight infections, reduce muscle spasms, increase immune response, promote sweating, increase the production of digestive fluids and decrease the thickness while increasing the production of mucosal fluid. Garlic has been used to treat colds, coughs, asthma, coronary heart disease, hypertension, atherosclerosis, infections, inflammatory skin conditions and hemorrhoids.

Yarrow flower contains aromatic compounds that shrink inflamed tissues and promote sweating. It also contains bitter compounds that relieve smooth muscle spasms, reduce blood pressure and stop bleeding. Yarrow has been used to treat hemorrhoids, fevers, nausea, and inflammatory skin conditions.

Capsicum fruit contains aromatic resins that increase blood circulation, promote sweating, increase the production of digestive fluids and reduce muscle spasms. It has been used to treat flatulence, colic, ulcers, rheumatic arthritis, cold hands and feet and dropsy.

Dandelion root contains bitter compounds that enhance the efficiency of the body's eliminative and detoxifying functions. These compounds help restore normal liver function, increase the production of digestive fluids and enzymes particularly bile, increase the flow of urine and have a laxative effect. Dandelion is an excellent herbal source of sodium, iron, and vitamin A. It has been used to treat jaundice, gallstones, dyspepsia, constipation, inflammatory skin conditions, frequent urination, hepatitis, gout and rheumatism.

Marshmallow root contains mucilaginous compounds that decrease the thickness while increasing the production of mucosal fluids, soothe inflamed tissue, heal wounds and increase the flow of urine. It is an excellent herbal source of trace minerals especially chromium, iron, magnesium and selenium. Marshmallow has been used to treat allergies, gastritis, gastric ulcers, enteritis, coughs, cystitis and hay fever.

Buchu leaf contains aromatic compounds that increase the production of urine and are antiseptic. It also contains astringent compounds that shrink inflamed tissues. Buchu has been used to treat dysuria, urinary tract infections, gout, nephritis, arthritis and rheumatism.

White Oak bark contains astringent compounds that are anitseptic, stop bleeding, and shrink inflamed tissues. It has been used to treat hemorrhoids, diarrhea and insect bites.

Licorice root contains bitter compounds that reduce inflammation, decrease the thickness and increase the production of mucosal fluids and relieve muscle spasms. In addition, licorice stimulates adrenal function, reduces the urge to cough, is mildly laxative and enhances immune response. It has been used to treat coughs, colds, arthritis, asthma, peptic ulcers, Addison's disease, dropsy and atherosclerosis.

Irish Moss and Kelp Combination

Composition

Irish Moss	Sarsaparilla
Kelp	Watercress
Black Walnut	Iceland Moss
Parsley	

Properties

Stimulant	Diuretic
Bulk laxative	Demulcent

General Description

Irish Moss and Kelp combination is used to balance hormonal indeficiency especially in the thyroid gland. It increases the metabolic rate, thyroid activity and the detoxifying function of the body. The herbs supply trace minerals, increase the flow of urine, absorb toxins from the bowel, increase blood circulation, provide bulk to the stool, soothe inflamed tissues and promote the growth of friendly colonic bacteria.

Chinese herbalists would describe this herbal combination as a fire enhancing formula. It also enhances the earth, metal, and water elements while reducing the wood element.

Irish Moss and Kelp combination has been used to treat **enlarged glands (thyroid, prostate, lymph), coughs, debility** and **convalescence.**

Imbalances indicating the use of this formula are commonly noted in the thyroid acupressure point located at the base of the neck, over the thyroid gland. Imbalances are often noted at the 9:30 position of the left iris and at the 2:30 position of the right iris. Use caution in cases of lung or sinus congestion.

This formula is commonly used in conjunction with pumpkin seeds, spirulina, the complex of B vitamins, vitamin A, vitamin C, calcium, manganese and zinc.

Individual Components

Irish Moss herb contains mucilaginous compounds that enhance the detoxifying and eliminative functions of the digestive system. These compounds absorb toxins from the bowel and provide bulk to the stool. Irish Moss is an excellent herbal source of the electrolyte minerals including calcium, magnesium, sodium and iodine. Iodine is essential to normal thyroid function. It is used to increase the metabolic rate and strengthen connective tissues including the hair, skin and nails. Irish moss has been used to treat enlarged

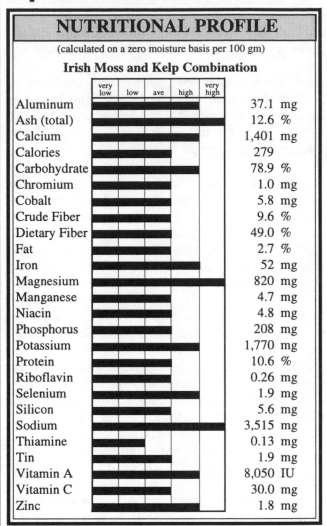

NUTRITIONAL PROFILE

(calculated on a zero moisture basis per 100 gm)

Irish Moss and Kelp Combination

	very low	low	ave	high	very high		
Aluminum						37.1	mg
Ash (total)						12.6	%
Calcium						1,401	mg
Calories						279	
Carbohydrate						78.9	%
Chromium						1.0	mg
Cobalt						5.8	mg
Crude Fiber						9.6	%
Dietary Fiber						49.0	%
Fat						2.7	%
Iron						52	mg
Magnesium						820	mg
Manganese						4.7	mg
Niacin						4.8	mg
Phosphorus						208	mg
Potassium						1,770	mg
Protein						10.6	%
Riboflavin						0.26	mg
Selenium						1.9	mg
Silicon						5.6	mg
Sodium						3,515	mg
Thiamine						0.13	mg
Tin						1.9	mg
Vitamin A						8,050	IU
Vitamin C						30.0	mg
Zinc						1.8	mg

glands, debility, fatigue, eczema, psoriasis, dry coughs and nosebleeds.

Kelp herb contains mucilaginous compounds that enhance the detoxifying and eliminative functions of the digestive system. These compounds absorb toxins from the bowel and provide bulk to the stool. Kelp is an excellent herbal source of calcium, magnesium, sodium and iodine. Iodine is essential to normal thyroid function. It is used to increase the metabolic rate and strengthen connective tissues including the hair, skin and nails. Kelp has been used to treat hypothyroidism, enlarged glands, debility, fatigue, eczema, psoriasis, arthritis and obesity.

Black Walnut hull contains astringent compounds that shrink inflamed tissues of the digestive system. It also contains bitter compounds that are antifungal and decrease the secretion of fluids in the digestive system. Black walnut has been used to treat hemorrhoids, inflammatory skin conditions, colitis, intestinal worms, parasites and fevers.

Parsley herb contains aromatic compounds that decrease the thickness and increase the production of mucosal fluids, increase the production of digestive fluids, increase menstrual and urine flow. It also contains bitter compounds that reduce muscle spasms and pains, reduce blood pressure and are antiseptic. Parsley is an excellent herbal source of trace minerals especially the electrolyte minerals including sodium, potassium, calcium and magnesium. It is also an excellent herbal source of vitamin A, vitamin C, and chlorophyllins. Parsley has been used to treat urinary tract infections, amenorrhea, dysmenorrhea, dyspepsia, bronchitis, allergies, arthritis, asthma, flatulence, dysuria and nephritis.

Sarsaparilla root contains bitter compounds that increase the production of urine and promote sweating. These compounds also relieve inflammation, muscle spasms and are antiseptic. Sarsaparilla is an excellent

herbal source of chromium, cobalt, iron and selenium. It has been used to treat rheumatism, gout, fevers, inflammatory skin conditions, prostatitis and impotence.

Watercress herb contains bitter compounds that increase blood circulation, increase the flow of urine and relieve smooth muscle spasms. It has been used to treat urinary tract infections, eczema, anemia, hepatitis and rheumatism.

Iceland Moss herb contains mucilaginous compounds that absorb toxins from the bowel, provide bulk to the stool and sooth inflamed tissues. It is an excellent herbal source of calcium, magnesium, sodium, potassium and iodine. Iodine increases the metabolic rate and thyroid activity. Iceland moss has been used to treat enlarged glands, inflammatory skin conditions, coughs, debility and chronic constipation.

Kelp Combination

Composition

Kelp	Hops
Irish Moss	Capsicum
Parsley	

Properties

Stimulant
Bulk laxative
Demulcent

General Description

Kelp combination is an iodine supplement. It increases the metabolic rate, thyroid activity and the detoxifying function of the body. The herbs increase body fluids and enrich them with minerals, absorb toxins from the bowel, increase blood circulation, provide bulk to the stool, sooth inflamed tissues and promote the growth of friendly colonic bacteria.

Chinese herbalists would describe this herbal combination as a fire enhancing formula. It also enhances the earth, metal and water elements, while reducing the wood element.

Kelp combination is indicated in cases of **enlarged glands (thyroid, prostate, lymph), coughs, debility** and **convalescence.**

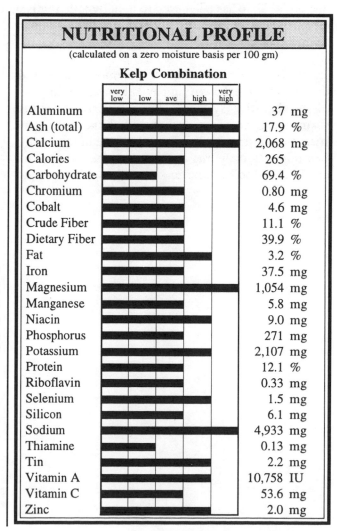

NUTRITIONAL PROFILE
(calculated on a zero moisture basis per 100 gm)
Kelp Combination

	very low	low	ave	high	very high		
Aluminum						37	mg
Ash (total)						17.9	%
Calcium						2,068	mg
Calories						265	
Carbohydrate						69.4	%
Chromium						0.80	mg
Cobalt						4.6	mg
Crude Fiber						11.1	%
Dietary Fiber						39.9	%
Fat						3.2	%
Iron						37.5	mg
Magnesium						1,054	mg
Manganese						5.8	mg
Niacin						9.0	mg
Phosphorus						271	mg
Potassium						2,107	mg
Protein						12.1	%
Riboflavin						0.33	mg
Selenium						1.5	mg
Silicon						6.1	mg
Sodium						4,933	mg
Thiamine						0.13	mg
Tin						2.2	mg
Vitamin A						10,758	IU
Vitamin C						53.6	mg
Zinc						2.0	mg

Imbalances indicating the use of this formula are commonly noted in the thyroid acupressure point located at the base of the neck over the thyroid gland. Imbalances are often noted at the 9:30 position of the left iris and at the 2:30 position of the right iris. Use caution in cases of lung or sinus congestion.

This formula is commonly used in conjunction with black walnut, pumpkin seeds, spirulina, the complex of B vitamins, vitamin A, vitamin C, calcium and zinc.

Individual Components

Kelp herb contains mucilaginous compounds that enhance the detoxifying and eliminative functions of the digestive system. These compounds absorb toxins from the bowel and provide bulk to the stool. Kelp is an excellent herbal source of calcium, magnesium, sodium and iodine. Iodine is essential to normal thyroid function. It is used to increase the metabolic rate and strengthen connective tissues including the hair, skin and nails. Kelp has been used to treat hypothyroidism, enlarged glands, debility, fatigue, eczema, psoriasis, arthritis and obesity.

Irish Moss herb contains mucilaginous compounds that enhance the detoxifying and eliminative functions of the digestive system. These compounds absorb toxins from the bowel and provide bulk to the stool. Irish moss is an excellent herbal source of the electrolyte minerals including calcium, magnesium, sodium and iodine. Iodine is essential to normal thyroid function. It is used to increase the metabolic rate and strengthen connective tissues including the hair, skin and nails. Irish moss has been used to treat enlarged glands, debility, fatigue, eczema, psoriasis, dry cough and nosebleeds.

Parsley herb contains aromatic compounds that decrease the thickness and increase the production of mucosal fluids, increase the production of digestive fluids and increase menstrual and urine flow. It contains bitter compounds that reduce muscle spasms and pains, reduce blood pressure and are antiseptic. Parsley is an excellent herbal source of trace minerals especially the electrolyte minerals including sodium, potassium, calcium, and magnesium. It is also an excellent herbal source of vitamin A, vitamin C, and chloropyllins. Parsley has been used to treat urinary tract infections, amenorrhea, dysmenorrhea, dyspepsia, bronchitis, allergies, arthritis, asthma, flatulence, dysuria and nephritis.

Hops flowers contain bitter compounds that have a sedative effect and relieve smooth muscle spasms, increase the flow of urine and are antiseptic. Hops is an excellent herbal source of niacin. It has been used to treat insomnia, painful urination, urinary tract infections, spastic colons and anxiety.

Capsicum fruit contains aromatic resins that increase blood circulation, promote sweating, increase the production of digestive fluids and reduce muscle spasms. It has been used to treat flatulence, colic, ulcers, rheumatic arthritis, cold hands and feet and dropsy.

Licorice and Red Beet Combination

Composition

Licorice	Hawthorn
Red beet	Fennel

Properties

Expectorant	Diuretic
Stimulant	Laxative

General Description

Licorice and Red Beet combination is an expectorant formula. It is used in conjunction with fasting cleanses to moisten mucous membranes and enhance the elimination of toxins. These fasts usually follow a laxative purge. The herbs decrease the thickness while increasing the production of mucosal fluids, increase blood circulation, promote the metabolism of toxins, increase the flow of urine and are mildly laxative.

Chinese herbalists would describe this herbal combination as a wood reducing formula. It also reduces the water and metal elements while enhancing the fire and earth elements.

Licorice and Red Beet combination has traditionally been used to treat **arthritis, rheumatism, obesity** and **constipation.**

Imbalances indicating the use of this formula are commonly noted in the liver acupressure point located approximately four inches to the right of the sternum between the 7th and 8th rib. Imbalances are often noted at the 7:30 position of the right iris. Use caution in cases of hypertension.

This formula is commonly used in conjunction with vitamin A, iron, the complex of B vitamins, the vitamin C family, yellow dock and horsetail.

Individual Components

Licorice root contains bitter compounds that reduce inflammation, decrease the thickness and increase the production of mucosal fluids and relieve muscle spasms. In addition, licorice stimulates adrenal function, reduces the urge to cough, is mildly laxative and enhances immune response. It has been used to treat coughs, colds, arthritis, asthma, peptic ulcers, Addison's disease, dropsy and atherosclerosis.

Red beet root contains bitter compounds that increase the flow of urine and increase the production of diges-

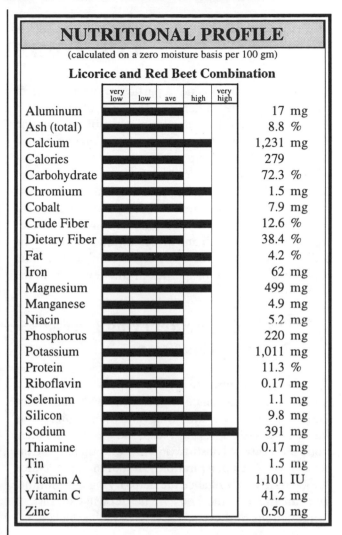

NUTRITIONAL PROFILE
(calculated on a zero moisture basis per 100 gm)

Licorice and Red Beet Combination

	very low	low	ave	high	very high	Value	
Aluminum						17	mg
Ash (total)						8.8	%
Calcium						1,231	mg
Calories						279	
Carbohydrate						72.3	%
Chromium						1.5	mg
Cobalt						7.9	mg
Crude Fiber						12.6	%
Dietary Fiber						38.4	%
Fat						4.2	%
Iron						62	mg
Magnesium						499	mg
Manganese						4.9	mg
Niacin						5.2	mg
Phosphorus						220	mg
Potassium						1,011	mg
Protein						11.3	%
Riboflavin						0.17	mg
Selenium						1.1	mg
Silicon						9.8	mg
Sodium						391	mg
Thiamine						0.17	mg
Tin						1.5	mg
Vitamin A						1,101	IU
Vitamin C						41.2	mg
Zinc						0.50	mg

tive fluids and enzymes. It also contains astringent compounds that shrink inflamed tissues. Red beet is an excellent herbal source of potassium. It has been used to treat liver congestion, menorrhagia, frequent urination and inflammatory skin conditions.

Hawthorn berries contain bitter compounds that increase coronary blood flow and myocardial metabolism allowing the heart to function with less oxygen. These compounds also lower blood pressure by decreasing cardiac output and dilating peripheral blood vessels. It has been used to treat hypertension, coronary heart disease, atherosclerosis, blood clots and insomnia.

Fennel seed contains aromatic compounds that stimulate the production of digestive fluids, relieve inflammation, are antiseptic, make one breathe deeply and more often, and increase the flow of urine. It has been used to treat indigestion, dyspepsia, anorexia, colic, flatulence, coughs and colds.

Chapter 8

The Immune System

The immune system is not a particular organ tissue or group of cells but rather it is the sum of the body's defense functions. It is made up of white blood cells and T-cells, macrophage, lymphokines and enzymes such as immune globins, superoxide dismutase and histamine. The overall function of these defenses is to correctly identify, metabolize and eliminate from the body metabolic waste, cell mutations and allergens that are popularly referred to as "toxins." Immune processes are a part of every cell and affect all the systems of the body. The names for the herbal combinations are chosen based on the properties of the key herbs in the formula.

Therapies for Relieving Excess Conditions

Long before the immune system was described, herbalists knew the importance of purifying the blood. Once a toxin is correctly identified and metabolized, the waste products end up in the blood to be eliminated from the body. These toxins are eliminated via the urine, feces or as perspiration. Herbal therapies called "blood purifiers" enhance the detoxifying and eliminative functions of the body. They consist of various combinations of diuretics, laxatives and stimulants.

Excess conditions in the immune system are often marked by patterns of minor aches, pains and ailments including: urticaria, dermatitis, acne, boils, carbuncles, psoriasis, eczema, food sensitivity, respiratory allergies, joint pains, red eyes and edema. If left unchecked, these ailments may develop into illnesses such as: inflammatory skin conditions, arthritis, lupus, muscular sclerosis, muscular dystrophy, scleroderma, vasculitis, cancers and allergies.

Early herbal therapies for these conditions consisted of single herbs like goldenseal which increases the release of bile. Goldenseal is not simply a cholagogue however, and with time and experience, herbalists recognized and recorded in their herbals the several properties of goldenseal. The British Herbal Pharmacopoeia

lists goldenseal as a stimulant to smooth muscle, stomachic, oxytocic, antihemorrhagic and laxative.

These lists of empirical properties of an herb are the key to understanding herbal combinations. Herbalists have found that they can enhance a particular property of a single herb by adding herbs that complement and support a given property. Conversely, the herbalist is also able to minimize an unwanted property by adding herbs that counteract to balance that property.

Therapies for Supplementing Deficient Conditions

Weaknesses in the immune system are characterized by chronic infections and general weaknesses. Herbalists use immunostimulants and antiseptics to assist the body in ridding itself of infections.

Weakened conditions of the immune system are often associated with patterns of minor aches, pains, and ailments including: candidiasis, ringworm, jock itch, athletes foot, chronic infections, anemia, herpes simplex and herpes zoster. If left unchecked, these ailments may develop into illnesses including: AIDS, herpes, poor wound healing, candidiasis, arthritis, allergies and cancers.

Early herbal therapies for these conditions consisted of single herbs like parthenium which increases immune response. Parthenium is not simply an immunostimulant however, and with time and experience, herbalists recognized and recorded in their herbals the several properties of parthenium. The British Herbal Pharmacopoeia lists parthenium as an antiseptic, antiviral and peripheral vasodilator.

These lists of empirical properties of an herb are the key to understanding herbal combinations. Herbalists have found that they can enhance a particular property of a single herb by adding herbs that complemented and supported that property. Conversely, the herbalist is also able to minimize an unwanted property by adding herbs that counteract or balance the property.

Therapies for Relieving Excess Conditions

Alfalfa and Dandelion Combination

Composition

Kelp
Dandelion
Alfalfa

Properties

Diuretic
Stimulant
Carminative
Cholagogue
Expectorant
Laxative
Demulcent
Nutritive

General Description

Alfalfa and Dandelion combination is a nutritive formula. It improves digestion and nutrient absorption by assisting the detoxifying and eliminative functions. The herbs increase the production of digestive fluids and enzymes, especially bile, soothe inflamed tissues, increase blood circulation, increase the flow of urine and are laxative.

Chinese herbalists would describe this herbal combination as a wood reducing formula. It also reduces the water and metal elements while enhancing the earth and fire elements.

Alfalfa and Dandelion combination has traditionally been used to treat **rheumatism, arthritis, obesity, loss of appetite, dyspepsia, jaundice and constipation.**

Imbalances indicating the use of this formula are commonly noted in the stomach acupressure point located to the left of the sternum. Imbalances are often noted at the 4:30 position of the left iris. Use caution in cases of hyperthyroidism.

This formula is commonly used in conjunction with goldenseal, echinacea, yellowdock, chickweed and the complex of B vitamins.

Individual Components

Kelp herb contains mucilaginous compounds that enhance the detoxifying and eliminative functions of the digestive system. These compounds absorb toxins from the bowel and provide bulk to the stool. Kelp is an excellent herbal source of calcium, magnesium, sodium and iodine. Iodine is essential to normal thyroid function. It is used to increase the metabolic rate and strengthen connective tissues including the hair, skin and nails. Kelp has been used to treat hypothyroidism, enlarged glands, debility, fatigue, eczema, psoriasis, arthritis and obesity.

Dandelion root contains bitter compounds that enhance the efficiency of the body's eliminative and detoxifying functions. These compounds help restore normal liver function, increase the production of digestive fluids and enzymes, particularly bile, increase the flow of urine and have a laxative effect. Dandelion is an excellent herbal source of sodium, iron, and vitamin A. It has been used to treat jaundice, gallstones, dyspepsia, constipation, inflammatory skin conditions, frequent urination, hepatitis, gout and rheumatism.

Alfalfa herb contains bitter compounds that enhance the efficiency of digestion by increasing appetite and the assimilation of nutrients. These compounds also lower blood pressure and balance oestrogenic hormones. Alfalfa is an excellent herbal source of vitamin A, vitamin C, niacin, and vitamin B-1. The herb has been used to treat debility, anorexia, arthritis, weak digestion, hypertension and gout.

Alfalfa and Yucca Combination

Composition

Hydrangea
Yucca
Horsetail
Chaparral
Alfalfa
Black Cohosh
Bromelain
Catnip

Yarrow
Capsicum
Valerian
White Willow
Burdock
Slippery Elm
Sarsaparilla

Properties

Diuretic
Expectorant
Anti-inflammatory
Antispasmodic
Sedative
Analgesic
Antiseptic
Diaphoretic

General Description

Alfalfa and Yucca combination is an arthritis formula. It is used to relieve pain and inflammation in connective tissues by enhancing the body's detoxifying and digestive functions. The herbs increase the flow of urine, decrease the thickness, while increasing the production of mucosal fluid and muscle spasms. The herbs also are sedative, promote sweating and are antiseptic.

Chinese herbalists would describe this herbal combination as a wood reducing or harmonizing formula. It also reduces the fire and metal elements while enhancing the earth and water elements.

Alfalfa and Yucca combination has traditionally been used to treat **arthritis, edema, skin inflammations, gout, rheumatism, gastritis, turbid urine, hypertension and general debility.**

Imbalances indicating the use of this formula are commonly noted in the liver acupressure point located approximately four inches to the right of the sternum between the 7th and 8th rib. Imbalances are often noted at the 7:30 position of the right iris. Use caution in cases of anemia, chronic chills and premenstrual syndrome.

This formula is commonly used in conjunction with the vitamin C family, vitamin B-6, zinc, and manganese, lobelia, schizandra and Chinese ephedra.

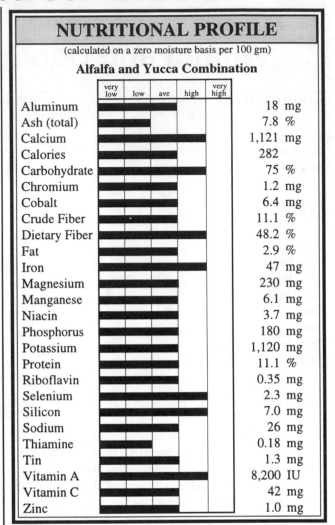

NUTRITIONAL PROFILE
(calculated on a zero moisture basis per 100 gm)

Alfalfa and Yucca Combination

	very low	low	ave	high	very high		
Aluminum						18	mg
Ash (total)						7.8	%
Calcium						1,121	mg
Calories						282	
Carbohydrate						75	%
Chromium						1.2	mg
Cobalt						6.4	mg
Crude Fiber						11.1	%
Dietary Fiber						48.2	%
Fat						2.9	%
Iron						47	mg
Magnesium						230	mg
Manganese						6.1	mg
Niacin						3.7	mg
Phosphorus						180	mg
Potassium						1,120	mg
Protein						11.1	%
Riboflavin						0.35	mg
Selenium						2.3	mg
Silicon						7.0	mg
Sodium						26	mg
Thiamine						0.18	mg
Tin						1.3	mg
Vitamin A						8,200	IU
Vitamin C						42	mg
Zinc						1.0	mg

Individual Components

Hydrangea root contains bitter compounds that increase the production of urine. It also contains astringent compounds that shrink inflamed tissues. Hydrangea has been used to treat urinary tract infections, arthritis, kidney stones, bladder stones, gout and rheumatism.

Yucca root contains bitter compounds that enhance the absorption of nutrients and promote the growth of friendly coloni bacteria. It has been used to treat yeast infections, arthritis, liver congestion and rheumatism.

Horsetail herb contains bitter compounds that increase the production of urine and shrink inflamed mucosal tissue, particularly the prostate. Horsetail is most noted for its trace mineral profile as it is an excellent herbal source of bioavailable silicon, calcium, magnesium, chromium, iron, manganese and potassium. It has been used to treat prostatitis, osteoporosis, enuresis, urinary tract infections and muscle cramps.

Chaparral contains bitter compounds that are antiseptic and increase immune response (anti-oxidant). It also contains aromatic compounds that increase the flow of urine and decrease the thickness while increasing the production of mucosal fluids. Chaparral is an excellent herbal source of vitamin A and vitamin C. It has been used to treat arthritis, blood diseases, allergies and inflammatory skin conditions.

Alfalfa herb contains bitter compounds that enhance the efficiency of digestion by increasing appetite and the assimilation of nutrients. These compounds also lower blood pressure and balance oestrogenic hormones. Alfalfa is an excellent herbal source of vitamin A, vitamin C, niacin and vitamin B-1. The herb has been used to treat debility, anorexia, arthritis, weak digestion, hypertension and gout.

Black Cohosh root contains bitter compounds that relieve smooth muscle spasms, reduce blood pressure and dilate peripheral blood vessels. It also contains astringent compounds that shrink inflamed tissue. Black cohosh has been employed in most inflammatory conditions associated with spasms or tension. It is an excellent herbal source of iron and vitamin A. Black cohosh has been used to treat menstrual cramps, nervous tension, anxiety, dysmenorrhea, hysteria, menopause, fevers and headaches.

Bromelain is a proteolytic enzyme found in pineapple and other plants. It enhances the efficiency of protein digestion. Bromelain has been used to treat dyspepsia, indigestion, bloating, nausea and arthritis.

Catnip herb contains aromatic compounds that have a sedative effect, relieve smooth muscle spasms and induce sweating. It has been used to treat coughs, colds, anxiety, colic, fevers, influenza, lung congestion and nausea.

Yarrow flower contains aromatic compounds that shrink inflamed tissues and promote sweating. It also contains bitter compounds that relieve smooth muscle spasms, reduce blood pressure and stop bleeding. Yarrow has been used to treat hemorrhoids, fevers, nausea and inflammatory skin conditions.

Capsicum fruit contains aromatic resins that increase blood circulation, promote sweating, increase the production of digestive fluids and reduce muscle spasms. It has been used to treat flatulence, colic, ulcers, rheumatic arthritis, cold hands and feet and dropsy.

Valerian root contains aromatic compounds that have a sedative effect, acting to decrease anxiety and aggression. These compounds also relieve smooth muscle spasms, lower blood pressure, and improve sleep quality in cases of insomnia. The herb is relatively inactive in normal sleepers. Valerian is the very best herbal source of calcium and an excellent herbal source of magnesium. It has been used to treat nervousness, anxiety, insomnia, stomach cramps, muscle spasms, hysteria and convulsions.

White Willow bark contains bitter compounds (salicylates) which are well known for their anti-inflammatory effects on connective tissues. These compounds relieve pain and reduce fevers. White willow also contains astringent compounds which shrink inflamed tissues. It is an excellent herbal source of magnesium. White willow has been used to treat rheumatism, arthritis, joint pains, fevers, headaches, influenza and earaches.

Burdock root contains mucilaginous compounds that decrease the thickness while increasing the production of mucosal fluids, soothe inflamed tissues and absorb toxins from the bowel. It also contains aromatic compounds that have an antiseptic effect and increase the flow of urine. The herb is an excellent herbal source of chromium, iron, magnesium, phosphorus, potassium, silicon and zinc. Burdock has been used to treat arthritis, allergies, eczema, bronchitis, urinary tract infections, gout and rheumatism.

Slippery Elm bark contains mucilaginous compounds that decrease the thickness while increasing the production of mucosal fluids. These compounds also soothe inflamed tissue, decrease bowel transit time and absorb toxins from the bowel. It also contains astringent compounds that shrink inflamed tissues. Slippery elm has been used to treat asthma, bronchitis, colitis, coughs, weak digestion and inflammatory bowel disease.

Sarsaparilla root contains bitter compounds that increase the production of urine and promote sweating. These compounds also relieve inflammation, muscle spasms and are antiseptic. Sarsaparilla is an excellent herbal source of chromium, cobalt, iron and selenium. It has been used to treat rheumatism, gout, fevers, inflammatory skin conditions, prostatitis and impotence.

Bupleurum and Peony Combination

Composition

Bupleurum	Licorice
Peony	Zhishi
Scute	Pinellia
Dong Quai	Cinnamon twig
Siberian Ginseng	Atractylodes
Ginger	Fushen

Properties

Diuretic
Carminative
Antidepressant
Diaphoretic
Cholagogue
Laxative

General Description

Bupleurum and Peony combination is used to relieve nervous tension and depression by restoring normal liver function. The herbs work to relieve depression and increase the production of digestive fluids and enzymes, especially bile. They also increase the flow of urine, promote sweating, increase peristaltic action and relieve muscle cramps.

Chinese herbalists would describe this herbal combination as a wood reducing formula. It also reduces the water element while enhancing the earth, metal and fire elements.

Bupleurum and Peony combination has traditionally been used to treat **depression, nervous tension, muscular tension, gallstones, hepatitis, hypoglycemia, anemia, gastric ulcers, inflammatory skin conditions, dysmenorrhea, migraine headaches** and **premenstrual syndrome.**

Imbalances indicating the use of this formula are commonly noted in the liver acupressure point located approximately four inches to the right of the sternum, between the 7th and 8th ribs. Imbalances are often noted at the 7:30 position of the left iris. Use caution in cases of inflammatory bowel disease.

This formula is commonly used in conjunction with evening primrose oil, vitamin E, the vitamin C family, the complex of B vitamins and goldenseal.

Individual Components

Bupleurum root contains bitter compounds that have an antidepressant effect, relieve pain and inflammation, reduce fevers, and have an antiseptic effect. In addition, these compounds reduce blood cholesterol and triglyceride levels, reduce fat cell production and inflammation in the liver. Bupleurum has been used to treat premenstrual syndrome, dysmenorrhea, lung congestion, malaria, muscle cramps, tumors, inflammatory skin conditions, angina pains, epilepsy and depression.

Peony root contains bitter compounds that are sedative, antiseptic and relieve pains. These compounds also lower blood pressure and decrease capillary permeability. It has been used to treat arthralgia, gastric pains, inflammatory skin conditions and dysmenorrhea.

Scute root contains bitter compounds that increase the flow of urine, are antiseptic, reduce capillary permeability and inflammation, increase the secretion of bile and relieve muscle spasms. It has been used to treat urinary tract infections, enteritis, coughs, colds, dysentery and jaundice.

Dong Quai root contains aromatic compounds that relieve smooth muscle spasms especially in the uterus, have a sedative effect and increase the production of digestive fluids. It also contains bitter compounds that regulate glycogen production in the liver, reduce pain and inflammation, increase blood flow especially to the heart, lower blood cholesterol, normalize uterine contractions and are antiseptic. Dong quai is an excellent herbal source of iron, magnesium and niacin. It has been used to treat anemia, abdominal pains, dysmenorrhea, amenorrhea, arthritis, coronary heart disease, atherosclerosis, angina pectoris, indigestion and headaches.

Siberian Ginseng root contains bitter compounds that help the body respond more quickly to stress. These compounds increase the production of DNA, RNA and proteins essential to all life processes. They stimulate the adrenal, pancreas, and pituitary glands to lower blood sugar and reduce inflammation. Ginseng also increases the production of digestive fluids and is a mild sedative. It had been used to treat anemia, impotence, insomnia, diarrhea, fatigue debility, weak digestion and failing memory.

Ginger root contains aromatic compounds that increase the production of digestive fluids and enzymes, lower blood pressure, lower blood sugar and cholesterol. It also contains bitter compounds that reduce muscle spasms, increase blood circulation and dilate blood vessels. Ginger is an excellent herbal source of trace minerals especially silicon, magnesium and manganese. It has been used to treat nausea, motion sickness, flatulence, colds, coughs, indigestion, fevers, vomiting, diarrhea, chronic bronchitis and cold hands and feet.

Licorice root contains bitter compounds that reduce inflammation, decrease the thickness and increase the production of mucosal fluids and relieve muscle spasms. In addition, licorice stimulates adrenal function, reduces the urge to cough, is mildly laxative and enhances immune response. It has been used to treat coughs, colds, arthritis, asthma, peptic ulcers, Addison's disease, dropsy and atherosclerosis.

Zhishi fruit (immature orange) contains aromatic compounds that decrease the thickness while increasing the production of mucosal fluids and increase the production of digestive fluids. It also contains bitter compounds that enhance vitamin C absorption and decrease capillary fragility. Zhishi has been used to treat constipation, indigestion, flatulence, dyspepsia and abdominal pains.

Pinellia root contains bitter compounds that decrease the thickness while increasing the production of mucosal fluids, relieve muscle spasms, increase the pro-duction of digestive fluids and absorb toxins. Pinellia root must be processed with alum or ginger root before ingestion since it is toxic. It has been used to treat morning sickness, nausea, vomiting, respiratory congestion, ulcers and blood poisoning.

Cinnamon twig contains aromatic compounds that promote sweating, increase blood circulation, increase the production of digestive fluids, relieve smooth muscle spasms, increase the flow of urine and are antiseptic. The herb is a general stimulant to the digestive, respiratory, urinary and circulatory systems. It has been used to treat colds, edema, dysuria, arthritis, amenorrhea, angina pain and dyspepsia.

Atractylodes root contains aromatic compounds that are antiseptic, increase the production of digestive fluids and enzymes, increase blood pressure, are laxative, stimulate liver function and increase the flow of urine. It has been used to treat dyspepsia, flatulence, loss of appetite, nausea, indigestion, rheumatic arthritis and night blindness.

Fushen herb contains bitter compounds that increase the flow of urine, decrease blood sugar and have a sedative effect. It has been used to treat dysuria, heart palpitations, insomnia and edema.

Dandelion and Barberry Combination

Composition

Dandelion	Parsley	Fennel
Barberry	Red beet	Horseradish
Rose hips		

Properties

Tonic	Diuretic
Cholagogue	Stimulant

General Description

Dandelion and Barberry combination is a liver tonic formula. It enhances liver function and tones the organs of the digestive system, especially the liver, stomach and gall bladder. The herbs increase bile production, relieve muscle spasms, relieve pain and increase the flow of urine.

Chinese herbalists would describe this herbal combination as a wood enhancing formula. It also enhances the water element while reducing the earth, metal and fire elements.

Dandelion and Barberry combination has traditionally been used to treat **liver congestion, gallstones, hepatitis, diabetes, ulcers, edema, congested lymphatic glands, amenorrhea, dysmenorrhea, kidney stones,** and **lumbago.**

Imbalances indicating the use of this formula are commonly noted in the liver acupressure point located approximately four inches to the right of the sternum between the seventh and eight rib. Imbalances are often noted at the 4:45 position of the right iris. Use caution in cases of impaired kidney function and inflammation in the female reproductive system.

This formula is commonly used in conjunction with vitamin A, lecithin, choline, the complex of B vitamins, methionine, vitamin D, vitamin E and the vitamin C family.

Individual Components

Dandelion root contains bitter compounds that enhance the efficiency of the body's eliminative and detoxifying functions. These compounds help restore normal liver function, increase the production of digestive fluids and enzymes, particularly bile, increase the flow of urine and have a laxative effect. Dandelion is an excellent herbal source of sodium, iron and vitamin A. It has been used to treat jaundice, gallstones, dyspepsia, constipation, inflammatory skin conditions, frequent urination, hepatitis, gout and rheumatism.

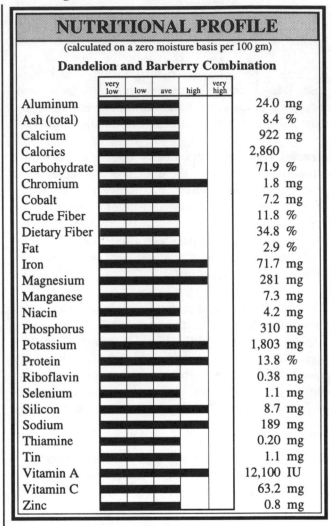

NUTRITIONAL PROFILE
(calculated on a zero moisture basis per 100 gm)

Dandelion and Barberry Combination

Nutrient	Level	Value	Unit
Aluminum	very low–low	24.0	mg
Ash (total)	very low–low	8.4	%
Calcium	very low–ave	922	mg
Calories	very low–ave	2,860	
Carbohydrate	very low–ave	71.9	%
Chromium	high	1.8	mg
Cobalt	very low–ave	7.2	mg
Crude Fiber	very low–low	11.8	%
Dietary Fiber	very low–ave	34.8	%
Fat	very low–low	2.9	%
Iron	very low–high	71.7	mg
Magnesium	very low–high	281	mg
Manganese	very low–ave	7.3	mg
Niacin	very low–ave	4.2	mg
Phosphorus	very low–low	310	mg
Potassium	very low–ave	1,803	mg
Protein	very low–ave	13.8	%
Riboflavin	very low–ave	0.38	mg
Selenium	very low–low	1.1	mg
Silicon	very low–high	8.7	mg
Sodium	very low–high	189	mg
Thiamine	very low–low	0.20	mg
Tin	very low–low	1.1	mg
Vitamin A	very low–ave	12,100	IU
Vitamin C	very low–ave	63.2	mg
Zinc	very low–low	0.8	mg

Barberry contains bitter compounds that improve the efficiency of digestion, stimulate the production of bile, dilate blood vessels and produce a mild laxative effect. It also contains astringent compounds that tighten inflamed tissues in the digestive system. Barberry has been used in cases of jaundice, dyspepsia, constipation and gallstones.

Rose hips contain bitter compounds called bioflavinoids which enhance the absorption of vitamin C and strengthen connective tissue. This results in decreased capillary fragility. It also contains astringent compounds which shrink inflamed tissues and reduce the secretion of mucosal fluids. Rose hips is an excellent herbal source of vitamin C. It has been used to treat the common cold, influenza, fevers, infections, inflammatory skin conditions, easy bruising, varicose veins, debility, capillary fragility and hemorrhoids.

Parsley herb contains aromatic compounds that decrease the thickness and increase the production of mucosal fluids, increase the production of digestive fluids, increase menstrual flow and increase urine flow. It also contains bitter compounds that reduce muscle spasms and pains, reduce blood pressure and are antiseptic. Parsley is an excellent herbal source of trace minerals especially the electrolyte minerals including sodium, potassium, calcium and magnesium. It is also an excellent herbal source of vitamin A, vitamin C and chlorophyllins. Parsley has been used to treat urinary tract infections, amenorrhea, dysmenorrhea, dyspepsia, bronchitis, allergies, arthritis, asthma, flatulence, dysuria and nephritis.

Red beet root contains bitter compounds that increase the flow of urine and increase the production of digestive fluids and enzymes. It also contains astringent compounds that shrink inflamed tissues. Red beet is an excellent herbal source of potassium. It has been used to treat liver congestion, menorrhagia, frequent urination and inflammatory skin conditions.

Fennel seed contains aromatic compounds that stimulate the production of digestive fluids, relieve inflammation, are antiseptic, make one breathe deeply and more often, and increase the flow of urine. It has been used to treat indigestion, dyspepsia, anorexia, colic, flatulence, coughs and colds.

Horseradish root contains aromatic compounds that increase circulation, are antiseptic and promote sweating. These compounds also decrease the thickness while increasing the production of mucosal fluid. Horseradish has been used to treat asthma, bronchitis, coughs, colds, fevers and rheumatism.

Dandelion and Parsley Combination

Composition

Red beet	Liverwort	Angelica
Dandelion	Black Cohosh	Chamomile
Parsley	Blessed Thistle	Gentain
Horsetail	Birch	Goldenrod

Properties

Cholagogue	Laxative
Diuretic	Analgesic
Antispasmodic	

General Description

Dandelion and Parsley Combination is used to restore normal liver function. The formula enhances the digestive and detoxifying functions working especially to increase the secretion and release of bile. The herbs increase bile production, increase the flow of urine, relieve muscle spasms, relieve pain and are mildly laxative.

Chinese herbalists would describe this herbal combination as a wood reducing formula. It also reduces the water element while enhancing the earth, metal, and fire elements.

Dandelion and Parsley combination has traditionally been used to treat **liver congestion, gallstones, hepatitis, diabetes, ulcers, edema, congested lymphatic glands, amenorrhea, dysmennorrhea, kidney stones** and **lumbago.**

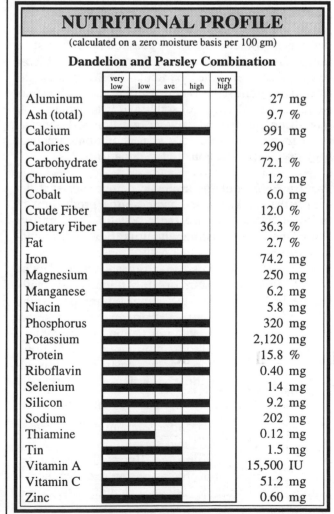

NUTRITIONAL PROFILE

(calculated on a zero moisture basis per 100 gm)

Dandelion and Parsley Combination

	very low	low	ave	high	very high	
Aluminum						27 mg
Ash (total)						9.7 %
Calcium						991 mg
Calories						290
Carbohydrate						72.1 %
Chromium						1.2 mg
Cobalt						6.0 mg
Crude Fiber						12.0 %
Dietary Fiber						36.3 %
Fat						2.7 %
Iron						74.2 mg
Magnesium						250 mg
Manganese						6.2 mg
Niacin						5.8 mg
Phosphorus						320 mg
Potassium						2,120 mg
Protein						15.8 %
Riboflavin						0.40 mg
Selenium						1.4 mg
Silicon						9.2 mg
Sodium						202 mg
Thiamine						0.12 mg
Tin						1.5 mg
Vitamin A						15,500 IU
Vitamin C						51.2 mg
Zinc						0.60 mg

Imbalances indicating the use of this formula are commonly noted in the liver acupressure point located approximately four inches to the right of the sternum between the 7th and 8th rib. Imbalances are often noted at the 4:45 position of the right iris. Use caution in cases of impaired kidney function and inflammation in the female reproductive system.

This formula is commonly used in conjunction with vitamin A, lecithin, choline, the compex of B vitamins, methionine, vitamin D, vitamin E and the vitamin C family.

Individual Components

Red beet root contains bitter compounds that increase the flow of urine and increase the production of digestive fluids and enzymes. It also contains astringent compounds that shrink inflamed tissues. Red beet is an excellent herbal source of potassium. It has been used to treat liver congestion,menorrhagia, frequent urination and inflammatory skin conditions.

Dandelion root contains bitter compounds that enhance the efficiency of the body's eliminative and detoxifying functions. These compounds help restore normal liver function, increase the production of digestive fluids and enzymes, particularly bile, increase the flow of urine and have a laxative effect. Dandelion is an excellent herbal source of sodium, iron and vitamin A. It has been used to treat jaundice, gallstones, dyspepsia, constipation, inflammatory skin conditions, frequent urination, hepatitis, gout and rheumatism.

Parsley herb contains aromatic compounds that decrease the thickness and increase the production of mucosal fluids, increase the production of digestive fluids, increase menstrual and urine flow. It also contains bitter compounds that reduce muscle spasms and pains, reduce blood pressure and are antiseptic. Parsley is an excellent herbal source of trace minerals especially the electrolyte minerals including sodium, potassium, calcium and magnesium. It is also an excellent herbal source of vitamin A, vitamin C and chlorophyllins. Parsley has been used to treat urinary tract infections, amenorrhea, dysmenorrhea, dyspepsia, bronchitis, allergies, arthritis, asthma, flatulence, dysuria and nephritis.

Horsetail herb contains bitter compounds that increase the production of urine and shrink inflamed mucosal tissue, particularly the prostate. Horsetail is most noted for its trace mineral profile as it is an excellent herbal source of bioavailable silicon, calcium, magnesium, chromium, iron, manganese and potassium. It has been used to treat prostatitis, osteoporosis, enuresis, urinary tract infections and muscle cramps.

Liverwort herb contains astringent alkaloids that increase the production of bile, shrink inflamed mucous membranes and increase the production of digestive fluids. It is an excellent herbal source of vitamin A and vitamin K. Liverwort has been used to treat hepatitis, cirrhosis, dyspepsia, gallstones and liver congestion.

Black Cohosh root contains bitter compounds that relieve smooth muscle spasms, reduce blood pressure and dilate peripheral blood vessels. It also contains astringent compounds that shrink inflamed tissue. Black cohosh has been employed in most inflammatory conditions associated with spasms or tension. It is an excellent herbal source of iron and vitamin A. Black cohosh has been used to treat menstrual cramps, nervous tension, anxiety, dysmenorrhea, hysteria, menopause, fevers and headaches.

Blessed Thistle contains bitter compounds that decrease the thickness while increasing the production of mucosal fluids particularly in the digestive and respiratory systems. It also contains astringent compounds that are antiseptic, dilate peripheral blood vessels and shrink inflamed tissue. Blessed thistle is an excellent herbal source of potassium and sodium. The herb has been used to treat dysmenorrhea, amenorrhea, arthritis, dysuria, jaundice, fevers and respiratory allergies.

Birch leaf contains aromatic compounds that relieve pains, are antiseptic and relieve muscle spasms. It also contains bitter compounds that enhance nutrient absorption and promote the growth of friendly colonic bacteria. Birch has been used to treat rheumatism, insomnia, inflammatory skin conditions and kidney infections.

Angelica root contains aromatic compounds that promote sweating, are antiseptic and decrease the thickness while increasing the production of mucosal fluids. It has been used to treat bronchitis, coughs, colds, indigestion, amenorrhea and inflammatory skin conditions.

Chamomile flowers contain aromatic compounds that increase the production of digestive fluids, reduce muscle spasms and pains, reduce inflammation and are antiseptic. In addition, these compounds have a sedative effect. Chamomile is one of the best herbal sources of niacin, magnesium and essential fatty acids. It has been used to treat dyspepsia, flatulence, nausea, vomiting, dysmenorrhea, bronchitis, urinary tract infections, insomnia, headaches and menstrual cramps.

Gentain root contains bitter compounds that increase appetite by enhancing the production of digestive fluids and enzymes, particularly bile. It is an excellent herbal source of vitamin B-1, niacin, magnesium, phosphorus, selenium and zinc. Gentain has been used to treat anorexia, dyspepsia, loss of appetite, indigestion and gallstones.

Goldenrod herb contains bitter compounds that decrease the thickness while increasing the production of mucosal fluids and sooth inflamed tissues. It has been used to treat asthma, rheumatism, arthritis and inflammatory skin conditions.

Eyebright Combination

Composition

Bayberry
Goldenseal
Eyebright
Red raspberry

Properties

Astringent
Anti-inflammatory
Analgesic
Antiseptic

General Description

Eyebright combination is an astringent formula. It is associated with inflammation in mucous membranes, particularly the eyes. It is often used as an eyewash. The herbs shrink inflamed tissues, are antiseptic and relieve pains.

Chinese herbalists would describe this herbal combination as a metal enhancing formula. It also enhances the earth and fire elements while reducing the water and wood elements.

Eyebright combination has been used to treat **eye infections, respiratory tract infections, diarrhea, inflammatory skin conditions, inflammatory conditions of the gastrointestinal tract, sinus congestion** and **edema.**

Imbalances indicating the use of this formula are commonly noted in the systemic allergy acupressure point located over the thymus gland in the middle of the sternum. Imbalances are often noted at the 11 o'clock position of the left iris and at the 1 o'clock position of the right iris. Use caution in cases of hyperacid stomaches or hypertension.

This formula is commonly used in conjunction with the complex of B vitamins, the vitamin C family, zinc and vitamin A.

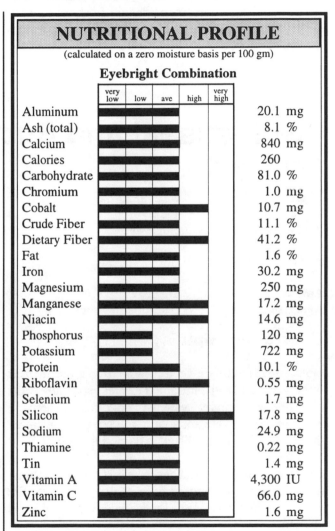

NUTRITIONAL PROFILE
(calculated on a zero moisture basis per 100 gm)

Eyebright Combination

	very low	low	ave	high	very high	
Aluminum						20.1 mg
Ash (total)						8.1 %
Calcium						840 mg
Calories						260
Carbohydrate						81.0 %
Chromium						1.0 mg
Cobalt						10.7 mg
Crude Fiber						11.1 %
Dietary Fiber						41.2 %
Fat						1.6 %
Iron						30.2 mg
Magnesium						250 mg
Manganese						17.2 mg
Niacin						14.6 mg
Phosphorus						120 mg
Potassium						722 mg
Protein						10.1 %
Riboflavin						0.55 mg
Selenium						1.7 mg
Silicon						17.8 mg
Sodium						24.9 mg
Thiamine						0.22 mg
Tin						1.4 mg
Vitamin A						4,300 IU
Vitamin C						66.0 mg
Zinc						1.6 mg

Individual Components

Bayberry bark contains astringent compounds that reduce the secretion of fluids, reduce pains and shrink inflamed tissues. These compounds also promote sweating, increase blood circulation and dilate peripheral blood vessels. It has been used to treat diarrhea, colds, intestinal flu, inflammatory conditions of the gastrointestinal tract, asthma, bronchitis, fevers and sinus congestion.

Goldenseal root contains bitter astringent alkaloids that normalize liver and spleen functions by increasing the production of digestive fluids and enzymes, particularly bile. The compounds are antiseptic, constrict peripheral blood vessels, especially in the uterus, are laxative and relieve pain and inflammation in mucosal tissue. Goldenseal is an excellent herbal source of trace minerals including cobalt, iron, magnesium, manganese, silicon and zinc. It is also an excellent herbal source of vitamin C. It has been used to treat hepatitis, gastritis, colitis, ulcers, menorrhagia, postpartum hemorrhages, dysmenorrhea, diabetes, infections, hemorrhoids, eczema, obesity and fevers.

Eyebright herb contains astringent compounds that shrink inflamed tissues. It also contains bitter compounds that relieve pains, are antiseptic and soothe inflamed mucous membranes. Eyebright is an excellent herbal source of vitamin B-1, vitamin B-2, niacin, calcium, cobalt, magnesium, manganese and zinc. It has been used to treat eye infections, colds, sinus congestion, allergies, jaundice and hepatitis.

Red Raspberry leaf contains astringent compounds that relieve pain and shrink inflamed tissues, especially in the female reproductive system. It also contains bitter compounds that relieve smooth muscle spasms. Red Raspberry is an excellent herbal source of manganese. It has been used to treat morning sickness, nausea, dysmenorrhea, false labor, colds, flu and fevers.

Goldenseal and Bugleweed Combination

Composition

Goldenseal	Marshmallow
Black Walnut	Plantain
Parthenium	Bugleweed

Properties

Antiseptic	Diruetic
Analgesic	Antiinflammatory

General Description

Goldenseal and Bugleweed combination is used to treat infections and soothe inflamed tissues especially in the digestive and urinary systems. Together the herbs in this combination are antiseptic, relieve pains, increase the flow of urine and shrink inflamed tissues.

Chinese herbalists would describe this herbal combination as a wood reducing formula. It also reduces the fire element while enhancing the metal, water and earth elements.

Goldenseal and Bugleweed combination has traditionally been used to treat **colitis, influenza, swollen glands, urinary tract infections, gastritis, abscesses and infectious fevers.**

Imbalances indicating the use of this formula are commonly noted in the colon acupressure point located approximately four inches to the right of the navel. Imbalances are often noted in the autonomic nerve wreath surrounding pupils. Use caution in cases of anemia, postpartum weakness and hypoglycemia.

NUTRITIONAL PROFILE
(calculated on a zero moisture basis per 100 gm)

Goldenseal and Bugleweed Combination

	very low	low	ave	high	very high	
Aluminum						40 mg
Ash (total)						7.2 %
Calcium						660 mg
Calories						289
Carbohydrate						79.2 %
Chromium						0.9 mg
Cobalt						7.8 mg
Crude Fiber						11.2 %
Dietary Fiber						40.1 %
Fat						2.3 %
Iron						49.8 mg
Magnesium						241 mg
Manganese						7.8 mg
Niacin						4.9 mg
Phosphorus						198 mg
Potassium						1,121 mg
Protein						11.4 %
Riboflavin						0.32 mg
Selenium						2.3 mg
Silicon						15.8 mg
Sodium						32.3 mg
Thiamine						0.22 mg
Tin						1.5 mg
Vitamin A						1,200 IU
Vitamin C						82.3 mg
Zinc						1.7 mg

This formula is commonly used in conjunction with myrrh gum, the vitamin C family, vitamin A, selenium, zinc, germanium, barley grass, alfalfa, asparagus and cabbage.

Individual Components

Goldenseal root contains bitter astringent alkaloids that normalize liver and spleen functions by increasing the production of digestive fluids and enzymes, particularly bile. The compounds are antiseptic, constrict peripheral blood vessels, especially in the uterus, are laxative and relieve pain and inflammation in mucosal tissue. Goldenseal is an excellent herbal source of trace minerals including cobalt, iron, magnesium, manganese, silicon and zinc. It is also an excellent herbal source of vitamin C. It has been used to treat hepatitis, gastritis, colitis, ulcers, menorrhagia, postpartum hemorrhage, dysmenorrhea, diabetes, infections, hemorrhoids, eczema, obesity and fevers.

Black Walnut hull contains astringent compounds that shrink inflamed tissues of the digestive system. It also contains bitter compounds that are antifungal and decrease the secretion of fluids in the digestive system. Black walnut has been used to treat hemorrhoids, inflammatory skin conditions, colitis, intestinal worms and parasites and fevers.

Parthenium root contains mucilaginous compounds that increase immune response, sequester infections and soothe inflamed tissues. Parthenium also contains bitter compounds that increase immune response by increasing the production of T-lymphocytes, phagocytic macrophages, interferons and lymphokines. Parthenium has been used to treat wounds infections, blood poisoning, inflammatory skin conditions and tonsillitis.

Marshmallow root contains mucilaginous compounds that decrease the thickness while increasing the production of mucosal fluids, soothe inflamed tissues, heal wounds and increase the flow of urine. It is an excellent herbal source of trace minerals especially chromium, iron, magnesium and selenium. Marshmallow has been used to treat allergies, gastritis, gastric ulcers, enteritis, coughs, cystitis and hay fevers.

Plantain seed contains mucilaginous compounds that absorb toxins from the bowel, soothe inflamed tissues and promote normal bowel function. Plantain has been used to treat chronic constipation, colitis, dysentery, coughs, ulcers and diarrhea.

Bugleweed herb contains astringent compounds that stop bleeding and shrink inflamed tissues. It also contains aromatic compounds that relieve pain and are mildly sedative. These compounds also lower heart rate while increasing cardiac output. Bugleweed has been used to treat arrhythmia, hemorrhage, angina pains, colitis and ulcers.

Pau d'arco and Yellow Dock Combination

Composition

Pau d'arco	Cascara Sagrada
Red Clover	Buckthorn
Yellow dock	Peach bark
Burdock	Oregon grape
Sarsaparilla	Stillengia
Dandelion	Prickly ash
Chaparral	Yarrow

Properties

Diuretic	Immunostimulant
Laxative	Carminative
Cholagogue	Antiseptic

General Description

Pau d'arco and Yellow Dock combination is a traditional blood purifier. The formula enhances the detoxifying and eliminative functions of the body. The herbs increase the flow of urine, are laxative, increase the production of digestive fluids and enzymes, are antiseptic and enhance immune response.

Chinese herbalists would describe this herbal combination as a wood reducing formula. It also reduces the metal and water element while enhancing the earth and fire elements.

Pau d'arco and Yellow Dock combination has traditionally been used to treat **arthritis, inflammatory skin conditions, constipation, jaundice, hepatitis, fevers** and **lymph infections.**

Imbalances indicating the use of this formula are commonly noted in the liver acupressure point located approximately four inches to the right of the sternum between the seventh and eighth ribs. Imbalances are often noted at the 7:30 position of the right iris. Also, a "lymphatic rosary" is often present. Use caution in cases of chronic weaknesses in the digestive system.

This formula is commonly used in conjunction with the vitamin C family, the complex of B vitamins, essential fatty acids, parsley, hydrangea, goldenseal, echinacea, pumpkin, vitamin A, zinc and spirulina.

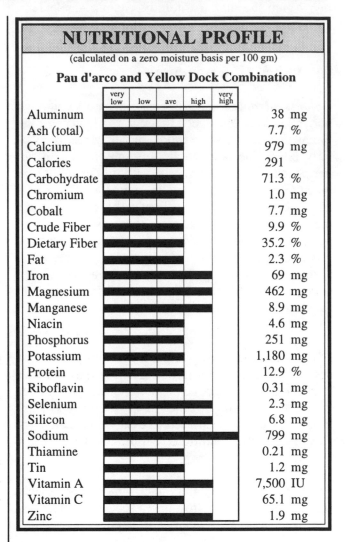

NUTRITIONAL PROFILE
(calculated on a zero moisture basis per 100 gm)

Pau d'arco and Yellow Dock Combination

	very low	low	ave	high	very high		
Aluminum						38	mg
Ash (total)						7.7	%
Calcium						979	mg
Calories						291	
Carbohydrate						71.3	%
Chromium						1.0	mg
Cobalt						7.7	mg
Crude Fiber						9.9	%
Dietary Fiber						35.2	%
Fat						2.3	%
Iron						69	mg
Magnesium						462	mg
Manganese						8.9	mg
Niacin						4.6	mg
Phosphorus						251	mg
Potassium						1,180	mg
Protein						12.9	%
Riboflavin						0.31	mg
Selenium						2.3	mg
Silicon						6.8	mg
Sodium						799	mg
Thiamine						0.21	mg
Tin						1.2	mg
Vitamin A						7,500	IU
Vitamin C						65.1	mg
Zinc						1.9	mg

Individual Components

Pau d'arco bark contains astringent compounds that shrink inflamed tissues and are anti-fungal. It also contains bitter compounds that have anti-tumor activity especially in certain blood and skin cancers. Pau d'arco is an excellent herbal source of calcium. It has been used to treat fungal infections, inflammatory skin conditions, leukemia, dysentery, jaundice, ulcers and rheumatism.

Red Clover flowers contain bitter compounds that increase the production of digestive fluids and enzymes, especially bile. These compounds also shrink inflammation and relieve pains. Red clover is an excellent herbal source of calcium, chromium, magnesium, phosphorus and potassium. It has been used to treat arthritis, jaundice, liver congestion, muscle cramps and inflammatory skin conditions.

Yellow dock contains bitter compounds that are laxative, increase the production of digestive fluids and enzymes, especially bile and increase the flow of urine. It also contains astringent compounds that shrink inflamed tissues. Yellow dock is an excellent herbal source of vitamin A, vitamin C, calcium, iron, magnesium, phosphorus and selenium. It has been used to treat liver congestion, constipation, arthritis, rheumatism, inflammatory bowel disorders and inflammatory skin conditions.

Burdock root contains mucilaginous compounds that decrease the thickness while increasing the production of mucosal fluids, soothe inflamed tissues and absorb toxins from the bowel. It also contains aromatic compounds that have an antiseptic effect and increase the flow of urine. The herb is an excellent herbal source of chromium, iron, magnesium, phosphorus, potassium, silicon and zinc. Burdock has been used to treat arthrits, allergies, eczema, bronchitis, urinary tract infections, gout and rheumatism.

Sarsaparilla root contains bitter compounds that increase the production of urine and promote sweating. These compounds also relieve inflammation, muscle spasms and are antiseptic. Sarsaparilla is an excellent herbal source of chromium, cobalt, iron and selenium. It has been used to treat rheumatism, gout, fevers, inflammatory skin conditions, prostatitis and impotence.

Dandelion root contains bitter compounds that enhance the efficiency of the body's eliminative and detoxifying functions. These compounds help restore normal liver function, increase the production of digestive fluids and enzymes, particularly bile, increase the flow of urine and have a laxative effect. Dandelion is an excellent herbal source of sodium, iron and vitamin A. It has been used to treat jaundice, gallstones, dyspepsia, constipation, inflammatory skin conditions, frequent urination, hepatitis, gout and rheumatism.

Chaparral contains bitter compounds that are antiseptic and increase immune response (antioxidant). It also contains aromatic compounds that increase the flow of urine and decrease the thickness while increasing the production of mucosal fluids. Chaparral is an excellent herbal source of vitamin A and vitamin C. It has been used to treat arthritis, blood diseases, allergies and inflammatory skin conditions.

Cascara Sagrada bark is perhaps the most famous herbal laxative. It contains bitter compounds that increase peristalsis, are purgative, increase the release of bile and promote the growth of friendly colonic bacteria. Cascara is used to treat constipation, dyspepsia, liver congestion, gallstones, hemorrhoids, jaundice and intestinal parasites.

Buckthorn bark contains bitter compounds that increase peristalsis, are purgative and increase the release of bile. It has been used to treat constipation, fevers, inflammatory skin conditions, rheumatism, hemorrhoids and intestinal parasites.

Peach bark contains bitter compounds that increase the flow of urine and relieve smooth muscle spasms. It also contains astringent compounds that shrink inflamed tissues and are antiseptic. Peach bark has been used to treat urinary tract infections, nephritis, jaundice, edema and inflammatory skin conditions.

Oregon grape root contains bitter alkaloids that constrict peripheral blood vessels, relieve pain and inflammation, are antiseptic, increase the release of bile and are laxative. It has been used to treat arthritis, jaundice, hepatitis, inflammatory skin conditions, fevers and constipation.

Stillengia herb contains bitter compounds that increase the release of bile. It also contains astringent compounds that are antiseptic and shrink inflamed tissues. Stillengia has been used to treat inflammatory skin conditions, infectious fevers and liver congestion.

Prickly Ash bark contains bitter compounds that reduce inflammation and pains, are sedative, increase the flow of urine, promote sweating and are mildly laxative. It has been used to treat rheumatism, lumbago and cold hands and feet.

Yarrow flower contains aromatic compounds that shrink inflamed tissues and promote sweating. It also contains bitter compounds that relieve smooth muscle spasms, reduce blood pressure and stop bleeding. Yarrow has been used to treat hemorrhoids, fevers, nausea and inflammatory skin conditions.

Red Beet and Yellow Dock Combination

Composition

Red beet	Burdock
Yellow dock	Nettle
Chickweed	Mullein
Strawberry	

Properties

Diuretic	Demulcent
Laxative	Vulnerary
Diaphoretic	

General Description

Red beet and Yellow dock combinations are used to treat chronic inflammatory conditions, especially skin problems, lymphatic infection and anemia. The formula works to enhance the detoxifying and eliminative functions, especially those marked by a sluggish bowel or liver disturbance. The herbs increase the flow of urine, are laxative, promote sweating and soothe inflamed tissues.

Chinese herbalists would describe this herbal combination as a wood reducing formula. It also reduces the water element while enhancing the metal fire and earth elements.

Red beet and Yellow dock combination has traditionally been used to treat **inflammatory skin conditions, chronic constipation, lymphatic infection** and **anemia due to parasites.**

Imbalances indicating the use of this formula are commonly noted in the thymus acupressure point located in the center of the sternum. Imbalances are often noted by the presence of a "lymphatic rosary" surrounding each iris. Use caution in cases of diarrhea and hepatitis.

This formula is commonly used in conjunction with vitamin A, zinc, red clover flowers and dandelion root.

Individual Components

Red beet root contains bitter compounds that increase the flow of urine and increase the production of digestive fluids and enzymes. It also contains astringent compounds that shrink inflamed tissues. Red beet is an excellent herbal source of potassium. It has been used to treat liver congestion, menorrhagia, frequent urination and inflammatory skin conditions.

Yellow dock contains bitter compounds that are laxative, increase the production of digestive fluids and enzymes, especially bile, and increase the flow of urine. It also contains astringent compounds that shrink inflamed tissues. Yellow dock is an excellent herbal source of vitamin A, vitamin C, calcium, iron, magnesium, phosphorus and selenium. It has been used to treat liver congestion, constipation, arthritis, rheumatism, inflammatory bowel disorders and inflammatory skin conditions.

Chickweed herb contains mucilaginous compounds that absorb toxins from the bowel, soothe inflamed tissues, give bulk to the stool and increase the flow of urine. These compounds also decrease the thickness while increasing the production of mucosal fluids.

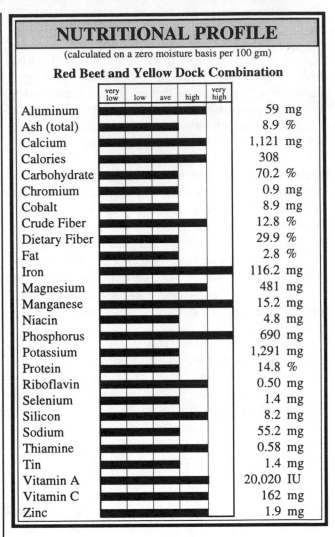

NUTRITIONAL PROFILE
(calculated on a zero moisture basis per 100 gm)

Red Beet and Yellow Dock Combination

Nutrient	Amount	Level
Aluminum	59 mg	low
Ash (total)	8.9 %	ave
Calcium	1,121 mg	high
Calories	308	ave
Carbohydrate	70.2 %	ave
Chromium	0.9 mg	ave
Cobalt	8.9 mg	low
Crude Fiber	12.8 %	high
Dietary Fiber	29.9 %	ave
Fat	2.8 %	low
Iron	116.2 mg	very high
Magnesium	481 mg	very high
Manganese	15.2 mg	high
Niacin	4.8 mg	ave
Phosphorus	690 mg	high
Potassium	1,291 mg	ave
Protein	14.8 %	low
Riboflavin	0.50 mg	high
Selenium	1.4 mg	ave
Silicon	8.2 mg	low
Sodium	55.2 mg	low
Thiamine	0.58 mg	ave
Tin	1.4 mg	low
Vitamin A	20,020 IU	high
Vitamin C	162 mg	low
Zinc	1.9 mg	low

Chickweed has been used to treat rheumatism, arthritis, inflammatory skin conditions and obesity.

Strawberry leaf contains astringent compounds that shrink inflamed tissues, decrease bleeding and relieve pains. it has been used to treat inflammatory skin conditions, hemorrhaging, fevers and diarrhea.

Burdock root contains mucilaginous compounds that decrease the thickness while increasing the production of mucosal fluids, soothe inflamed tissues and absorb toxins from the bowel. It also contains aromatic compounds that have an antiseptic effect and increase the flow of urine. The herb is an excellent herbal source of chromium, iron, magnesium, phosphorus, potassium, silicon and zinc. Burdock has been used to treat arthritis, allergies, eczema, bronchitis, urinary tract infections, gout and rheumatism.

Nettle leaf contains bitter compounds that increase the flow of urine, are antiseptic and relieve pains. It also contains astringent compounds that shrink inflamed tissues and stop bleeding. Nettle has been used to treat urinary tract infections, respiratory tract infections, inflammatory skin conditions, diarrhea and asthma.

Mullein leaves contain mucilaginous compounds that decrease the thickness and increase the production of mucosal fluids. These compounds soothe inflamed tissues. Mullein also contains aromatic compounds that increase the flow of urine. The herb has been used to treat bronchitis, coughs, colds, hay fever, dysuria, nephritis and sinus congestion.

Therapies for Supplementing Deficient Conditions

Astragalus and Ganoderma Combination

Composition

Astragalus	Schizandra	Siberian Ginseng
Ganoderma	Atractylodes	Epimedium
Dong Quai	Hoelen	Ligustrum
Peony	Eucommia	Ophiopogon
Rehmannia	Achyranthes	Licorice
Polygala	Lycium	Citrus

Properties

Immune Stimulant	Adaptogen
General Tonic	Stimulant

General Description

Astragalus and Ganoderma combination is a general tonic formula. The herbs work to stimulate immune response, enhance the body's response to stress, improve blood circulation and promote healing due to trauma and chronic degenerative conditions.

Chinese herbalists would describe this herbal combination as a metal enhancing formula. It also enhances the wood earth fire and water elements.

Astragalus and Ganoderma combination has traditionally been used to treat **fatigue, impaired immune response, chronic poor health, backaches, impotence, general debility, recovery from trauma** and **weak muscles.**

Imbalances indicating the use of this formula are commonly noted in the thymus acupressure point located in the center of the sternum. Imbalances are often noted at the 4:30 position of the left iris.

This formula is used in conjunction with parthenium, myrrh, goldenseal, germanium, the vitamin C family, the complex of B vitamins, bee pollen and vitamin E.

Individual Components

Astragalus root contains bitter compounds that increase the flow of urine, are antiseptic, increase the production of digestive fluids, including bile, and relieve muscle spasms. Astragalus also contains muci-laginous compounds that enhance immune response, increasing the production of lymphocytes and macrophages. The herb also increases heart action, lowers blood pressure and blood sugar. It has been used to treat fatigue, debility, urinary tract infections, edema, nephritis, ulcers, prolapse of organs and night sweats.

Ganoderma herb contains bitter compounds that increase coronary blood flow, lower blood pressure, lower blood cholesterol and allow the heart to function more efficiently on less oxygen These compounds also calm the nerves, relieve pain and are antiseptic. Ganoderma also contains mucilaginous compounds that improve immune response and decrease the thickness while increasing the production of mucosal fluids. The herb has been used to treat insomnia, atherosclerosis, asthma, bronchitis, angina pains, hypertension and immune deficiency.

Dong Quai root contains aromatic compounds that relieve smooth muscle spasms especially in the uterus, have a sedative effect and increase the production of digestive fluids. It also contains bitter compounds that regulate glycogen production in the liver, reduce pain and inflammation, increase blood flow, especially to the heart, lower blood cholesterol, normalize uterine contractions and are antiseptic. Dong quai is an excellent herbal source of iron, magnesium and niacin. It has been used to treat anemia, abdominal pains, dysmenorrhea, amenorrhea, arthritis, coronary heart disease, atherosclerosis, angina pectoris, indigestion and headaches.

Peony root contains bitter compounds that are sedative, antiseptic and relieve pains. These compounds also lower blood pressure and decrease capillary permeability. It has been used to treat arthralgia, gastric pains, inflammatory skin conditions and dysmenorrhea.

Rehmannia root contains astringent compounds that stop bleeding and reduce inflammation especially in the digestive system. The herb also contains bitter compounds that reduce capillary fragility. It has been used to treat ulcers, menorrhagia, thirst diabetes, constipation, anemia and infertility.

Polygala root contains bitter compounds that decrease the thickness and increase the production of mucosal fluids, have a sedative effect and are antiseptic. These compounds also lower blood pressure and increase uterine tension. Polygala has been used to treat insomnia, heart palpitations, ulcers, inflammatory skin conditions, bronchitis and nervous tension.

Schizandra fruit contains bitter compounds that allow the body to more quickly respond to stress. This increases the body's capacity for work and decreases fatigue. These compounds increase blood circulation, blood sugar and bile production while lowering blood pressure. Schizandra also contains astringent compounds that increase the contraction of the heart muscle and the uterus and are antiseptic. The herb has been used to treat heart palpitations, dropsy, nervous exhaustion, asthma, diabetes, chronic diarrhea, night sweats, seminal emissions, insomnia, frequent urination and anxiety.

Atractylodes root contains aromatic compounds that are antiseptic, increase the production of digestive fluids and enzymes, increase blood pressure, are laxative, stimulate liver function and increase the flow of urine. It has been used to treat dyspepsia, flatulence, loss of appetite, nausea, indigestion, rheumatic arthritis and night blindness.

Hoelen herb contains bitter compounds that increase the flow of urine, decrease blood sugar and have a sedative effect. It has been used to treat edema, dropsy, diarrhea, insomnia, frequent urination and heart palpitations.

Eucommia bark contains bitter compounds that reduce blood pressure, relieve muscle spasms, especially in the uterus and calm the mind. It also contains mucilaginous compounds that absorb toxins from the bowel, lower cholesterol absorption and enhance the production of mucosal fluids especially in the urinary system. Eucommia has been used to treat backache, dysuria, impotence, muscular weakness, osteoporosis and to prevent miscarriage.

Achyranthes root contains bitter compounds that increase the production of urine, relieve pains, lower blood pressure and decrease peristalsis. These compounds also increase the contraction of the uterus and promote menstruation. It also contains mucilaginous compounds that sooth inflamed tissue and increase the production of mucosal fluids. Achyranthes has been used to treat amenorrhea, backache, hypertension, muscle aches and dysuria.

Lycium fruit contains bitter compounds that lower blood sugar, promote the regeneration of liver cells and lower blood cholesterol. It has been used to treat atherosclerosis, backache, impotence, vertigo, poor eyesight and diabetes.

Siberian Ginseng root contains bitter compounds that help the body respond more quickly to stress. These compounds increase the production of DNA, RNA and proteins essential to all life processes. They stimulate the adrenal, pancreas and pituitary glands to lower blood sugar and reduce inflammation. Ginseng also increases the production of digestive fluids and is a mild sedative. It had been used to treat anemia, impotence, insomnia, diarrhea, fatigue debility, weak digestion and failing memory.

Epimedium herb contains bitter compounds that are antiseptic, lower blood pressure, relieve inflammation, increase the flow of urine and decrease the thickness while increasing the production of mucosal fluids. It has been used to treat impotence, lumbago, arthritic hypertension and bronchitis.

Ligustrum fruit contains bitter compounds that are cardiotonic, relieve pains, increase the flow of urine and are laxative. In addition, these compounds are antiseptic, increase immune response by stimulating the production of white blood cells and reduce inflammation in the eye. Ligustrum has been used to treat lumbago, constipation, cataracts, retinitis, pneumonia, bronchitis, urinary tract infections, gastroenteritis, colds, flu and dysmenorrhea.

Ophiopogon root contains bitter compounds that have a sedative effect, promote the production of mucosal fluids, reduce muscle spasms and have an antiseptic effect. In addition, the herb lowers blood sugar and regenerates beta cells in the islets of langerhorn of the pancreas. Ophiopogon has been used to treat insomnia, coronary heart disease, heart palpitations, fear and dry coughs.

Licorice root contains bitter compounds that reduce inflammation, decrease the thickness and increase the production of mucosal fluids and relieve muscle spasms. In addition, licorice stimulates adrenal function, reduces the urge to cough, is mildly laxative and enhances immune response. It has been used to treat coughs, colds, arthritis, asthma, peptic ulcers, Addison's disease, dropsy and atherosclerosis.

Citrus peel contains aromatic compounds that are antiseptic, reduce muscle spasms and decrease the thickness while increasing the production of mucosal fluids. It also contains bitter compounds that are anti-inflammatory, reduce muscle spasms, increase the production of digestive fluid and increase blood circulation. Citrus peel has been used to treat coughs, colds, flu, fevers and bronchitis.

Dandelion and Purslane Combination

Composition

Dandelion	Scute	Thalaspi
Purslane	Pinellia	Siberian Ginseng
Indigo	Licorice	Cinnamon twig
Indigo root	Bupleurum	

Properties

Immune stimulant
Tonic
Antiviral

General Description

Dandelion and Purslane combination is used to fight chronic infections. The herbs work to stimulate immune response, enhance the body's response to stress, reduce glandular inflammation and protect the liver from common organic poisons.

Chinese herbalists would describe this herbal combination as a metal enhancing formula. It also enhances the wood and earth elements while reducing the fire and water elements.

Dandelion and Purslane combination has traditionally been used to treat **viral infections, hepatitis, candidiasis, inflammatory skin conditions, inflammation of the lymph glands, adenitis** and **tonsillitis.**

Imbalances indicating the use of this formula are commonly noted in the thymus acupressure point located in the center of the sternum. Imbalances are often noted at the 4:30 position of the left iris.

This formula is commonly used in conjunction with parthenium, germanium, vitamin E, the vitamin C family, the complex of B vitamins and myrrh.

Individual Components

Dandelion root contains bitter compounds that enhance the efficiency of the body's eliminative and detoxifying functions. These compounds help restore normal liver function, increase the production of digestive fluids and enzymes, particularly bile, increase the flow of urine and have a laxative effect. Dandelion is an excellent herbal source of sodium, iron and vitamin A. It has been used to treat jaundice, gallstones, dyspepsia, constipation, inflammatory skin conditions, frequent urination, hepatitis, gout and rheumatism.

Purslane herb contains mucilaginous compounds that enhance digestion and absorb toxins from the digestive tract. Purslane also contains essential fatty acids that help maintain a healthy circulatory system. This herb has been used to treat dyspepsia, enteritis, high blood pressure, candidiasis and digestive tract infections.

Indigo herb contains bitter compounds that reduce inflammation, staunch bleeding and are antiseptic. Indigo is an excellent herbal source of potassium. It has been used to treat glandular inflammation of the lymph nodes, tonsils and adenoids, hepatitis and inflammatory skin conditions.

Indigo root contains bitter compounds that protect the liver from common organic poisons and reduce fevers. Indigo root is an excellent herbal source of potassium. It has been used to treat hepatitis and leukemia.

Scute root contains bitter compounds that increase the flow of urine, are antiseptic, reduce capillary permeability and inflammation, increase the secretion of bile and relieve muscle spasms. It has been used to treat urinary tract infections, enteritis, coughs, colds, dysentery and jaundice.

Pinellia root contains bitter compounds that decrease the thickness while increasing the production of mucosal fluids, relieve muscle spasms, increase the production of digestive fluids and absorb toxins. Pinellia root must be processed with alum or ginger root before ingestion as it is toxic. It has been used to treat morning sickness, nausea, vomiting, respiratory congestion, ulcers and blood poisoning.

Licorice root contains bitter compounds that reduce inflammation, decrease the thickness and increase the production of mucosal fluids and relieve muscle spasms. In addition, licorice stimulates adrenal function, reduces the urge to cough, is mildly laxative and enhances immune response. It has been used to treat coughs, colds, arthritis, asthma, peptic ulcers, Addison's disease, dropsy and atherosclerosis.

Bupleurum root contains bitter compounds that have an antidepressant effect, relieve pain and inflammation, reduce fevers and have an antiseptic effect. In addition, these compounds reduce blood cholesterol and triglyceride levels and reduce fat cell production and inflammation in the liver Bupleurum has been used to treat premenstrual syndrome, dysmenorrhea, lung congestion, malaria, muscle cramps, tumors, inflammatory skin conditions, angina pains, epilepsy and depression.

Thlaspi herb contains bitter compounds that reduce fevers and enhance the elimination of toxins from the blood. It has been used to treat fevers, inflammatory skin conditions and hepatitis.

Siberian Ginseng root contains bitter compounds that help the body respond more quickly to stress. These compounds increase the production of DNA, RNA and proteins essential to all life processes. They stimulate the adrenal, pancreas, and pituitary glands to lower blood sugar and reduce inflammation. Ginseng also increases the production of digestive fluids and is a mild sedative. It has been used to treat anemia, impotence, insomnia, diarrhea, fatigue, debility, weak digestion and failing memory.

Cinnamon twig contains aromatic compounds that promote sweating, increase bloods circulation, increase the production of digestive fluids, relieve smooth muscle spasms, increase the flow of urine and are antiseptic. The herb is a general stimulant to the digestive, respiratory, urinary and circulatory systems. It has been used to treat colds, edema, dysuria, arthritis, amenorrhea, angina pain and dyspepsia.

Ginseng and Phaffia Combination

Composition

Siberian Ginseng	Astragalus
Phaffia	Gotu Kola
Ginkgo	

Properties

Adaptogen	Tonic
Nervine	Vulnerary

General Description

Ginseng and Phaffia combination is used to assist the recuperative powers of the body. All the herbs are noted as tonics and have been used to increase endurance and longevity. In the short term, this formula is an adaptogen used to overcome the effects of anxiety and stress. With long term use, Ginseng and Phaffia combination enhances the function of the reproductive system as a tonic and vulnerary.

Chinese herbalists would describe this herbal combination as an earth enhancing or yin tonic formula. It also enhances the water and metal elements, while reducing the fire and wood elements.

Ginseng and Phaffia combination has traditionally been used to treat **stress disorders, prolonged illnesses, failing memory, epilepsy, senility, premature aging, sexual dysfunction** and **venereal diseases.**

Imbalances indicating the use of this formula are commonly noted in the stress acupressure point located on the forehead and the genital acupressure point located on the lower abdomen. Imbalances are often noted at the 5:00 position of the left iris.

This formula is commonly used in conjunction with the vitamin C family, the complex of B vitamins, licorice, fenugreek, alfalfa, calcium, magnesium, manganese and iron.

Individual Components

Siberian Ginseng root contains bitter compounds that help the body respond more quickly to stress. These compounds increase the production of DNA, RNA and proteins essential to all life processes. They stimulate the adrenal, pancreas, and pituitary glands to lower blood sugar and reduce inflammation. Ginseng also increases the production of digestive fluids and is a mild sedative. It has been used to treat anemia, impotence, insomnia, diarrhea, fatigue, debility, weak digestion and failing memory.

Phaffia root contains bitter compounds (saponins) that are adaptogens. The compounds have non-specific immune strengthening properties. Suma has been used to treat stress disorders, diabetes, skin inflammations and sexual dysfunction.

Ginkgo leaves contain bitter compounds (flavonoids) that decrease capillary permeability, thrombosis and platelet aggregation. These compounds increase peripheral blood flow and reduce inflammation. Ginkgo is an excellent herbal source of iron, calcium and vitamin C. It has been used to treat poor circulation, deafness, Alzheimer's disease and atherosclerosis.

Astragalus root contains bitter compounds that increase the flow of urine, are antiseptic, increase the production of digestive fluids including bile and relieve muscle spasms. Astragalus also contains mucilaginous compounds that enhance immune response, increasing the production of lymphocytes and macrophages. The herb also increases heart action, lowers blood pressure and blood sugar. It has been used to treat fatigue, debility, urinary tract infections, edema, nephritis, ulcers, prolapse of organs and night sweats.

Gotu Kola herb contains bitter compounds that have a sedative effect, dilate peripheral blood vessels and increase the flow of urine. It is an excellent herbal source of niacin, calcium, magnesium, manganese, silicon and sodium. Gotu kola has been used to treat insomnia, failing memory, schizophrenia, fevers, headaches and inflammatory skin conditions.

Parthenium and Goldenseal Combination

Composition

Parthenium	Yarrow
Goldenseal	Capsicum

Properties

Antiseptic
Immunostimulant
Anti-inflammatory
Carminative

General Description

Parthenium and Goldenseal combination is used to fight infections especially of the digestive tract. The herbs are antiseptic and increase immune response. They also increase the production of digestive fluids and soothe inflamed tissue.

Chinese herbalists would describe this combination as a wood reducing formula. It also reduces the fire element while enhancing the metal, fire and earth elements.

Parthenium and Goldenseal combination has traditionally been used to treat **jaundice, influenza, ulcers, infectious fevers, swollen glands, excess bile, gastritis, enteritis** and **abscesses.**

Imbalances indicating the use of this formula are commonly noted in the liver acupressure point located approximately four inches to the right of the sternum between the seventh and eight rib. Imbalances are often noted in the lymphatic wreaths of both irises. Use caution in cases of anemia, postpartum weakness and hypoglycemia.

This formula is commonly used in conjunction with the vitamin C family, vitamin A, vitamin E, selenium, zinc,

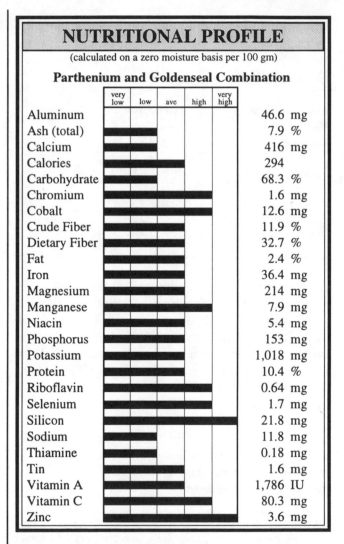

NUTRITIONAL PROFILE
(calculated on a zero moisture basis per 100 gm)
Parthenium and Goldenseal Combination

Nutrient	Value
Aluminum	46.6 mg
Ash (total)	7.9 %
Calcium	416 mg
Calories	294
Carbohydrate	68.3 %
Chromium	1.6 mg
Cobalt	12.6 mg
Crude Fiber	11.9 %
Dietary Fiber	32.7 %
Fat	2.4 %
Iron	36.4 mg
Magnesium	214 mg
Manganese	7.9 mg
Niacin	5.4 mg
Phosphorus	153 mg
Potassium	1,018 mg
Protein	10.4 %
Riboflavin	0.64 mg
Selenium	1.7 mg
Silicon	21.8 mg
Sodium	11.8 mg
Thiamine	0.18 mg
Tin	1.6 mg
Vitamin A	1,786 IU
Vitamin C	80.3 mg
Zinc	3.6 mg

germanium, barley grass, wheat grass, alfalfa, asparagus, broccoli, cauliflower and cabbage.

Individual Components

Parthenium root contains mucilaginous compounds that increase immune response, sequester infections and soothe inflamed tissues. Parthenium also contains bitter compounds that increase immune response by increasing the production of T-lymphocytes, phagocytic macrophages, interferons and lymphokines. Parthenium has been used to treat wounds, infections, blood poisoning, inflammatory skin conditions and tonsillitis.

Goldenseal root contains bitter astringent alkaloids that normalize liver and spleen functions by increasing the production of digestive fluids and enzymes, particularly bile. The compounds are antiseptic, constrict peripheral blood vessels, especially in the uterus, are laxative and relieve pain and inflammation in mucosal tissue. Goldenseal is an excellent herbal source of trace minerals including cobalt, iron, magnesium, manganese, silicon and zinc. It is also an excellent herbal source of vitamin C. It has been used to treat hepatitis,

gastritis, colitis, ulcers, menorrhagia, postpartum hemorrhages, dysmenorrhea, diabetes, infections, hemorrhoids, eczema, obesity and fevers.

Yarrow flower contains aromatic compounds that shrink inflamed tissues and promote sweating. It also contains bitter compounds that relieve smooth muscle spasms, reduce blood pressure and stop bleeding. Yarrow has been used to treat hemorrhoids, fevers, nausea and inflammatory skin conditions.

Capsicum fruit contains aromatic resins that increase blood circulation, promote sweating, increase the production of digestive fluids and reduce muscle spasms. It has been used to treat flatulence, colic, ulcers, rheumatic arthritis, cold hands and feet and dropsy.

Parthenium and Myrrh Combination

Composition

Parthenium	Yarrow
Myrrh	Capsicum

Properties

Antiseptic	Expectorant
Immunostimulant	Analgesic

General Description

Parthenium and Myrrh combination is used to fight infections, particularly of the lymphatic and respiratory systems. The herbs are antiseptic, increase immune response, relieve pain and decrease the thickness while increasing the production of mucosal fluids.

Chinese herbalists would describe this herbal combination as a metal enhancing formula. It also enhances the fire and water elements while reducing the wood and earth elements.

Parthenium and Myrrh combination has traditionally been used to treat **blood poisoning, eczema, infections, fevers, earaches, swollen glands, wounds** and **abscesses.**

Imbalances indicating the use of this formula are commonly noted in the liver acupressure point located approximately four inches to the right of the sternum, between the seventh and eighth rib. Imbalances are often noted in the lymphatic wreaths of both irises. Use caution in cases of anemia, postpartum weakness and hypertension.

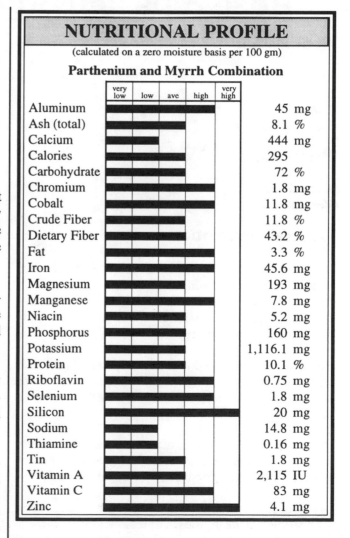

NUTRITIONAL PROFILE
(calculated on a zero moisture basis per 100 gm)

Parthenium and Myrrh Combination

	very low	low	ave	high	very high	
Aluminum						45 mg
Ash (total)						8.1 %
Calcium						444 mg
Calories						295
Carbohydrate						72 %
Chromium						1.8 mg
Cobalt						11.8 mg
Crude Fiber						11.8 %
Dietary Fiber						43.2 %
Fat						3.3 %
Iron						45.6 mg
Magnesium						193 mg
Manganese						7.8 mg
Niacin						5.2 mg
Phosphorus						160 mg
Potassium						1,116.1 mg
Protein						10.1 %
Riboflavin						0.75 mg
Selenium						1.8 mg
Silicon						20 mg
Sodium						14.8 mg
Thiamine						0.16 mg
Tin						1.8 mg
Vitamin A						2,115 IU
Vitamin C						83 mg
Zinc						4.1 mg

This formula is commonly used in conjunction with the vitamin C family, vitamin A, betacarotene, vitamin E, selenium, zinc, germanium, barley grass, wheat grass, alfalfa, asparagus, broccoli, cauliflower and cabbage.

Individual Components

Parthenium root contains mucilaginous compounds that increase immune response, sequester infections and sooth inflamed tissues. Parthenium also contains bitter compounds that increase immune response by increasing the production of T-lymphocytes, phagocytic macrophages, interferons and lymphokines. Parthenium has been used to treat wounds, infections, blood poisoning, inflammatory skin conditions and tonsillitis.

Myrrh gum contains astringent resins that promote the healing of sores. These compounds shrink inflamed tissue, are antiseptic and reduce pain in mucous membranes. Myrrh also decreases the thickness while increasing the production of mucosal fluids. It has been used to treat colds, coughs, bronchitis, asthma, dysmenorrhea, rheumatism and arthritis.

Yarrow flower contains aromatic compounds that shrink inflamed tissues and promote sweating. It also contains bitter compounds that relieve smooth muscle spasms, reduce blood pressure and stop bleeding. Yarrow has been used to treat hemorrhoids, fevers, nausea, and inflammatory skin conditions.

Capsicum fruit contains aromatic resins that increase blood circulation, promote sweating, increase the production of digestive fluids and reduce muscle spasms. It has been used to treat flatulence, colic, ulcers, rheumatic arthritis, cold hands and feet and dropsy.

Rose Hips and Broccoli Combination

Composition

Rose hips	Red clover
Broccoli	Parsley
Cabbage	Wheat grass
Siberian Ginseng	Horseradish

Properties

Antioxidant	Nervine
Vulnerary	Tonic

General Description

Rose hips and Broccoli combination is an antioxidant formula designed to combat the effects of stress on the immune system. The herbs work to scavenge free radicals, improve blood circulation, promote healing and improve immune response.

Chinese herbalists would describe this herbal combination as a metal enhancing formula. It also enhances the fire and water elements, while reducing the wood and earth elements.

Rose hips and Broccoli combination has traditionally been used to treat **stress disorders, poor digestion, debility, fatigue, infections, nausea** and **earaches.**

Imbalances indicating the use of this formula are commonly noted in the thymus acupressure point located in the center of the sternum. Imbalances are often noted at the 4:30 position of the left iris.

NUTRITIONAL PROFILE
(calculated on a zero moisture basis per 100 gm)

Rose Hips and Broccoli Combination

Nutrient	Value
Aluminum	22 mg
Ash (total)	6.2 %
Calcium	854 mg
Calories	279
Carbohydrate	64.2 %
Chromium	3.2 mg
Cobalt	8.3 mg
Crude Fiber	11.4 %
Dietary Fiber	34.0 %
Fat	1.9 %
Iron	21 mg
Magnesium	289 mg
Manganese	12.0 mg
Niacin	8.2 mg
Phosphorus	502 mg
Potassium	2,400 mg
Protein	14.1 %
Riboflavin	0.62 mg
Selenium	1.9 mg
Silicon	5.4 mg
Sodium	95 mg
Thiamine	0.71 mg
Tin	1.1 mg
Vitamin A	2,620 IU
Vitamin C	135 mg
Zinc	2.3 mg

This formula is commonly used in conjunction with parthenium, goldenseal, myrrh, germanium, the vitamin C family, the complex of B vitamins, pollen and vitamin E.

Individual Components

Rose hips contain bitter compounds called bioflavinoids which enhance the absorption of vitamin C and strengthen connective tissue. This results in decreased capillary fragility. It also contains astringent compounds which shrink inflamed tissues and reduce the secretion of mucosal fluids. Rosehips is an excellent herbal source of vitamin C. It has been used to treat the common cold, influenza, fevers, infections, inflammatory skin conditions, easy bruising, varicose veins, debility, capillary fragility and hemorrhoids.

Broccoli herb contains bitter compounds (ascorbigens) that have antioxidant and healing properties. Broccoli is an excellent food source of many nutrients including vitamin C, beta carotene, protein, potassium and riboflavin. Broccoli has been used to treat dysuria, constipation and as a preventative measure to strengthen immune response.

Cabbage leaves contain bitter compounds (ascorbigens) that have antioxidant and healing properties. Cabbage is an excellent food source of many nutrients including potassium, protein, riboflavin, thiamine, beta-carotene, and vitamin C. Cabbage has been used to treat skin disorders, constipation and as a preventative measure to strengthen immune response.

Siberian Ginseng root contains bitter compounds that help the body respond more quickly to stress. These compounds increase the production of DNA, RNA and proteins essential to all life processes. They also stimulate the adrenal, pancreas, and pituitary glands to lower blood sugar and reduce inflammation. Ginseng also increases the production of digestive fluids and is a mild sedative. It has been used to treat anemia, impotence, insomnia, diarrhea, fatigue, debility, weak digestion and failing memory.

Red clover flowers contain bitter compounds that increase the production of digestive fluids and enzymes, especially bile. These compounds also shrink inflammation and relieve pains. Red clover is an excellent herbal source of calcium, chromium, magnesium, phosphorus and potassium. It has been used to treat arthritis, jaundice, liver congestion, muscle cramps and inflammatory skin conditions.

Parsley herb contains aromatic compounds that decrease the thickness and increase the production of mucosal fluids, increase the production digestive fluids, increase menstrual flow and increase urine flow. It contains bitter compounds that reduce muscle spasms and pains, reduce blood pressure and are antiseptic. Parsley is an excellent herbal source of trace minerals, especially the electrolyte minerals including sodium, potassium, calcium, and magnesium. It is also an excellent herbal source of vitamin A, vitamin C and chlorophyllins. Parsley has been used to treat urinary tract infections, amenorrhea, dysmenorrhea, dyspepsia, bronchitis, allergies, arthritis, asthma, flatulence, dysuria and nephritis.

Wheat grass is the young shoots of wheat. It contains bitter compounds that enhance digestion. It is an excellent herbal source of trace nutrients and enzymes, especially superoxide dismutase, a natural antioxidant. Wheatgrass has been used to treat general debility, fatigue, arthritis and to enhance immune response.

Horseradish root contains aromatic compounds that increase circulation, are antiseptic and promote sweating. These compounds also decrease the thickness while increasing the production of mucosal fluid. Horseradish has been used to treat asthma, bronchitis, coughs, colds, fevers and rheumatism.

Eyebright herb contains astringent compounds that shrink inflamed tissues. It also contains bitter compounds that relieve pains, are antiseptic and sooth inflamed mucous membranes. Eyebright is an excellent herbal source of vitamin B-1, vitamin B-2, niacin, calcium, cobalt, magnesium, manganese and zinc. It has been used to treat eye infections, colds, sinus congestion, allergies, jaundice and hepatitis.

Chapter 9

The Nervous System

The nervous system consists of the central nervous system (including the brain and spinal cord), the peripheral nervous system and the sensory system including the eyes, ears, nose and tongue. Its prime function is to communicate responses between internal and external stimuli. The names for the herbal combinations are chosen based on the properties of the key herbs in the formula.

Therapies for Relieving Excess Conditions

Insomnia or fitful sleep is typical of an excess condition of the nervous system. It is often accompanied by anxiety, restlessness and weakness in the sexual organs. Herbalists use aromatic herbs and astringent herbs to calm the mind and the heart.

Excess conditions in the nervous system are marked by patterns of minor aches, pains and ailments including: anxiety, restlessness, fidgeting, muscle spasms, failing memory, neurosis, excitability, nightmares, emotional instability, rapid speech, abnormal laughing, angina pains, inflammatory skin conditions, red eyes, hypertension, heart palpitations, frequent urination and dizziness. If left unchecked, these ailments may develop into illnesses including: epilepsy, stroke, insomnia, heart disease, autism, carpal tunnel syndrome, glaucoma, migraine headaches, hyperkinesis, pains, neuralgia and neuropathy, tinnitis, vertigo and schizophrenia.

Early herbal therapies for these conditions consisted of single herbs like valerian which has a sedative effect. Valerian is not simply a sedative herb however, and with time and experience, herbalists recognized and recorded in their herbals the several properties of valerian. The British Herbal Pharmacopoeia lists valerian as a sedative, anadyne, hypnotic, antispasmodic, carminative and hypotensive.

These lists of empirical properties of an herb are the key to understanding herbal combinations. Herbalists have found that they can enhance a particular property of a single herb by adding herbs that complement and support that given property. Conversely, the herbalist is able to minimize the effects of an unwanted property by adding herbs that counteract and balance the unwanted property.

Therapies for Supplementing Deficient Conditions

Weakness in the nervous system is characterized by a lack of energy and a sense of tension. This often results in headaches and various degrees of depression.

Weakened conditions of the nervous system are often associated with patterns of minor aches, pains and ailments including: hypochondria, fatigue, vertigo, neurosis, hysteria, nightmares, worry, migrating pains, menstrual pains, backaches, abdominal pains, chronic respiratory infections, insomnia, angina pains, chronic coughs, fright, edema and chronic sore throats. If left unchecked, these ailments may develop into the following illnesses: depression, insomnia, premenstrual syndrome, allergies, bronchitis, asthma, colds and influenza.

Early herbal therapies for these conditions were of great importance to the Chinese herbalist. Western herbalists often tried to "sweat the evil spirit" out of a depressed individual, often leaving the victim weaker and more depressed. The Chinese, on the other hand, were blessed with herbs such as bupleurum root which increases one's sense of well being. The properties of bupleurum include: antidepressant, analgesic, antiinflammatory antipyretic and cholagogue.

These empirical properties of an herb are the key to understanding herbal combinations. Herbalists have found that they can enhance a particular property of a single herb by adding herbs that complement and support a given property. Conversely, the herbalist is able to minimize an unwanted property by adding herbs that counteract and balance the unwanted property.

Chamomile and Passionflower Combination

Composition

Chamomile
Passionflower
Hops

Feverfew
Fennel
Marshmallow

Properties

Sedative
Analgesic
Antispasmodic

General Description

Chamomile and Passionflower combination is a sedative and tranquilizing formula used to relieve the effects of everyday stresses. The herbs work to relieve nervous tension and anxiety.

Chinese herbalists would describe this herbal combination as a fire reducing formula. It also reduces the earth and wood elements while enhancing the metal and water elements.

Chamomile and Passionflower combination has traditionally been used to treat **anxiety, muscle tension, insomnia, muscle spasms, nervous headache** and **premenstrual syndrome.**

Imbalances indicating the use of this formula are commonly noted in the stress acupressure point located above the left clavicle. Imbalances are often noted in the nerve wreath surrounding each pupil. Use caution as overdoses may cause nausea.

This formula is commonly used in conjunction with the complex of B vitamins, the vitamin C family, schizandra, ginseng, bee pollen and wheat germ.

Individual Components

Chamomile flowers contain aromatic compounds that increase the production of digestive fluids, reduce muscle spasms and pains, reduce inflammation and are antiseptic. In addition, these compounds have a sedative effect. Chamomile is one of the best herbal sources of niacin,

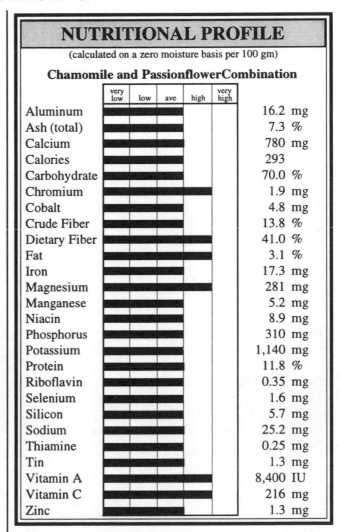

NUTRITIONAL PROFILE

(calculated on a zero moisture basis per 100 gm)

Chamomile and Passionflower Combination

	very low	low	ave	high	very high	
Aluminum						16.2 mg
Ash (total)						7.3 %
Calcium						780 mg
Calories						293
Carbohydrate						70.0 %
Chromium						1.9 mg
Cobalt						4.8 mg
Crude Fiber						13.8 %
Dietary Fiber						41.0 %
Fat						3.1 %
Iron						17.3 mg
Magnesium						281 mg
Manganese						5.2 mg
Niacin						8.9 mg
Phosphorus						310 mg
Potassium						1,140 mg
Protein						11.8 %
Riboflavin						0.35 mg
Selenium						1.6 mg
Silicon						5.7 mg
Sodium						25.2 mg
Thiamine						0.25 mg
Tin						1.3 mg
Vitamin A						8,400 IU
Vitamin C						216 mg
Zinc						1.3 mg

magnesium and essential fatty acids. It has been used to treat dyspepsia, flatulence, nausea, vomiting, dysmenorrhea, bronchitis, urinary tract infections, insomnia, headaches and menstrual cramps.

Passionflower contains bitter compounds that have a sedative effect and relieve muscle spasms. It has been used to treat insomnia, coughs, headaches and dysmenorrhea.

Hops flowers contain bitter compounds that have a sedative effect and relieve smooth muscle spasms, increase the flow of urine and are antiseptic. Hops is an excellent herbal source of niacin. It has been used to treat insomnia, painful urination, urinary tract infections, spastic colon and anxiety.

Feverfew herb contains bitter compounds that reduce inflammation and pain and dilate peripheral blood vessels. Feverfew is an excellent herbal source of niacin. It has been used to treat migraine headaches and arthritis.

Fennel seed contains aromatic compounds that stimulate the production of digestive fluids, relieve inflammation, are antiseptic, make one breath deeply and more often, and increase the flow of urine. It has been used to treat indigestion, dyspepsia, anorexia, colic, flatulence, coughs, and colds.

Marshmallow root contains mucilaginous compounds that decrease the thickness while increasing the production of mucosal fluids, soothe inflamed tissue, heal wounds and increase the flow of urine. It is an excellent herbal source of trace minerals, especially chromium, iron, magnesium, and selenium. Marshmallow has been used to treat allergies, gastritis, gastric ulcers, enteritis, coughs, cystitis and hay fevers.

Fushen and Dragon Bone Combination

Composition

Fushen	Cinnamon Bark	Zizyphus
Dragon bone	Polygala	Polygonum
Oyster shell	Acorus	Licorice
Haliotis	Saussurea	Ginger
Albizia	Siberian Ginseng	Curcuma
Coptis		

Properties

Sedative	Antispasmodic
Carminative	Diuretic

General Description

Fushen and Dragon Bone combination is a sedative formula. It combines herbs with sedative properties with natural sources of calcium to calm the nervous and circulatory systems. The herbs have a sedative effect and improve digestion by increasing the production of digestive fluids, increasing the flow of urine, and relieving muscle spasms often associated with anxiety. In addition, calcium is a natural tranquilizer that also calms muscle spasms.

Chinese herbalists describe this herbal combination as a fire reducing formula. It also reduces the earth element while enhancing the water, wood and metal elements.

Fushen and Dragon Bone combination has traditionally been used to treat **insomnia, indigestion, paranoia, neurosis, fright, excitability, angina pains, hyperventilation** and **heart palpitations.**

Imbalances indicating the use of this formula are commonly noted in the stress acupressure point located on the forehead between the eyes. Imbalances are often noted in the nerve wreath surrounding each pupil.

This formula is commonly used in conjunction with the complex of B vitamins, the vitamin C family, passionflower, chamomile, scullcap and hops.

Individual Components

Fushen herb contains bitter compounds that increase the flow of urine, decrease blood sugar and have a sedative effect. It has been used to treat dysuria, heart palpitations, insomnia and edema.

Dragon bone is fossilized bone material consisting of calcium carbonate and calcium phosphate. These compounds are astringent and act to reduce sweating, neutralize gastric acidity, relax muscle cramps and have a mild sedative effect. Dragon bone has been used to treat insomnia, heart palpitations, hypertension, night sweats, hyperacid stomaches and headaches.

Oyster shell is primarily calcium carbonate. It is astringent and reduces sweating, neutralizes stomach acid, relaxes muscle cramps and has a mild sedative effect. It has been used to treat insomnia, heart palpitations, hypertension, night sweats, hyperacid stomaches and headaches.

Haliotis shell or abalone shell is primarily calcium carbonate. It is astringent and reduces sweating, neutralizes stomach acid, relaxes muscle cramps and has a mild sedative effect. It has been used to treat insomnia, heart palpitations, hypertension, night sweats, hyperacid stomaches and headaches.

Albizia bark contains astringent compounds that shrink inflamed tissue especially in the uterus. It also contains bitter compounds that relieve pains, have a sedative effect, increase blood circulation and increase the flow of urine. Albizia has been used to treat insomnia, heart palpitations, anxiety and inflammatory skin conditions.

Coptis root contains bitter astringent alkaloids similar to those found in goldenseal. These compounds normalize liver and spleen function by increasing the production of digestive fluids and enzymes, particularly bile. These compounds are antiseptic, constrict peripheral blood vessels, especially in the uterus, are laxative and relieve pain and inflammation in mucosal tissue. Coptis has been used to treat hepatitis, gastritis, colitis, ulcers, menorrhagia, postpartum hemorrhages, dysmenorrhea, diabetes, infections, hemorrhoids, eczema, obesity and fevers.

Cinnamon bark contains aromatic compounds that promote sweating, increase blood circulation, increase the production of digestive fluids, relieve smooth muscle spasms, increase the flow of urine and are antiseptic. It has been used to treat colds, edema, dysuria, arthritis, amenorrhea, angina, pains, dyspepsia and hypochondria.

Polygala root contains bitter compounds that decrease the thickness and increase the production of mucosal fluids, have a sedative effect and are antiseptic. These compounds also lower blood pressure and increase uterine tension. Polygala has been used to treat insomnia, heart palpitations, ulcers, inflammatory skin conditions, bronchitis and nervous tension.

Acorus root contains aromatic compounds that have a sedative effect, increase the production of digestive fluids, relieve muscle spasms, lower blood pressure, reduce fevers and are antiseptic. Acorus has been used to treat nervous tension, depression, epilepsy, poor appetite, gastritis and flatulence.

Saussurea root contains aromatic compounds that increase the production of digestive fluids, increase blood circulation and are antiseptic. It also contains bitter compounds that relieve smooth muscle spasms, lower blood pressure and relieve pains. Saussurea has been used to treat gastritis, chest pains, jaundice, gall stones and diarrhea.

Siberian Ginseng root contains bitter compounds that help the body respond more quickly to stress. These compounds increase the production of DNA, RNA and proteins essential to all life processes. They stimulate the adrenal, pancreas, and pituitary glands to lower blood sugar and reduce inflammation. Ginseng also increases the production of digestive fluids and is a mild sedative. It had been used to treat anemia, impotence, insomnia, diarrhea, fatigue, debility, weak digestion and failing memory.

Zizyphus seed contains bitter compounds that have a sedative effect, relieve pains, reduce fevers and lower blood pressure. It has been used to treat insomnia, heart palpitation , night sweats and nervous tension.

Polygonum herb contains bitter compounds that increase the flow of urine, increase the production of bile and lower blood pressure. It also contains astringent compounds that are antiseptic, shrink inflamed tissue, especially in the uterus, and constrict peripheral blood vessels. Polygonum has been used to treat urinary tract infections, dysuria, jaundice, inflammatory skin conditions and as an anthelmintic.

Licorice root contains bitter compounds that reduce inflammation, decrease the thickness and increase the production of mucosal fluids and relieve muscle spasms. In addition, licorice stimulates adrenal function, reduces the urge to cough, is mildly laxative and enhances immune response. It has been used to treat coughs, colds, arthritis, asthma, peptic ulcers, Addison's disease, dropsy and atherosclerosis.

Ginger root contains aromatic compounds that increase the production of digestive fluids and enzymes, lower blood pressure, lower blood sugar and cholesterol. It also contains bitter compounds that reduce muscle spasms, increase blood circulation and dilate blood vessels. Ginger is an excellent herbal source of trace minerals especially silicon, magnesium and manganese. It has been used to treat nausea, motion sickness, flatulence, colds, coughs, indigestion, fevers, vomiting, diarrhea, chronic bronchitis and cold hands and feet.

Curcuma root contains bitter compounds that relieve pain and inflammation in mucosal tissue and increase the production of bile. It also contains aromatic compounds that increase the production of digestive fluids and are antiseptic. It has been used to treat angina pains, anxiety, hepatitis, gall stones and dysmenorrhea.

Ginseng and Gota Kola Combination

Composition

Siberian Ginseng	Capsicum
Gotu Kola	

Properties

Nervine	Vulnerary
Tonic	

General Description

Ginseng and Gota Kola combination is used to assist the recuperative powers of the body. All the herbs are noted as tonics and have been used to increase endurance and longevity. In the short term, this formula is a nervine used to overcome the effects of anxiety and stress. With long term use, Ginseng and Gota Kola combination enhances the function of the reproductive system as a tonic and vulnerary.

Chinese herbalists would describe this herbal combination as an earth enhancing or yin tonic formula. It also enhances the water and metal elements while reducing the fire and wood elements.

Ginseng and Gota Kola combination has traditionally been used to treat **nervous disorders, prolonged illness, failing memory, epilepsy, senility, premature aging, sexual dysfunction** and **venereal disease.**

Imbalances indicating the use of this formula are commonly noted in the stress acupressure point located on the forehead and the genital acupressure point located on the lower abdomen. Imbalances are often noted at the 5 o'clock position of the left iris. Use caution when using this formula as large doses may cause headaches.

This formula is commonly used in conjunction with the vitamin C family, the complex of B vitamins, licorice, fenugreek, alfalfa, calcium, magnesium, manganese and iron.

Individual Components

Siberian Ginseng root contains bitter compounds that helps the body respond more quickly to stress. These compounds increase the production of DNA, RNA and proteins essential to all life processes. They stimulate the adrenal, pancreas, and pituitary glands to lower blood sugar and reduce inflammation. Ginseng also

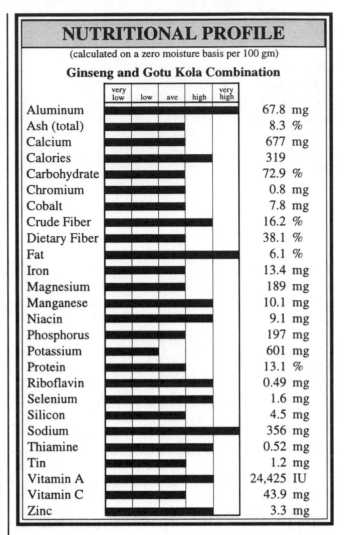

NUTRITIONAL PROFILE

(calculated on a zero moisture basis per 100 gm)

Ginseng and Gotu Kola Combination

	very low	low	ave	high	very high	
Aluminum						67.8 mg
Ash (total)						8.3 %
Calcium						677 mg
Calories						319
Carbohydrate						72.9 %
Chromium						0.8 mg
Cobalt						7.8 mg
Crude Fiber						16.2 %
Dietary Fiber						38.1 %
Fat						6.1 %
Iron						13.4 mg
Magnesium						189 mg
Manganese						10.1 mg
Niacin						9.1 mg
Phosphorus						197 mg
Potassium						601 mg
Protein						13.1 %
Riboflavin						0.49 mg
Selenium						1.6 mg
Silicon						4.5 mg
Sodium						356 mg
Thiamine						0.52 mg
Tin						1.2 mg
Vitamin A						24,425 IU
Vitamin C						43.9 mg
Zinc						3.3 mg

increases the production of digestive fluids and is a mild sedative. It had been used to treat anemia, impotence, insomnia, diarrhea, fatigue, debility, weak digestion and failing memory.

Gotu Kola herb contains bitter compounds that have a sedative effect, dilate peripheral blood vessels and increase the flow of urine. It is an excellent herbal source of niacin, calcium, magnesium, manganese, silicon and sodium. Gotu kola has been used to treat insomnia, failing memory, schizophrenia, fevers, headache and inflammatory skin conditions.

Capsicum fruit contains aromatic resins that increase blood circulation, promote sweating, increase the production of digestive fluids and reduce muscle spasms. It has been used to treat flatulence, colic, ulcers, rheumatic arthritis, cold hands and feet and dropsy.

Pollen and Ginseng Combination

Composition

Siberian Ginseng   Yellow dock
Gotu Kola   Schizandra
Pollen   Barley grass
Kelp   Rose hips
Licorice   Capsicum

Properties

Stimulant

Tonic

General Description

Pollen and Ginseng combination is an energy release formula. All the herbs are used to increase endurance and stamina by relieving nervous tension and eliminating the products of metabolism. Formerly, herbal combinations of this type were called "spring tonics."

Chinese herbalists would describe this herbal combination as a fire enhancing formula. It also enhances the earth and metal elements while reducing the water and wood elements.

Pollen and Ginseng combination has traditionally been used to treat **fatigue, depression, dysmenorrhea, post-partum depression, prolonged illnesses** and **sexual dysfunction.**

Imbalances indicating the use of this formula are commonly noted in the stress acupressure point located above the forehead. Imbalances are often noted at the 5:00 position of the left iris.

This formula is commonly used in conjunction with the vitamin C family, the complex of B vitamins, calcium, magnesium and iron.

Individual Components

Siberian Ginseng root contains bitter compounds that help the body respond more quickly to stress. These compounds increase the production of DNA, RNA and proteins essential to all life processes. They also stimulate the adrenal, pancreas, and pituitary glands to lower blood sugar and reduce inflammation. Ginseng also increases the production of digestive fluids and is a mild

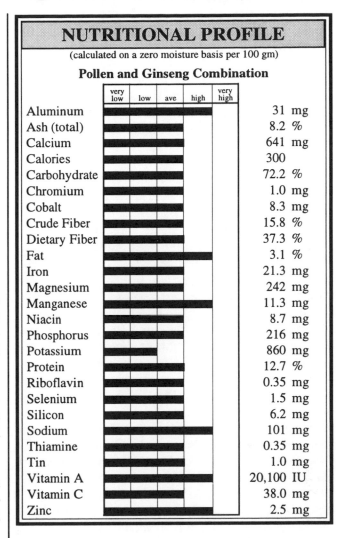

NUTRITIONAL PROFILE
(calculated on a zero moisture basis per 100 gm)
Pollen and Ginseng Combination

	very low	low	ave	high	very high	
Aluminum						31 mg
Ash (total)						8.2 %
Calcium						641 mg
Calories						300
Carbohydrate						72.2 %
Chromium						1.0 mg
Cobalt						8.3 mg
Crude Fiber						15.8 %
Dietary Fiber						37.3 %
Fat						3.1 %
Iron						21.3 mg
Magnesium						242 mg
Manganese						11.3 mg
Niacin						8.7 mg
Phosphorus						216 mg
Potassium						860 mg
Protein						12.7 %
Riboflavin						0.35 mg
Selenium						1.5 mg
Silicon						6.2 mg
Sodium						101 mg
Thiamine						0.35 mg
Tin						1.0 mg
Vitamin A						20,100 IU
Vitamin C						38.0 mg
Zinc						2.5 mg

sedative. It has been used to treat anemia, impotence, insomnia, diarrhea, fatigue, debility, weak digestion and failing memory.

Gotu Kola herb contains bitter compounds that have a sedative effect, dilate peripheral blood vessels and increase the flow of urine. It is an excellent herbal source of niacin, calcium, magnesium, manganese, silicon and sodium. Gotu kola has been used to treat insomnia, failing memory, schizophrenia, fevers, headaches and inflammatory skin conditions.

Pollen is gathered by bees from a variety of flowers. It is an excellent source of carbohydrates which may in part account for its reputation as an energy booster. Pollen has been used to treat fatigue, sexual dysfunction, poor memory and convalescence.

Kelp herb contains mucilaginous compounds that enhance the detoxifying and eliminative functions of the digestive system. These compounds absorb toxins from the bowel and provide bulk to the stool. Kelp is an excellent herbal source of calcium, magnesium, sodium and iodine. Iodine is essential to normal thyroid function. It is used to increase the metabolic rate and strengthen connective tissues including the hair, skin and nails. Kelp has been used to treat hypothyroidism, enlarged glands, debility, fatigue, eczema, psoriasis, arthritis and obesity.

Licorice root contains bitter compounds that reduce inflammation, decrease the thickness and increase the production of mucosal fluids and relieve muscle spasms. In addition, licorice stimulates adrenal function, reduces the urge to cough, is mildly laxative and enhances immune response. It has been used to treat coughs, colds, arthritis, asthma, peptic ulcers, Addison's disease, dropsy and atherosclerosis.

Yellow dock contains bitter compounds that are laxative, increase the production of digestive fluids and enzymes, especially bile, and increase the flow of urine. It also contains astringent compounds that shrink inflamed tissues. Yellow dock is an excellent herbal source of vitamin A, vitamin C, calcium, iron, magnesium, phosphorus and selenium. It has been used to treat liver congestion, constipation, arthritis, rheumatism, inflammatory bowel disorders and inflammatory skin conditions.

Schizandra fruit contains bitter compounds that allow the body to more quickly respond to stress. This increases the body's capacity for work and decreases fatigue. These compounds increase blood circulation, blood sugar and bile production while lowering blood pressure. Schizandra also contains astringent compounds that increase the contraction of the heart muscle and the uterus and are antiseptic. The herb has been used to treat heart palpitations, dropsy, nervous exhaustion, asthma, diabetes, chronic diarrhea, night sweats, seminal emissions, insomnia, frequent urination and anxiety.

Barley grass is the young shoots of barley. It contains bitter compounds that enhance digestion. It is an excellent source of trace nutrients and enzymes, especially super oxide dismutase, a natural antioxidant. Barley grass has been used to treat general debility, fatigue, arthritis and to enhance immune response.

Rose hips contain bitter compounds called bioflavinoids which enhance the absorption of vitamin C and strengthen connective tissue. This results in decreased capillary fragility. It also contains astringent compounds which shrink inflamed tissues and reduce the secretion of mucosal fluids. Rosehips is an excellent herbal source of vitamin C. It has been used to treat the common cold, influenza, fevers, infections, inflammatory skin conditions, easy bruising, varicose veins, debility, capillary fragility and hemorrhoids.

Capsicum fruit contains aromatic resins that increase blood circulation, promote sweating, increase the production of digestive fluids and reduce muscle spasms. It has been used to treat flatulence, colic, ulcers, rheumatic arthritis, cold hands and feet and dropsy.

Scullcap Combination

Composition

Scullcap
Valerian
Hops

Properties

Sedative
Antispasmodic
Diuretic

General Description

Scullcap combination is a sedative and tranquillizing formula. Used in combination, the herbs have a sedative effect and relieve smooth muscle spasms, especially in the digestive and urinary systems. In addition, the formula increases the flow of urine. Unlike conventional sedatives, this formula only induces drowsiness in poor sleepers.

Chinese herbalists would describe this herbal combination as a fire reducing formula. It also reduces earth and wood elements while enhancing the metal and water elements.

Scullcap combination has traditionally been used to treat **insomnia, muscle spasms, epilepsy, nervous headaches, hypertension, nocturnal emissions, arthritis, menstrual disorders** and **flatulence.**

Imbalances indicating the use of this formula are commonly noted in the stress acupressure point located on the forehead and in the stress acupressure point located above the left clavicle. Imbalances are often noted in the nerve wreath surrounding each pupil. Use caution as extreme doses can cause nausea and paralysis.

This formula is commonly used in conjunction with the complex of B vitamins, the vitamin C family, schizandra fruit, ginseng, bee pollen and wheat germ.

Individual Components

Scullcap herb contains bitter compounds that have a sedative effect and relieve smooth muscle spasms. This herb is particularly useful in calming the nervous and circulatory systems. Scullcap is an excellent herbal source of vitamin C and bioflavonoids. It has been used

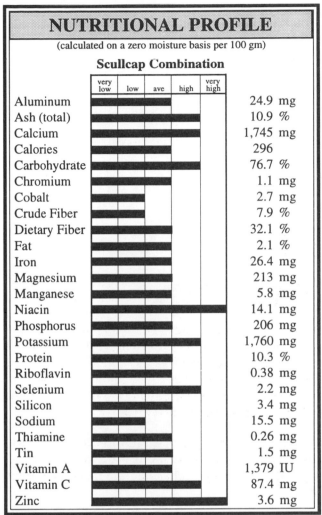

NUTRITIONAL PROFILE
(calculated on a zero moisture basis per 100 gm)

Scullcap Combination

	very low	low	ave	high	very high	
Aluminum						24.9 mg
Ash (total)						10.9 %
Calcium						1,745 mg
Calories						296
Carbohydrate						76.7 %
Chromium						1.1 mg
Cobalt						2.7 mg
Crude Fiber						7.9 %
Dietary Fiber						32.1 %
Fat						2.1 %
Iron						26.4 mg
Magnesium						213 mg
Manganese						5.8 mg
Niacin						14.1 mg
Phosphorus						206 mg
Potassium						1,760 mg
Protein						10.3 %
Riboflavin						0.38 mg
Selenium						2.2 mg
Silicon						3.4 mg
Sodium						15.5 mg
Thiamine						0.26 mg
Tin						1.5 mg
Vitamin A						1,379 IU
Vitamin C						87.4 mg
Zinc						3.6 mg

to treat insomnia, anxiety, nervous tension, headaches, enuresis and muscle twitching.

Valerian root contains aromatic compounds that have a sedative effect, acting to decrease anxiety and aggression. These compounds also relieve smooth muscle spasms, lower blood pressure and improve sleep quality in cases of insomnia. The herb is relatively inactive in normal sleepers. Valerian is the very best herbal source of calcium and an excellent herbal source of magnesium. It has been used to treat nervousness, anxiety, insomnia, stomach cramps, muscle spasms, hysteria and convulsions.

Hops flowers contain bitter compounds that have a sedative effect and relieve smooth muscle spasms, increase the flow of urine and are antiseptic. Hops is an excellent herbal source of niacin. It has been used to treat insomnia, painful urination, urinary tract infections, spastic colon and anxiety.

Valerian and Black Cohosh Combination

Composition

Black Cohosh	Lady's Slipper
Capsicum	Scullcap
Valerian	Hops
Passionflower	Wood Betony

Properties

Sedative
Antispasmodic
Analgesic

General Description

Valerian and Black Cohosh combination is a sedative and tranquillizing formula. The herbs in this formula work to relieve nervous tension often associated with anxiety and tense muscles. In addition, reaction time and reflexes are not impaired by this formula as peripheral blood circulation is increased.

Chinese herbalists would describe this herbal combination as a fire reducing formula. It also reduces earth and wood elements while enhancing the metal and water elements.

Valerian and Black Cohosh combination has traditionally been used to treat **menstrual cramps, nervous headaches, muscle spasms, arthritis** and **insomnia.**

Imbalances indicating the use of this formula are commonly noted in the stress acupressure point located above the left clavicle. Imbalances are often noted in the nerve wreath surrounding each pupil. Use caution as overdoses can cause nausea.

This formula is commonly used in conjunction with the complex of B vitamins, the vitamin C family, schizandra, ginseng, bee pollen and wheat germ.

Individual Components

Black Cohosh root contains bitter compounds that relieve smooth muscle spasms, reduce blood pressure and dilate peripheral blood vessels. It also contains astringent compounds that shrink inflamed tissue. Black cohosh has been employed in most inflammatory conditions associated with spasms or tension. It is an excellent herbal source of iron and vitamin A. Black cohosh has been used to treat menstrual cramps, nervous tension, anxiety, dysmenorrhea, hysteria, menopause, fevers and headaches.

Capsicum fruit contains aromatic resins that increase blood circulation, promote sweating, increase the production of digestive fluids and reduce muscle spasms. It has been used to treat flatulence, colic, ulcers, rheumatic arthritis, cold hands and feet and dropsy.

Valerian root contains aromatic compounds that have a sedative effect, acting to decrease anxiety and aggression. These compounds also relieve smooth muscle

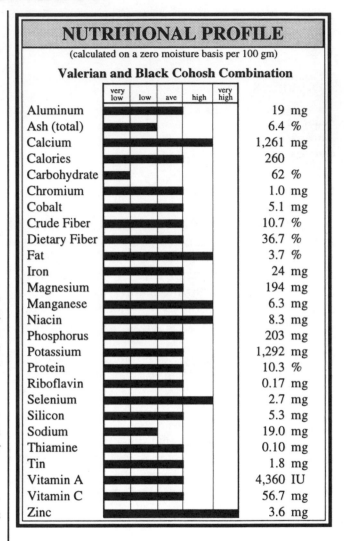

NUTRITIONAL PROFILE

(calculated on a zero moisture basis per 100 gm)

Valerian and Black Cohosh Combination

	very low	low	ave	high	very high		
Aluminum						19	mg
Ash (total)						6.4	%
Calcium						1,261	mg
Calories						260	
Carbohydrate						62	%
Chromium						1.0	mg
Cobalt						5.1	mg
Crude Fiber						10.7	%
Dietary Fiber						36.7	%
Fat						3.7	%
Iron						24	mg
Magnesium						194	mg
Manganese						6.3	mg
Niacin						8.3	mg
Phosphorus						203	mg
Potassium						1,292	mg
Protein						10.3	%
Riboflavin						0.17	mg
Selenium						2.7	mg
Silicon						5.3	mg
Sodium						19.0	mg
Thiamine						0.10	mg
Tin						1.8	mg
Vitamin A						4,360	IU
Vitamin C						56.7	mg
Zinc						3.6	mg

spasms, lower blood pressure, and improve sleep quality in cases of insomnia. The herb is relatively inactive in normal sleepers. Valerian is the very best herbal source of calcium and an excellent herbal source of magnesium. It has been used to treat nervousness, anxiety, insomnia, stomach cramps, muscle spasms, hysteria and convulsions.

Passionflower contains bitter compounds that have a sedative effect and relieve muscle spasms. It has been used to treat insomnia, coughs, headaches and dysmenorrhea.

Lady's Slipper herb contains bitter compounds that have a sedative effect and relieve muscle spasms. It also contains astringent compounds that relieve pain and inflammation. Lady's Slipper has been used to treat dysmenorrhea, headaches, abdominal cramps, anxiety, nervous tension and colic.

Scullcap herb contains bitter compounds that have a sedative effect and relieve smooth muscle spasms. This herb is particularly useful in calming the nervous and circulatory systems. Scullcap is an excellent herbal source of vitamin C and bioflavonoids. It has been used to treat insomnia, anxiety, nervous tension, headaches, enuresis and muscle twitching.

Hops flowers contain bitter compounds that have a sedative effect and relieve smooth muscle spasms, increase the flow of urine and are antiseptic. Hops is an excellent herbal source of niacin. It has been used to treat insomnia, painful urination, urinary tract infections, spastic colons and anxiety.

Wood Betony contains bitter compounds that relieve muscle spasms, increase the flow of urine and dilate peripheral blood vessels. It has been used to treat arthritis, rheumatism, jaundice, epilepsy, fevers, headaches and muscle twitching.

Therapies for Supplementing Deficient Conditions

Bupleurum and Cyperus Combination

Composition

Bupleurum	Pinellia
Cyperus	Aurantium
Bamboo	Zhishi
Coptis	Ophiopogon
Hoelen	Dong Quai
Gambir	Saussurea
Licorice	Perilla leaf
Ginger	Ligusticum
Siberian Ginseng	Platycodon

Properties

Antidepressant	Anti-inflammatory
Stimulant	Diuretic
Expectorant	

General Description

Bupleurum and Cyperus combination is an antidepressant formula that works to relieve aches, pains and congestion. The herbs increase peripheral blood circulation, lymphatic flow, decrease the thickness while increasing the production of mucosal fluid, reduce inflammation, and increase the flow of urine. These combined actions result in an increased sense of well being.

Chinese herbalists describe this herbal combination as a fire enhancing formula. It also enhances the earth element while reducing the metal, water and wood elements.

Bupleurum and Cyperus combination has traditionally been used to treat **depression, fatigue, insomnia, neurosis, tinnitis, postpartum depression, dysmenorrhea, morning sickness, menopause, lung congestion** and **premenstrual syndrome.**

Imbalances indicating the use of this formula are commonly noted in the thymus acupressure point located in the center of the sternum. Imbalances are often noted at the 5 o'clock position of the left iris.

This formula is commonly used in conjunction with l-glutamine, l-tryptophan, manganese, potassium and the vitamin C family.

Individual Components

Bupleurum root contains bitter compounds that have an antidepressant effect, relieve pain and inflammation, reduce fever, and have an antiseptic effect. In addition, these compounds reduce blood cholesterol and triglyceride levels and reduce fat cell production and inflammation in the liver. Bupleurum has been used to treat premenstrual syndrome, dysmenorrhea, lung congestion, malaria, muscle cramps, tumors, inflammatory skin conditions, angina pains, epilepsy and depression.

Cyperus root contains aromatic compounds that relieve smooth muscle spasms especially in the uterus, increase the production of digestive fluids and relieve pains. It has been used to treat dyspepsia, dysmenorrhea, nausea, flatulence, abdominal pain and menorrhagia.

Bamboo sap contains mucilaginous compounds that decrease the thickness while increasing the production of mucosal fluid and are antiseptic. It has been used to treat respiratory tract infections, lung congestion, vomiting and gastritis.

Coptis root contains bitter astringent alkaloids similar to those found in goldenseal. These compounds normalize liver and spleen function by increasing the production of digestive fluids and enzymes, particularly bile. These compounds are antiseptic, constrict peripheral blood vessels, especially in the uterus, are laxative and relieve pain and inflammation in mucosal tissue. Coptis has been used to treat hepatitis, gastritis, colitis, ulcers, menorrhagia, postpartum hemorrhage, dysmenorrhea, diabetes, infections, hemorrhoids, eczema, obesity and fevers.

Hoelen herb contains bitter compounds that increase the flow of urine, decrease blood sugar and have a sedative effect. It has been used to treat edema, dropsy, diarrhea, insomnia, frequent urination and heart palpitations.

Gambir herb contains bitter compounds that have a sedative effect, relieve muscle spasms, lower blood pressure, slow respiration, dilate peripheral blood vessels and decrease heart rate. It has been used to treat epilepsy, hypertension, convulsion, dizziness and anxiety.

Licorice root contains bitter compounds that reduce inflammation, decrease the thickness and increase the production of mucosal fluids and relieve muscle spasms. In addition, licorice stimulates adrenal function, reduces the urge to cough, is mildly laxative and enhances immune response. It has been used to treat coughs, colds, arthritis, asthma, peptic ulcers, Addison's disease, dropsy and atherosclerosis.

Ginger root contains aromatic compounds that increase the production of digestive fluids and enzymes, lower blood pressure, lower blood sugar and cholesterol. It also contains bitter compounds that reduce muscle spasms, increase blood circulation and dilate blood vessels. Ginger is an excellent herbal source of trace minerals especially silicon, magnesium, and manganese. It has been used to treat nausea, motion sickness, flatulence, colds, coughs, indigestion, fevers, vomiting, diarrhea, chronic bronchitis and cold hands and feet.

Siberian Ginseng root contains bitter compounds that help the body respond more quickly to stress. These compounds increase the production of DNA, RNA and proteins essential to all life processes. They also stimulate the adrenal, pancreas, and pituitary glands to lower blood sugar and reduce inflammation. Ginseng also increases the production of digestive fluids and is a mild sedative. It had been used to treat anemia, impotence, insomnia, diarrhea, fatigue debility, weak digestion and failing memory.

Pinellia root contains bitter compounds that decrease the thickness while increasing the production of mucosal fluids, relieve muscle spasms, increase the production of digestive fluids and absorb toxins. Pinellia root must by processed with alum or ginger root before ingestion since it is toxic. It has been used to treat morning sickness, nausea, vomiting, respiratory congestion, ulcers and blood poisoning.

Aurantium herb contains bitter compounds that decrease the thickness while increasing the production of mucosal fluids. It also contains aromatic compounds that increase blood circulation. It has been used to treat angina pains, coughs, colds, hiccups, vomiting and lung congestion.

Zhishi fruit (immature orange) contains aromatic compounds that decrease the thickness while increasing the production of mucosal fluids and increase the production of digestive fluids. It also contains bitter compounds that enhance vitamin C absorption, and decrease capillary fragility. Zhishi has been used to treat constipation, indigestion, flatulence, dyspepsia and abdominal pains.

Ophiopogon root contains bitter compounds that have a sedative effect, promote the production of mucosal fluids, reduce muscle spasms and have an antiseptic effect. In addition, the herb lowers blood sugar and regenerates beta cells in the islets of langerhorn of the pancreas. Ophiopogon has been used to treat insomnia, coronary heart disease, heart palpitations, fear and dry coughs.

Dong Quai root contains aromatic compounds that relieve smooth muscle spasms, especially in the uterus, have a sedative effect and increase the production of digestive fluids. It also contains bitter compounds that regulate glycogen production in the liver, reduce pain and inflammation, increase blood flow especially to the heart, lower blood cholesterol, normalize uterine contractions and are antiseptic. Dong quai is an excellent herbal source of iron, magnesium and niacin. It has been used to treat anemia, abdominal pains, dysmenorrhea, amenorrhea, arthritis, coronary heart disease, atherosclerosis, angina pectoris, indigestion and headaches.

Saussurea root contains aromatic compounds that increase the production of digestive fluids, increase blood circulation and are antiseptic. It also contains bitter compounds that relieve smooth muscle spasms, lower blood pressure and relieve pains. Saussurea has been used to treat gastritis, chest pains, jaundice, gall stones and diarrhea.

Perilla leaf contains aromatic compounds that decrease the thickness while increasing the production of mucosal fluid and reduce smooth muscle spasms especially of the bronchiole. These compounds also promote sweating, reduce fevers, increase blood sugar and are antiseptic. Perilla leaf has been used to treat asthma, vomiting, diarrhea, coughs, colds, lung congestion, bronchitis and nausea due to food poisoning.

Ligusticum root contains aromatic compounds that promote sweating, increase blood circulation, relieve pain and inflammation and relieve muscle spasms. It has been used to treat headaches, migraine headaches, arthritis, rheumatism, dysmenorrhea, flu, colds, inflammatory skin conditions and anemia.

Platycodon root contains bitter compounds that decrease the thickness while increasing the production of mucosal fluids, lower blood sugar, lower blood cholesterol and are antiseptic. It is used to treat coughs, weak digestion, inflammatory skin conditions and respiratory tract infections.

Chapter 10

The Respiratory System

The respiratory system is made up of the lungs, trachea, throat, mouth and sinuses. Its prime function is to supply oxygen to the blood. It also functions to trap and expel airborne toxins in its mucosa. Imbalances of the respiratory system often affect the immune, circulatory and nervous systems. The names for the herbal combinations are chosen based on the properties of the key herbs in the formula.

Therapies for Relieving Excess Conditions

Sinus and lung congestion resulting from infection or allergy are typical of excess conditions of the respiratory system. The production of mucous sequesters toxins and assists in their elimination.

Excess conditions in the respiratory system are often marked by patterns of minor aches, pains and ailments including: earaches, sore throats, diarrhea, coughs, sinus congestion, hay fever, edema, sinus headaches, numbness in arms, lymphatic swelling, chest pains, grief, sadness, stiff neck, stiff shoulders, wheezing, obesity, difficulty digesting fats, stubbornness, defensive attitude and cold hands and feet. If left unchecked these ailments may develop into illnesses including: bronchitis, asthma, lymphoma skin cysts, colitis, colds, coughs, influenza, pneumonia, tuberculosis and emphysema.

Early herbal therapies for these conditions consisted of single herbs like fenugreek which decrease the thickness while increasing the production of mucosal fluids. Fenugreek is not simply an expectorant however, and with time and experience, herbalists recognized and recorded in their herbals the several properties of fenugreek. The British Herbal Pharmacopoeia lists fenugreek as a mucilaginous, demulcent, laxative, nutritive expectorant, orexigenic, emollient and vulnerary.

These lists of empirical properties are the key to understanding herbal combinations. Herbalists have found that they can enhance a particular property of a single herb by adding herbs that compliment and support the given property. Conversely, the herbalist is also able to minimize the effect of an unwanted property by adding herbs that counteract or balance that property.

Therapies for Supplementing Deficient Conditions

Weaknesses in the respiratory system are marked by chronic infection and congestion. Herbalists use herbs that reduce inflammation and strengthen immune response to overcome illnesses such as chronic bronchitis and asthma.

Weakened conditions of the respiratory system are often associated with patterns of minor aches, pains and ailments including: shortness of breath, weak muscles, poor appetite, fatigue, grief, frequent crying, pain in chest, chronic coughs, chronic colds, dry coughs, thirst, anemia, dry skin, wheezing, emaciation recurring infections, fever and difficulty in breathing. If left unchecked, these ailments may develop into illnesses including: emphysema, chronic bronchitis, colds, flu, tuberculosis, chronic pneumonia and diabetes.

Early herbal therapies for these conditions consisted of single herbs such as Chinese ephedra which dilates the bronchiole and enhances peripheral blood circulation. Chinese ephedra is not simply a bronchodilator however, and with time and experience, herbalists recognized and recorded in their herbals the several properties of Chinese ephedra. The British Herbal Pharmacopoeia lists Chinese ephedra as an antiasthmatic bronchodilator, hypertensive, peripheral vasoconstrictor, adrenal stimulant, cerebral stimulant and cardiac stimulant.

These empirical properties of an herb are the key to understanding herbal combinations. Herbalists have found that they can enhance a particular property of single herbs by adding herbs that complement and support a given property. Conversely, the herbalist is also able to minimize the effect of an unwanted property by adding herbs that counteract or balance that property.

Chamomile and Rose Hips Combination

Composition

Rose hips	Goldenseal
Chamomile	Myrrh
Yarrow	Peppermint
Slippery Elm	Sage
Capsicum	Lemongrass

Properties

Carminative
Antiseptic
Analgesic
Antispasmodic
Stimulant
Diaphoretic

General Description

Chamomile and Rosehips combination is used to treat the common cold, especially those associated with nausea, muscle aches, headaches, stuffy nose, chills and fevers. The herbs work to increase the production of digestive fluids, calm muscle spasms, fight infections, improve blood circulation and promote sweating.

Chinese herbalists would describe this herbal combination as an earth enhancing formula. It also enhances the fire and metal elements while reducing the wood and water elements.

Chamomile and Rosehips combination has traditionally been used to treat **the common cold, headaches, influenza, muscle aches, nausea, vomiting, fevers and chills.**

Imbalances indicating the use of this formula are commonly noted in the stomach acupressure point located approximately one inch below and one inch to the left of the sternum. Imbalances are often noted by the presence of a "lymphatic rosary" surrounding each iris.

This formula is commonly used in conjunction with the vitamin C family, echinacea, zinc, licorice and germanium.

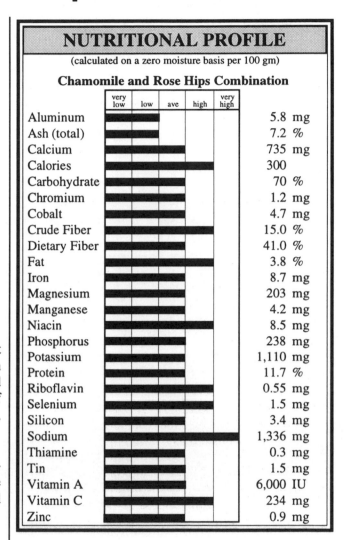

NUTRITIONAL PROFILE
(calculated on a zero moisture basis per 100 gm)
Chamomile and Rose Hips Combination

	very low	low	ave	high	very high	
Aluminum						5.8 mg
Ash (total)						7.2 %
Calcium						735 mg
Calories						300
Carbohydrate						70 %
Chromium						1.2 mg
Cobalt						4.7 mg
Crude Fiber						15.0 %
Dietary Fiber						41.0 %
Fat						3.8 %
Iron						8.7 mg
Magnesium						203 mg
Manganese						4.2 mg
Niacin						8.5 mg
Phosphorus						238 mg
Potassium						1,110 mg
Protein						11.7 %
Riboflavin						0.55 mg
Selenium						1.5 mg
Silicon						3.4 mg
Sodium						1,336 mg
Thiamine						0.3 mg
Tin						1.5 mg
Vitamin A						6,000 IU
Vitamin C						234 mg
Zinc						0.9 mg

Individual Components

Rose hips contains bitter compounds called bioflavonoids which enhance the absorption of vitamin C and strengthen connective tissue. This results in decreased capillary fragility. It also contains astringent compounds which shrink inflamed tissue and reduce the secretion of mucosal fluid. Rose hips is an excellent herbal source of vitamin C. It has been used to treat the common cold, influenza, fevers, infections, inflammatory skin conditions, easy bruising varicose veins, debility, capillary fragility and hemorrhoids.

Chamomile flowers contain aromatic compounds that increase the production of digestive fluids, reduce muscle spasms and pains, reduce inflammation and are antiseptic. In addition, these compounds have a sedative effect. Chamomile is one of the best herbal sources of niacin, magnesium and essential fatty acids. It has been used to treat dyspepsia, flatulence, nausea, vomiting, dysmenorrhea, bronchitis, urinary tract infections, insomnia, headaches and menstrual cramps.

Yarrow flower contains aromatic compounds that shrink inflamed tissues and promote sweating. It also contains bitter compounds that relieve smooth muscle spasms, reduce blood pressure and stop bleeding. Yarrow has been used to treat hemorrhoids, fevers, nausea and inflammatory skin conditions.

Slippery Elm bark contains mucilaginous compounds that decrease the thickness while increasing the production of mucosal fluids. These compounds soothe inflamed tissue, decrease bowel transit time and absorb toxins from the bowel. It also contains astringent compounds that shrink inflamed tissues. Slippery elm has been used to treat asthma, bronchitis, colitis, coughs, weak digestion and inflammatory bowel disease.

Capsicum fruit contains aromatic resins that increase blood circulation, promote sweating, increase the production of digestive fluids and reduce muscle spasms. It has been used to treat flatulence, colic, ulcers, rheumatic arthritis, cold hands and feet and dropsy.

Goldenseal root contains bitter astringent alkaloids that normalize liver and spleen functions by increasing the production of digestive fluids and enzymes, particularly bile. The compounds are antiseptic, constrict peripheral blood vessels, especially in the uterus, are laxative and relieve pain and inflammation in mucosal tissue. Goldenseal is an excellent herbal source of trace minerals including cobalt, iron, magnesium, manganese, silicon and zinc. It is also an excellent herbal source of vitamin C. It has been used to treat hepatitis, gastritis, colitis, ulcers, menorrhagia, postpartum hemorrhages, dysmenorrhea, diabetes, infections, hemorrhoids, eczema, obesity and fevers.

Myrrh gum contains astringent resins that promote the healing of sores. These compounds shrink inflamed tissue, are antiseptic and reduce pain in mucous membranes. Myrrh also decreases the thickness while increasing the production of mucosal fluids. It has been used to treat colds, coughs, bronchitis, asthma, dysmenorrhea, rheumatism and arthritis.

Peppermint leaf contains aromatic compounds that increase the production of digestive fluids, relieve muscle spasms, increase blood circulation, reduce pains, promote sweating and are antiseptic. It also contains astringent compounds which shrink inflamed tissues. Peppermint has been used to treat indigestion, flatulence, mouth sores, loss of appetite, muscle cramps, nausea, morning sickness and dysmenorrhea.

Sage leaf contains aromatic compounds that increase the production of digestive fluids, are antiseptic and are powerful antioxidants. It also contains astringent compounds that shrink inflamed tissue and decrease perspiration. Sage has been used to treat dyspepsia, sore throats, night sweats, headaches, colds and influenza.

Lemongrass herb contains aromatic compounds that have a sedative effect, decrease the secretion of fluids and are antiseptic. It has been used to treat colds, flu, nausea, indigestion and anxiety.

Fenugreek Combination

Composition

Boneset	Horseradish
Fennel	Mullein
Fenugreek	

Properties

Expectorant	Antiseptic
Stimulant	Demulcent
Diaphoretic	Diuretic

General Description

Fenugreek combination is used to treat bronchitis and congestion in the respiratory system. The herbs work to decrease the thickness while increasing the production of mucosal fluid, soothe inflamed tissue and fight infections. In addition, the formula promotes sweating and increases blood circulation.

Chinese herbalists would describe this combination as a metal reducing formula. It also reduces the water and earth elements while enhancing the fire and wood elements.

Fenugreek combination has traditionally been used to treat **bronchitis, asthma, hay fevers, coughs, nasal drainage, swollen glands, earache, insomnia, diarrhea** and **dyspepsia.**

Imbalances indicating the use of this formula are commonly noted in the respiratory allergy acupressure point located on the nose. Imbalances are often noted at the 3:30 position of the left iris and at the 10:30 position of the right iris. Also, a "lymphatic rosary" is common in both irises.

This formula is commonly used in conjunction with the vitamin C family, thyme, lobelia, passionflower, vitamin A, licorice and vitamin E.

Individual Components

Boneset herb contains aromatic compounds that promote sweating, are antiseptic and decrease the thickness while increasing the production of mucosal fluid. It has been used to treat bronchitis, coughs, colds, fevers and respiratory tract infections.

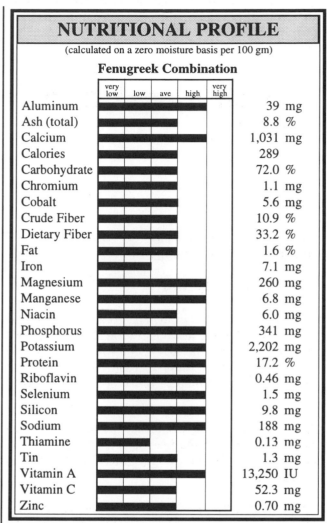

NUTRITIONAL PROFILE
(calculated on a zero moisture basis per 100 gm)

Fenugreek Combination

	very low	low	ave	high	very high		
Aluminum						39	mg
Ash (total)						8.8	%
Calcium						1,031	mg
Calories						289	
Carbohydrate						72.0	%
Chromium						1.1	mg
Cobalt						5.6	mg
Crude Fiber						10.9	%
Dietary Fiber						33.2	%
Fat						1.6	%
Iron						7.1	mg
Magnesium						260	mg
Manganese						6.8	mg
Niacin						6.0	mg
Phosphorus						341	mg
Potassium						2,202	mg
Protein						17.2	%
Riboflavin						0.46	mg
Selenium						1.5	mg
Silicon						9.8	mg
Sodium						188	mg
Thiamine						0.13	mg
Tin						1.3	mg
Vitamin A						13,250	IU
Vitamin C						52.3	mg
Zinc						0.70	mg

Fennel seed contains aromatic compounds that stimulate the production of digestive fluids, relieve inflammation, are antiseptic, make one breathe deeply and more often, and increase the flow of urine. It has been used to treat indigestion, dyspepsia, anorexia, colic, flatulence, coughs and colds.

Fenugreek seed contains mucilaginous compounds that decrease the thickness while increasing the production of mucosal fluids and sooth inflamed tissue. It also contains bitter compounds that increase the production of digestive fluids and enzymes and have a mild laxative effect. Fenugreek is an excellent herbal source of iron and selenium. It has been used to treat bronchitis, dyspepsia, fevers, ulcers, respiratory tract infections, anorexia and gastritis.

Horseradish root contains aromatic compounds that increase circulation, are antiseptic and promote sweating. These compounds also decrease the thickness while increasing the production of mucosal fluid. Horseradish has been used to treat asthma, bronchitis, coughs, colds, fevers and rheumatism.

Mullein leaves contain mucilaginous compounds that decrease the thickness and increase the production of mucosal fluids. These compounds soothe inflamed tissue. Mullein also contains aromatic compounds that increase the flow of urine. The herb has been used to treat bronchitis, coughs, colds, hay fever, dysuria, nephritis and sinus congestion.

Fenugreek and Thyme Combination

Composition

Fenugreek
Thyme

Properties

Expectorant	**Antispasmodic**
Antiseptic	**Anti-inflammatory**

General Description

Fenugreek and Thyme is an expectorant formula used to treat inflammations and congestion in the respiratory system. The herbs work to render the respiratory fluids less viscous, reduce muscle spasms and help clear infections. These combined actions reduce the urge to cough.

Chinese herbalists would describe this herbal combination as a metal reducing formula. It also reduces the water and earth elements while enhancing the fire and wood elements.

Fenugreek and Thyme combination has traditionally been used to treat **bronchitis, indigestion, sinus congestion, fevers, coughs, colds, headaches** and **worms**.

Imbalances indicating the use of this formula are commonly noted in the sinus acupressure point located on the nose and forehead. Imbalances are often noted at the 3:30 position of the left iris. Also a "lymphatic rosary" is common surrounding both irises. Use caution in cases of pregacy and menstrual hemorrhaging.

This formula is commonly used in conjunction with vitamin A, the vitamin C family, lobelia, licorice and zinc.

Individual Components

Fenugreek seed contains mucilaginous compounds that decrease the thickness while increasing the production of mucosal fluids and sooth inflamed tissues. It also contains bitter compounds that increase the production of digestive fluids and enzymes and have a mild

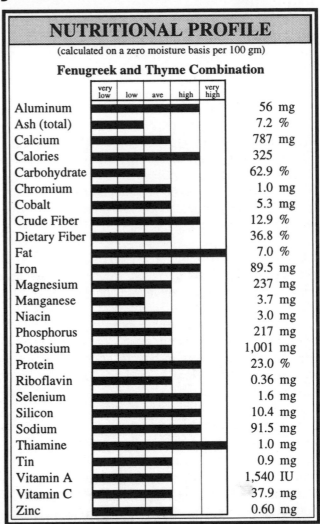

NUTRITIONAL PROFILE
(calculated on a zero moisture basis per 100 gm)
Fenugreek and Thyme Combination

	very low	low	ave	high	very high		
Aluminum						56	mg
Ash (total)						7.2	%
Calcium						787	mg
Calories						325	
Carbohydrate						62.9	%
Chromium						1.0	mg
Cobalt						5.3	mg
Crude Fiber						12.9	%
Dietary Fiber						36.8	%
Fat						7.0	%
Iron						89.5	mg
Magnesium						237	mg
Manganese						3.7	mg
Niacin						3.0	mg
Phosphorus						217	mg
Potassium						1,001	mg
Protein						23.0	%
Riboflavin						0.36	mg
Selenium						1.6	mg
Silicon						10.4	mg
Sodium						91.5	mg
Thiamine						1.0	mg
Tin						0.9	mg
Vitamin A						1,540	IU
Vitamin C						37.9	mg
Zinc						0.60	mg

laxative effect. Fenugreek is an excellent herbal source of iron and selenium. It has been used to treat bronchitis, dyspepsia, fevers, ulcers, respiratory tract infections, anorexia and gastritis.

Thyme herb contains aromatic compounds that are antiseptic, dilate the bronchioles and increase ciliary movements in the lungs. These compounds also decrease the thickness while increasing the production of mucosal fluid. It also contains bitter compounds that relieve smooth muscle spasms. Thyme has been used to treat bronchitis, asthma, coughs, colds, fevers, infections and rheumatism.

Marshmallow and Fenugreek Combination

Composition

Marshmallow
Fenugreek

Properties

Expectorant
Anti-inflammatory
Vulnerary

General Description

Marshmallow and Fenugreek combination is an expectorant formula. The herbs work to decrease the thickness while increasing the production of mucosal fluid, reduce inflammation, relieve smooth muscle spasms and assist the healing process.

Chinese herbalists would describe this herbal combination as a metal reducing formula. It also reduces the water and earth elements while enhancing the fire and wood elements.

Marshmallow and Fenugreek combination has traditionally been used to treat **bronchitis, asthma, hay fever, coughs, colds, earaches** and **sinus congestion.**

Imbalances indicating the use of this formula are commonly noted in the respiratory allergy acupressure point located on the nose. Imbalances are often noted at the 3:30 position of the left iris and at the 10:30 position of the right iris. Also, a "lymphatic rosary" is common in both irises.

This formula is commonly used in conjunction with the vitamin C family, comfrey, zinc, thyme, lobelia, vitamin A and germanium.

Individual Components

Marshmallow root contains mucilaginous compounds that decrease the thickness while increasing the production of mucosal fluids, soothe inflamed tissue, heal wounds and increase the flow of urine. It is an excellent herbal source of trace minerals especially chromium, iron, magnesium and selenium. Marshmallow has been used to treat allergies, gastritis, gastric ulcers, enteritis, coughs, cystitis and hay fever.

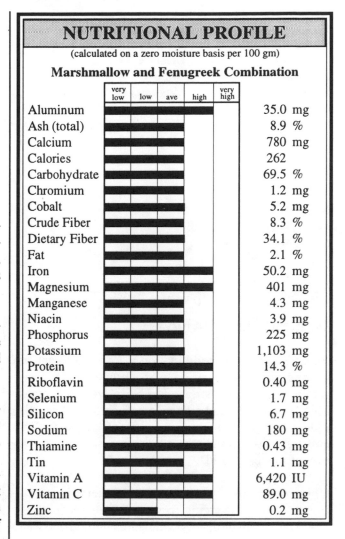

NUTRITIONAL PROFILE
(calculated on a zero moisture basis per 100 gm)

Marshmallow and Fenugreek Combination

	very low	low	ave	high	very high	
Aluminum						35.0 mg
Ash (total)						8.9 %
Calcium						780 mg
Calories						262
Carbohydrate						69.5 %
Chromium						1.2 mg
Cobalt						5.2 mg
Crude Fiber						8.3 %
Dietary Fiber						34.1 %
Fat						2.1 %
Iron						50.2 mg
Magnesium						401 mg
Manganese						4.3 mg
Niacin						3.9 mg
Phosphorus						225 mg
Potassium						1,103 mg
Protein						14.3 %
Riboflavin						0.40 mg
Selenium						1.7 mg
Silicon						6.7 mg
Sodium						180 mg
Thiamine						0.43 mg
Tin						1.1 mg
Vitamin A						6,420 IU
Vitamin C						89.0 mg
Zinc						0.2 mg

Fenugreek seed contains mucilaginous compounds that decrease the thickness while increasing the production of mucosal fluids and sooth inflamed tissue. It also contains bitter compounds that increase the production of digestive fluids and enzymes and have a mild laxative effect. Fenugreek is an excellent herbal source of iron and selenium. It has been used to treat bronchitis, dyspepsia, fevers, ulcers, respiratory tract infections, anorexia and gastritis.

Pinellia and Citrus Combination

Composition

Pinellia	Hoelen
Citrus	Ginger
Frittilaria	Licorice
Bamboo	Bupleurum
Platycodon	Magnolia bark
Ophiopogon	Apricot seed
Schizandra	Chinese ephedra
Tussilago	Morus bark

Properties

Expectorant
Decongestant
Stimulant
Diuretic
Diaphoretic
Antidepressant

General Description

Pinellia and Citrus combination is an expectorant and decongestant formula used to treat bronchitis and respiratory system congestion. The herbs work to increase blood circulation and dilate the bronchioles. They also induce sweating, increase the flow of lymphatic fluid and decrease the thickness while increasing the production of mucosal fluid.

Chinese herbalists would describe this herbal combination as a metal reducing formula. It also reduces the water and earth elements while enhancing the fire and wood elements.

Pinellia and Citrus combination has traditionally been used to treat **sinus congestion, bronchitis, sinusitis, headaches, asthma, persistent coughs, emphysema, tuberculosis, croup, sore throats** and **the common cold.**

Imbalances indicating the use of this formula are commonly noted in the respiratory allergy acupressure point located on the nose. Imbalances are often noted at the 10:00 position of the right iris and the 2 o'clock position of the left iris. Use caution in cases of hypertension and insomnia.

This formula is commonly used in conjunction with lobelia, licorice, comfrey, mullein, the vitamin C family, vitamin A, vitamin E and zinc.

Individual Components

Pinellia root contains bitter compounds that decrease the thickness while increasing the production of mucosal fluids, relieve muscle spasms, increase the production of digestive fluids and absorb toxins. Pinellia root must by processed with alum or ginger root before ingestion since it is toxic. It has been used to treat morning sickness, nausea, vomiting, respiratory congestion, ulcers and blood poisoning.

Citrus peel contains aromatic compounds that are antiseptic, reduce muscle spasms and decrease the thickness while increasing the production of mucosal fluids. It also contains bitter compounds that are antiinflammatory, reduce muscle spasms, increase the production of digestive fluid and increase blood circulation. Citrus peel has been used to treat coughs, colds, flu, fever, and bronchitis.

Frittilaria root contains bitter compounds that dilate the bronchioles, relieve smooth muscle spasms, dilate peripheral blood vessels especially in the uterus and lower blood pressure. It has been used to treat coughs, asthma, bronchitis, pneumonia and tuberculosis.

Bamboo sap contains mucilaginous compounds that decrease the thickness while increasing the production of mucosal fluid and are antiseptic. It has been used to treat respiratory tract infections, lung congestion, vomiting and gastritis.

Platycodon root contains bitter compounds that decrease the thickness while increasing the production of mucosal fluids, lower blood sugar, lower blood cholesterol and are antiseptic. It is used to treat coughs, weak digestion, inflammatory skin conditions and respiratory tract infections.

Ophiopogon root contains bitter compounds that have a sedative effect, promote the production of mucosal fluids, reduce muscle spasms and have an antiseptic effect. In addition, the herb lowers blood sugar and regenerates beta cells in the islets of langerhorn of the pancreas. Ophiopogon has been used to treat insomnia, coronary heart disease, heart palpitations, fear and dry coughs.

Schizandra fruit contains bitter compounds that allow the body to more quickly respond to stress. This increases the body's capacity for work and decreases fatigue. These compounds also increase blood circulation, blood sugar and bile production while lowering blood pressure. Schizandra also contains astringent compounds that increase the contraction of the heart muscle and the uterus and are antiseptic. The herb has been used to treat heart palpitations, dropsy, nervous exhaustion, asthma, diabetes, chronic diarrhea, night sweats, seminal emissions, insomnia, frequent urination and anxiety.

Tussilago flower contains bitter compounds that decrease the thickness while increasing the production of mucosal fluids, relieve smooth muscle spasms and dilate the bronchioles. It is used to treat chronic coughs, asthma and bronchitis.

Hoelen herb contains bitter compounds that increase the flow of urine, decrease blood sugar and have a sedative effect. It has been used to treat edema, dropsy, diarrhea, insomnia, frequent urination and heart palpitations.

Ginger root contains aromatic compounds that increase the production of digestive fluids and enzymes, lower blood pressure, lower blood sugar and cholesterol. It also contains bitter compounds that reduce muscle spasms, increase blood circulation and dilate blood vessels. Ginger is an excellent herbal source of trace minerals, especially silicon, magnesium and manganese. It has been used to treat nausea, motion sickness, flatulence, colds, coughs, indigestion, fevers, vomiting, diarrhea, chronic bronchitis and cold hands and feet.

Licorice root contains bitter compounds that reduce inflammation, decrease the thickness and increase the production of mucosal fluids and relieve muscle spasms. In addition, licorice stimulates adrenal function, reduces the urge to cough, is mildly laxative and enhances immune response. It has been used to treat coughs, colds, arthritis, asthma, peptic ulcers, Addison's disease, dropsy and atherosclerosis.

Bupleurum root contains bitter compounds that have an antidepressant effect, relieve pain and inflammation, reduce fevers and have an antiseptic effect. In addition, these compounds reduce blood cholesterol and triglyceride levels and reduce fat cell production and inflammation in the liver. Bupleurum has been used to treat premenstrual syndrome, dysmenorrhea, lung congestion, malaria, muscle cramps, tumors, inflammatory skin conditions, angina pains, epilepsy and depression.

Magnolia bark contains bitter compounds that relieve muscle cramps, are antiseptic and have sedative properties. It has been used to treat gastritis, coughs, asthma, diarrhea, vomiting and flatulence.

Apricot seed contains bitter compounds (Amygdalin) that relieve smooth muscle spasms, relieve pains, are antiseptic and anthelmintic, decrease the production of gastric fluids and have a laxative effect. It has been used to treat coughs, asthma, bronchitis and constipation.

Chinese ephedra herb contains bitter alkaloids that dilate the bronchioles, enhance adrenal function, shrink inflamed tissue and enhance peripheral blood circulation. These compounds also decrease the secretion of mucosal fluids, increase heart rate and blood pressure and induce sweating. The herb is an excellent herbal source of vitamin B-1, B-2 and C. Ephedra has been used to treat asthma, bronchitis, respiratory tract infections, sinus congestion, colds, coughs and arthritis.

Morus bark contains bitter compounds that increase the flow of urine, reduce blood pressure, decrease the thickness while increasing the production of mucosal fluids, reduce muscle spasms and have a sedative effect. It has been used to treat coughs, colds, asthma, hypertension and edema.

Yerba Santa Combination

Composition

Blessed Thistle   Scullcap
Pleurisy root   Yerba Santa

Properties

Expectorant   Antispasmodic
Bronchodilator   Antitussive

General Description

Yerba Santa combination is an expectorant formula. Together, the herbs in this formula increase the fluidity of mucous in the respiratory system, dilate peripheral blood vessels and bronchioles, and relax muscle spasms, especially those associated with the urge to cough.

Chinese herbalists would describe this combination as a metal reducing formula. It also reduces the fire and earth elements while enhancing the wood and water elements.

Yerba Santa combination has traditionally been used to treat **rheumatism, arthritis, menstrual cramping, insomnia, hysteria, headaches and fevers.**

Imbalances indicating the use of this formula are commonly noted in the respiratory allergy acupressure point located on the nose. Imbalances are often noted at the 3:30 position of the left iris and in the 10:30 position of the right iris. Use caution in cases of high fevers and night sweats.

This formula is commonly used in conjunction with the vitamin C family, thyme, comfrey, lobelia, vitamin A, licorice, vitamin E and zinc.

Individual Components

Blessed Thistle contains bitter compounds that decrease the thickness while increasing the production of mucosal fluids, particularly in the digestive and respiratory systems. It also contains astringent compounds that are antiseptic, dilate peripheral blood vessels and shrink inflamed tissue. Blessed thistle is an excellent herbal source of potassium and sodium. The herb has been used to treat dysmenorrhea, amenorrhea, arthritis, dysuria, jaundice, fevers and respiratory allergies.

Pleurisy root contains bitter compounds that promote sweating, relieve smooth muscle spasms, decrease the

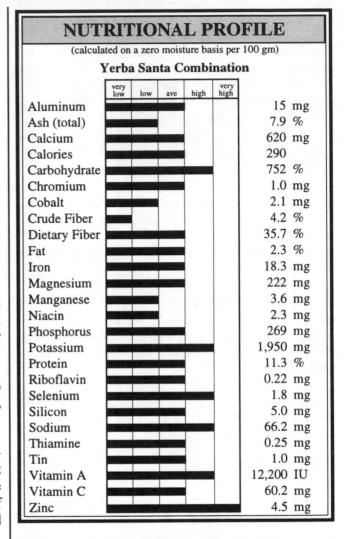

NUTRITIONAL PROFILE
(calculated on a zero moisture basis per 100 gm)

Yerba Santa Combination

	very low	low	ave	high	very high	
Aluminum						15 mg
Ash (total)						7.9 %
Calcium						620 mg
Calories						290
Carbohydrate						752 %
Chromium						1.0 mg
Cobalt						2.1 mg
Crude Fiber						4.2 %
Dietary Fiber						35.7 %
Fat						2.3 %
Iron						18.3 mg
Magnesium						222 mg
Manganese						3.6 mg
Niacin						2.3 mg
Phosphorus						269 mg
Potassium						1,950 mg
Protein						11.3 %
Riboflavin						0.22 mg
Selenium						1.8 mg
Silicon						5.0 mg
Sodium						66.2 mg
Thiamine						0.25 mg
Tin						1.0 mg
Vitamin A						12,200 IU
Vitamin C						60.2 mg
Zinc						4.5 mg

thickness while increasing the production of mucosal fluid and dilate peripheral blood vessels. It has been used to treat bronchitis, croup, pneumonia, dry coughs, influenza and pleurisy.

Scullcap herb contains bitter compounds that have a sedative effect and relieve smooth muscle spasms. This herb is particularly useful in calming the nervous and circulatory systems. Scullcap is an excellent herbal source of vitamin C and bioflavonoids. It has been used to treat insomnia, anxiety, nervous tension, headaches, enuresis and muscle twitching.

Yerba Santa herb contains aromatic compounds that decrease the thickness while increasing the production of mucosal fluids and are antiseptic. It also contains astringent compounds that shrink inflamed tissues. Yerba santa has been used to treat asthma, bronchitis, respiratory allergies, coughs, colds, influenza and rheumatism.

Anemarrhena and Astragalus Combination

Composition

Anemarrhena	Siberian Ginseng
Astragalus	Blue Citrus
Bupleurum	Platycodon
Qinjiao	Dong Quai
Aster	Schizandra
Lycium bark	Ophiopogon
Pinellia	Citrus
Licorice	Atractylodes

Properties

Immunostimulant
Antiseptic
Antiviral
Antispasmodic
Stimulant
Expectorant
Antispasmodic
Antitussive
Anti-inflammatory

General Description

Anemarrhena and Astragalus combination is a tonic formula used to increase immune response and enhance the body's response to stress. The herbs work to stimulate blood circulation, relieve muscle spasms, enhance immunoresponse, soothe inflamed tissues and fight infections, especially chronic weaknesses of the respiratory system.

Chinese herbalists would describe this herbal combination as a metal enhancing formula. It also enhances the fire and wood elements while reducing the earth and water elements.

Anemarrhena and Astragalus combination has traditionally been used to treat **chronic bronchitis, asthma, wheezing, chronic respiratory infections, emphysema, thirst, constipation, chest tightness, fevers, debility, pneumonia** and **chronic coughs.**

Imbalances indicating the use of this formula are commonly noted in the thymus acupressure point located in the center of the sternum. Imbalances are often noted at the 5 o'clock position of the right iris.

This formula is commonly used in conjunction with echinacea, zinc, germanium, the vitamin C family, vitamin A and goldenseal.

Individual Components

Anemarrhena root contains bitter compounds that reduce fevers, lower blood sugar, are antiseptic and increase the production of urine. These compounds also decrease the thickness while increasing the production of mucosal fluids. It has been used to treat fevers, thirst, respiratory tract infections, bronchitis, lumbago, constipation and dysuria.

Astragalus root contains bitter compounds that increase the flow of urine, are antiseptic, increase the production of digestive fluids, including bile, and relieve muscle spasms. Astragalus also contains mucilaginous compounds that enhance immune response, increase the production of lymphocytes and macrophages. The herb also increases heart action and lowers blood pressure and blood sugar. It has been used to treat fatigue, debility, urinary tract infections, edema, nephritis, ulcers, prolapse of organs and night sweats.

Bupleurum root contains bitter compounds that have an antidepressant effect, relieve pain and inflammation, reduce fevers and have an antiseptic effect. In addition, these compounds reduce blood cholesterol and triglyceride levels, reduce fat cell production and inflammation in the liver. Bupleurum has been used to treat premenstrual syndrome, dysmenorrhea, lung congestion, malaria, muscle cramps, tumors, inflammatory skin conditions, angina pains, epilepsy and depression.

Qinjiao root contains bitter compounds that relieve inflammation and pains, have a sedative effect, increase blood sugar, lower blood pressure and are antiseptic. It has been used to treat rheumatism, fevers, debility, allergic inflammations, jaundice and hepatitis.

Aster root contains bitter compounds that are antiseptic and antifungal, decrease the thickness while increasing the production of mucosal fluid and relieve smooth muscle spasms. It has been used to treat coughs, respiratory tract congestion, bronchitis, tuberculosis and colds.

Lycium bark contains bitter compounds, particularly betaine which supplement the hydrochloric acid content of gastric fluid. It also contains astringent compounds that dilate peripheral blood vessels, lower blood sugar, lower blood cholesterol, reduce fevers and are antiseptic. It has been used to treat diabetes, weak digestion and respiratory tract allergies.

Pinellia root contains bitter compounds that decrease the thickness while increasing the production of mucosal fluids, relieve muscle spasms, increase the production of digestive fluids and absorb toxins. Pinellia root must by processed with alum or ginger root before ingestion since it is toxic. It has been used to treat morning sickness, nausea, vomiting, respiratory congestion, ulcers and blood poisoning.

Licorice root contains bitter compounds that reduce inflammation, decrease the thickness and increase the production of mucosal fluids and relieve muscle spasms. In addition, licorice stimulates adrenal function, reduces the urge to cough, is mildly laxative and enhances immune response. It had been used to treat coughs, colds, arthritis, asthma, peptic ulcers, Addison's disease, dropsy and atherosclerosis.

Siberian Ginseng root contains bitter compounds that help the body respond more quickly to stress. These compounds increase the production of DNA, RNA and proteins essential to all life processes. They also stimulate the adrenal, pancreas, and pituitary glands to lower blood sugar and reduce inflammation. Ginseng also increases the production of digestive fluids and is a mild sedative. It had been used to treat anemia, impotence, insomnia, diarrhea, fatigue, debility, weak digestion and failing memory.

Blue Citrus contains aromatic compounds that increase the production of digestive fluids. It also contains bioflavonoids which enhance the bioavailability of vitamin C, strengthen connective tissue and decrease capillary fragility. It has been used to treat indigestion, weak digestion, flatulence, hepatitis, cirrhosis and gastritis.

Platycodon root contains bitter compounds that decrease the thickness while increasing the production of mucosal fluids, lower blood sugar, lower blood choles-terol and are antiseptic. It is used to treat coughs, weak digestion, inflammatory skin conditions and respiratory tract infections.

Dong Quai root contains aromatic compounds that relieve smooth muscle spasms, especially in the uterus, have a sedative effect and increase the production of digestive fluids. It also contains bitter compounds that regulate glycogen production in the liver, reduce pain and inflammation, increase blood flow, especially to the heart, lower blood cholesterol, normalize uterine contractions and are antiseptic. Dong quai is an excellent herbal source of iron, magnesium and niacin. It has been used to treat anemia, abdominal pains, dysmenorrhea, amenorrhea, arthritis, coronary heart disease, atherosclerosis, angina pectoris, indigestion and headaches.

Schizandra fruit contains bitter compounds that allow the body to more quickly respond to stress. This increases the body's capacity for work and decreases fatigue. These compounds also increase blood circulation, blood sugar and bile production while lowering blood pressure. Schizandra also contains astringent compounds that increase the contraction of the heart muscle and the uterus and are antiseptic. The herb has been used to treat heart palpitations, dropsy, nervous exhaustion, asthma, diabetes, chronic diarrhea, night sweats, seminal emissions, insomnia, frequent urination and anxiety.

Ophiopogon root contains bitter compounds that have a sedative effect, promote the production of mucosal fluids, reduce muscle spasms and have an antiseptic effect. In addition, the herb lowers blood sugar and regenerates beta cells in the islets of langerhorn of the pancreas. Ophiopogon has been used to treat insomnia, coronary heart disease, heart palpitations, fear and dry coughs.

Citrus peel contains aromatic compounds that are antiseptic, reduce muscle spasms and decrease the thickness while increasing the production of mucosal fluids. It also contains bitter compounds that are anti-inflammatory, reduce muscle spasms, increase the production of digestive fluid and increase blood circulation. Citrus peel has been used to treat coughs, colds, flu, fevers and bronchitis.

Atractylodes root contains aromatic compounds that are antiseptic, increase the production of digestive fluids and enzymes, increase blood pressure, are laxative, stimulate liver function and increase the flow of urine. It has been used to treat dyspepsia, flatulence, loss of appetite, nausea, indigestion, rheumatic arthritis and night blindness.

Bayberry and Ginger Combination

Composition

Bayberry	Clove
Ginger	Capsicum
White pine	

Properties

Diaphoretic	Antiseptic
Stimulant	Antipyretic
Expectorant	Carminative

General Description

Bayberry and Ginger combination is used to treat colds and flu characterized by a combination of respiratory tract congestion, and digestive system inflammation and fevers. The herbs work to induce sweating, expel mucous, soothe inflamed mucous membranes, relieve diarrhea, increase blood circulation and reduce fevers in the abdomen.

Chinese herbalists would describe this herbal combination as a wood enhancing formula. It also enhances the fire and metal elements while reducing the water and earth elements.

Bayberry and Ginger combination has traditionally been used to treat **the common cold, influenza, gastric distress, nausea, stomachaches, dysentery, diarrhea** and **hemorrhoids.**

Imbalances indicating the use of this formula are commonly noted in the stomach acupressure point located approximately one inch below and one inch to the left of the sternum. Imbalances are often noted by the presence of a "lymphatic rosary" surrounding each iris. Use caution in cases of hypertension, gastric ulcers and constipation.

This formula is commonly used in conjunction with the vitamin C family, vitamin A, zinc, echinacea, goldenseal and licorice.

Individual Components

Bayberry bark contains astringent compounds that reduce the secretion of fluids, reduce pain and shrink inflamed tissues. These compounds also promote sweating, increase blood circulation and dilate peripheral blood vessels. It has been used to treat diarrhea, colds, intestinal flu, inflammatory conditions of the gastrointestinal tract, asthma, bronchitis, fevers and sinus congestion.

Ginger root contains aromatic compounds that increase the production of digestive fluids and enzymes, lower blood pressure, lower blood sugar and cholesterol. It also contains bitter compounds that reduce muscle

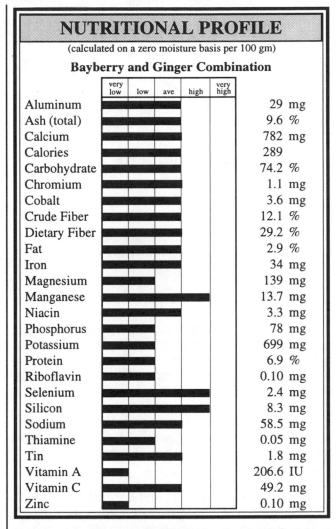

NUTRITIONAL PROFILE
(calculated on a zero moisture basis per 100 gm)
Bayberry and Ginger Combination

	very low	low	ave	high	very high		
Aluminum						29	mg
Ash (total)						9.6	%
Calcium						782	mg
Calories						289	
Carbohydrate						74.2	%
Chromium						1.1	mg
Cobalt						3.6	mg
Crude Fiber						12.1	%
Dietary Fiber						29.2	%
Fat						2.9	%
Iron						34	mg
Magnesium						139	mg
Manganese						13.7	mg
Niacin						3.3	mg
Phosphorus						78	mg
Potassium						699	mg
Protein						6.9	%
Riboflavin						0.10	mg
Selenium						2.4	mg
Silicon						8.3	mg
Sodium						58.5	mg
Thiamine						0.05	mg
Tin						1.8	mg
Vitamin A						206.6	IU
Vitamin C						49.2	mg
Zinc						0.10	mg

spasms, increase blood circulation and dilate blood vessels. Ginger is an excellent herbal source of trace minerals, especially silicon, magnesium and manganese. It has been used to treat nausea, motion sickness, flatulence, colds, coughs, indigestion, fevers, vomiting, diarrhea, chronic bronchitis and cold hands and feet.

White pine bark contains aromatic compounds that decrease the thickness while increasing the production of mucosal fluids. These compounds also relieve pain and muscle spasms and are antiseptic. It also contains astringent compounds that shrink inflamed tissues. White pine has been used to treat coughs, colds, sinus congestion, influenza, croup, rheumatism, tonsillitis and bronchitis.

Clove fruit contains aromatic compounds that relieve pains, increase blood circulation, are antiseptic, decrease the thickness while increasing the production of mucosal fluids and increase the production of digestive fluids. Clove has been used to treat toothaches, earaches, colds, flu, backaches, bronchitis, dysentery, muscle aches, nausea and vomiting.

Capsicum fruit contains aromatic resins that increase blood circulation, promote sweating, increase the production of digestive fluids and reduce muscle spasms.

It has been used to treat flatulence, colic, ulcers, rheumatic arthritis, cold hands and feet and dropsy.

Ephedra and Passionflower Combination

Composition

Marshmallow	Catnip
Chinese ephedra	Senega
Mullein	Slippery Elm
Passionflower	

Properties

Decongestant	Antispasmodic
Stimulant	Expectorant
Analgesic	

General Description

Ephedra and Passionflower combination is a decongestant formula. The herbs in this combination work together to relieve headaches, sinus pressure and the urge to cough. Unlike conventional decongestants, this formula improves concentration.

Chinese herbalists would describe this herbal combination as a metal reducing formula. It also reduces the water and earth elements while enhancing the fire and wood elements.

Ephedra and Passionflower combination has traditionally been used to treat **rhinitis, nasal congestion, nasal drainage, sneezing, respiratory allergies, headaches, sinus headaches, common colds, coughs, bronchitis** and **asthma.**

Imbalances indicating the use of this formula are commonly noted in the respiratory allergy acupressure point located on the nose. Imbalances are often noted at the 10:30 position of the left iris and 2 o'clock position of the right iris. Use caution in cases of hypertension, palpitations, insomnia and weak digestion.

This formula is commonly used in conjunction with lobelia, comfrey, licorice, the vitamin C family, vitamin A, vitamin E and zinc.

Individual Components

Marshmallow root contains mucilaginous compounds that decrease the thickness while increasing the production of mucosal fluids, soothe inflamed tissue, heal wounds and increase the flow of urine. It is an excellent herbal source of trace minerals especially chromium,

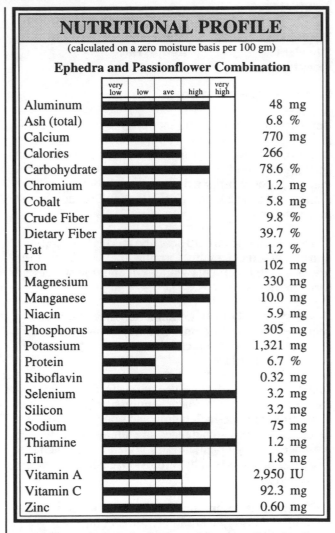

NUTRITIONAL PROFILE
(calculated on a zero moisture basis per 100 gm)
Ephedra and Passionflower Combination

	very low	low	ave	high	very high	
Aluminum						48 mg
Ash (total)						6.8 %
Calcium						770 mg
Calories						266
Carbohydrate						78.6 %
Chromium						1.2 mg
Cobalt						5.8 mg
Crude Fiber						9.8 %
Dietary Fiber						39.7 %
Fat						1.2 %
Iron						102 mg
Magnesium						330 mg
Manganese						10.0 mg
Niacin						5.9 mg
Phosphorus						305 mg
Potassium						1,321 mg
Protein						6.7 %
Riboflavin						0.32 mg
Selenium						3.2 mg
Silicon						3.2 mg
Sodium						75 mg
Thiamine						1.2 mg
Tin						1.8 mg
Vitamin A						2,950 IU
Vitamin C						92.3 mg
Zinc						0.60 mg

iron, magnesium and selenium. Marshmallow has been used to treat allergies, gastritis, gastric ulcers, enteritis, coughs, cystitis and hay fever.

Chinese ephedra herb contains bitter alkaloids that dilate the bronchioles, enhance adrenal function, shrink inflamed tissue and enhance peripheral blood circulation. These compounds also decrease the secretion of mucosal fluids, increase heart rate and blood pressure and induce sweating. The herb is an excellent herbal source of vitamin B-1, B-2 and C. Ephedra has been used to treat asthma, bronchitis, respiratory tract infections, sinus congestion, colds, coughs and arthritis.

Mullein leaves contain mucilaginous compounds that decrease the thickness and increase the production of mucosal fluids. These compounds also soothe inflamed tissue. Mullein also contains aromatic compounds that increase the flow of urine. The herb has been used to treat bronchitis, coughs, colds, hay fever, dysuria, nephritis and sinus congestion.

Passionflower contains bitter compounds that have a sedative effect and relieve muscle spasms. It has been used to treat insomnia, coughs, headaches and dysmenorrhea.

Catnip herb contains aromatic compounds that have a sedative effect, relieve smooth muscle spasms and induce sweating. It has been used to treat coughs, colds, anxiety, colic, fevers, influenza, lung congestion and nausea.

Senega root contains mucilaginous compounds that decrease the thickness while increasing the production of mucosal fluids. These compounds also soothe inflamed tissue and absorb toxins from the bowel. It has been used to treat asthma, bronchitis, croup pneumonia and respiratory tract infections.

Slippery Elm bark contains mucilaginous compounds that decrease the thickness while increasing the production of mucosal fluids. These compounds soothe inflamed tissue, decrease bowel transit time and absorb toxins from the bowel. It also contains astringent compounds that shrink inflamed tissues. Slippery elm has been used to treat asthma, bronchitis, colitis, coughs, weak digestion and inflammatory bowel disease.

Ephedra and Senega Combination

Composition

Ephedra	Parsley
Senega	Chaparral
Goldenseal	Burdock
Capsicum	

Properties

Expectorant	Antiseptic
Decongestant	Diuretic
Anti-inflammatory	Stimulant

General Description

Ephedra and Senega combination is an expectorant and decongestant formula used to treat inflammations of the respiratory system resulting from allergies and infections. Together, the herbs in this combination soothe inflamed mucous membranes, fight infection and eliminate excess fluids.

Chinese herbalists would describe this herbal combination as a metal reducing formula. It also reduces the water and wood elements while enhancing the fire and earth elements.

Ephedra and Senega combination has traditionally been used to treat **hay fevers, allergies of the respiratory system, coughs, colds, itching eyes, nose and throats, wheezing, asthma, sinus, congestion and respiratory tract infections.**

Imbalances indicating the use of this formula are commonly noted in the respiratory allergy acupressure point located on the nose. Imbalances are often noted at the 2 o'clock position of the right iris. Use caution in cases of hypertension, palpitations, insomnia and weak digestion.

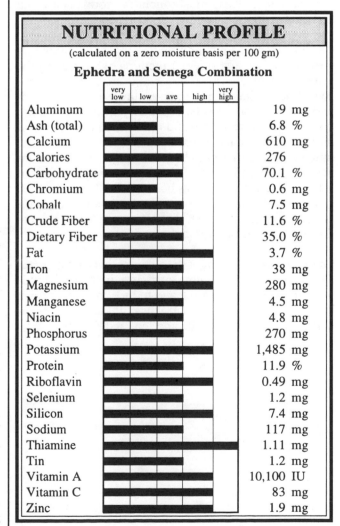

NUTRITIONAL PROFILE
(calculated on a zero moisture basis per 100 gm)

Ephedra and Senega Combination

	very low	low	ave	high	very high		
Aluminum						19	mg
Ash (total)						6.8	%
Calcium						610	mg
Calories						276	
Carbohydrate						70.1	%
Chromium						0.6	mg
Cobalt						7.5	mg
Crude Fiber						11.6	%
Dietary Fiber						35.0	%
Fat						3.7	%
Iron						38	mg
Magnesium						280	mg
Manganese						4.5	mg
Niacin						4.8	mg
Phosphorus						270	mg
Potassium						1,485	mg
Protein						11.9	%
Riboflavin						0.49	mg
Selenium						1.2	mg
Silicon						7.4	mg
Sodium						117	mg
Thiamine						1.11	mg
Tin						1.2	mg
Vitamin A						10,100	IU
Vitamin C						83	mg
Zinc						1.9	mg

This formula is commonly used in conjunction with lobelia, licorice, the vitamin C family, vitamin A, vitamin E and zinc.

Individual Components

Ephedra herb contains bitter alkaloids that dilate the bronchioles, enhance adrenal function, shrink inflamed tissue and enhance peripheral blood circulation. These compounds also decrease the secretion of mucosal fluids, increase heart rate and blood pressure and induce sweating. The herb is an excellent herbal source of vitamin B-1, B-2 and C. Ephedra has been used to treat asthma, bronchitis, respiratory tract infections, sinus congestion, colds, coughs and arthritis.

Senega root contains mucilaginous compounds that decrease the thickness while increasing the production of mucosal fluids. These compounds also sooth inflamed tissue and absorb toxins from the bowel. It has been used to treat asthma, bronchitis, croup pneumonia and respiratory tract infections.

Goldenseal root contains bitter astringent alkaloids that normalize liver and spleen functions by increasing the production of digestive fluids and enzymes, particularly bile. The compounds are antiseptic, constrict peripheral blood vessels, especially in the uterus, are laxative and relieve pain and inflammation in mucosal tissue. Goldenseal is an excellent herbal source of trace minerals including cobalt, iron, magnesium, manganese, silicon and zinc. It is also an excellent herbal source of vitamin C. It has been used to treat hepatitis, gastritis, colitis, ulcers, menorrhagia, postpartum hemorrhages, dysmenorrhea, diabetes, infections, hemorrhoids, eczema, obesity and fevers.

Capsicum fruit contains aromatic resins that increase blood circulation, promote sweating, increase the production of digestive fluids and reduce muscle spasms. It has been used to treat flatulence, colic, ulcers, rheumatic arthritis, cold hands and feet and dropsy.

Parsley herb contains aromatic compounds that decrease the thickness and increase the production of mucosal fluids, increase the production of digestive fluids and increase menstrual and urine flow. It contains bitter compounds that reduce muscle spasms and pains, reduce blood pressure and are antiseptic. Parsley is an excellent herbal source of trace minerals especially the electrolyte minerals including sodium, potassium, calcium and magnesium. It is also an excellent herbal source of vitamin A, vitamin C and chlorophyllins. Parsley has been used to treat urinary tract infections, amenorrhea, dysmenorrhea, dyspepsia, bronchitis, allergies, arthritis, asthma, flatulence, dysuria and nephritis.

Chaparral contains bitter compounds that are antiseptic and increase immune response (antioxidant). It also contains aromatic compounds that increase the flow of urine and decrease the thickness while increasing the production of mucosal fluids. Chaparral is an excellent herbal source of vitamin A and vitamin C. It has been used to treat arthritis, blood diseases, allergies and inflammatory skin conditions.

Burdock root contains mucilaginous compounds that decrease the thickness while increasing the production of mucosal fluids, soothe inflamed tissues and absorb toxins from the bowel. It also contains aromatic compounds that have an antiseptic effect and increase the flow of urine. The herb is an excellent herbal source of chromium, iron, magnesium, phosphorus, potassium, silicon and zinc. Burdock has been used to treat arthritis, allergies, eczema, bronchitis, urinary tract infections, gout and rheumatism.

Chapter 11

The Structural System

The structural system is made up of the bones, teeth, voluntary muscles and connective tissues of the body. Its prime function is to provide the bony framework for our bodies and give them the ability to move and work. Imbalances in the structural system often affect the nervous, circulatory and urinary systems. The names for the herbal combinations are chosen based on the properties of the key herbs in the formula.

Therapies for Relieving Excess Conditions

Excesses in the structural system are commonly marked by painful inflammations that restrict mobility. These conditions are often preceded by patterns of minor aches, pains and ailments including: headaches, hypertension, constipation, eczema, allergies, joint pains, painful skin eruptions, mouth sores, cysts, anger, eye infections and ear infections. If left unchecked, these ailments may develop into illnesses including: arthritis, gout, gingivitis, periodontal disease, bursitis and rheumatism.

Early herbal therapies for these conditions consisted of single herbs like white willow bark that relieves pain and inflammation in connective tissues. White willow is not simply an analgesic however, and with time and experience, herbalists recognized and recorded in their herbals the several properties of white willow. The British Herbal Pharmacopoeia lists white willow as an antiinflammatory, antirheumatic, antihidrotic, analgesic, antiseptic and astringent.

These lists of empirical properties are the key to understanding herbal combinations. Herbalists have found that they can enhance a particular property of a single herb by adding herbs that complement and support the given property. Conversely, the herbalist is also able to minimize the effects of an unwanted property by adding herbs that counteract or balance that property.

Therapies for Supplementing Deficient Conditions

Weaknesses in the structural system are marked by chronic fatigue, pain and dysfunction, particularly around joints. Also, imbalances are often noted in the kidneys as this eliminative organ is stressed. These conditions are often marked by patterns of minor aches, pains and ailments including: fatigue, lumbago, backaches, unusual fear, thirst, forgetfulness, greying of hair, constipation, frequent urination, insomnia and muscle cramps. If left unchecked, these ailments may develop into illnesses including: rickets, osteoporosis, osteomalacia, nephritis, diabetes, kidney stones, prostatitis and deafness.

Early herbal therapies for these conditions consisted of single herbs, like comfrey, for the healing of wounds and fractures. Comfrey is not only a vulnerary however, and with time and experience, herbalists recognized and recorded in their herbals the several properties of comfrey. The British Herbal Pharmacopoeia lists comfrey as a vulnerary, cell proliferant, astringent, antihemorrhagic and demulcent.

These lists of empirical properties are the key to understanding herbal combinations. Herbalists have found that they can enhance a particular property of a single herb by adding herbs that complement and support the given property. Conversely, the herbalist is also able to minimize the effects of an unwanted property by adding herbs that counteract or balance that property.

Forsythia and Schizonepeta Combination

Composition

Forsythia	Bupleurum
Schizonepeta	Licorice
Phellodendron	Coptis
Lonicera	Dong Quai
Carthamus	Peony
Platycodon	Chrysanthemum
Scute	Arctium
Siler	Vitex
Ligusticum	Gardenia

Properties

Diuretic
Sedative
Laxative
Anti-inflammatory
Analgesic

General Description

Forsythia and Schizonepeta combination is a blood purifying formula that assists the detoxifying and eliminative functions of the body. The herbs work to increase the flow of urine, relieve pain and soothe inflamed tissues. In addition, the herbs provide a laxative effect and relieve nervous tension.

Chinese herbalists would describe this herbal combination as a wood reducing formula. It also reduces the fire element while enhancing the water, metal and earth elements.

Forsythia and Schizonepeta combination has traditionally been used to treat **premenstrual syndrome, menopause, dry eyes, hemorrhoids, gallstones, hepatitis, anemia, insomnia, chipping nails and depression.**

Imbalances indicating the use of this formula are commonly noted in the calcium acupressure point located just above the left clavicle. Imbalances are often noted at the 4:00 position of the left iris. Use caution in cases of diarrhea.

This formula is commonly used in conjunction with the complex of B vitamins, evening primrose oil and vitamin E.

Individual Components

Forsythia fruit contains bitter compounds that increase the flow of urine, increase blood circulation, are antiseptic and suppress the urge to vomit. These compounds also reduce fevers and soothe inflamed tissue. Forsythia has been used to treat colds, fevers, flu, urinary tract infections, inflammatory skin conditions and constipation.

Schizonepeta herb contains aromatic compounds that promote sweating, reduce inflammation and muscle spasms, reduce fevers and are antiseptic. It has been used to treat colds, headaches, measles, uterine bleeding, inflammatory skin conditions and influenza.

Phellodendron bark contains bitter compounds that increase the production of digestive fluids and enzymes, particularly bile. These compounds are also antiseptic and laxative, relieve pain and inflammation in mucosal tissue and constrict peripheral blood vessels. Phellodendron has been used to treat diarrhea, jaundice, urinary tract infections, eczema, boils, fevers and night sweats.

Lonicera herb contains bitter compounds that relieve smooth muscle spasms, increase the flow of urine, shrink inflamed tissue and are antiseptic. It has been used to treat colds, dysentery, hepatitis and rheumatic arthritis.

Carthamus flower contains aromatic compounds that increase blood circulation, relieve pains and stimulate peristalsis and uterine contractions. It has been used to treat amenorrhea and dysmenorrhea.

Platycodon root contains bitter compounds that decrease the thickness while increasing the production of mucosal fluids, lower blood sugar, lower blood cholesterol and are antiseptic. It is used to treat coughs, weak digestion, inflammatory skin conditions and respiratory tract infections.

Scute root contains bitter compounds that increase the flow of urine, are antiseptic, reduce capillary permeability and inflammation, increase the secretion of bile and relieve muscle spasms. It has been used to treat urinary tract infection, enteritis, coughs, colds, dysentery and jaundice.

Siler root contains aromatic compounds that promote sweating, reduce fevers and are antiseptic. It has been used to treat colds, headaches, rheumatism and arthritis.

Ligusticum root contains aromatic compounds that promote sweating, increase blood circulation, relieve pain and inflammation and relieve muscle spasms. It has been used to treat headaches, migraine headaches, arthritis, rheumatism, dysmenorrhea, flu, colds, inflammatory skin conditions and anemia.

Bupleurum root contains bitter compounds that have an anti-depressant effect, relieve pain and inflammation, reduce fevers and have an antiseptic effect. In addition, these compounds reduce blood cholesterol and triglyceride levels and reduce fat cell production and inflammation in the liver. Bupleurum has been used to treat premenstrual syndrome, dysmenorrhea, lung congestion, malaria, muscle cramps, tumors, inflammatory skin conditions, angina pains, epilepsy and depression.

Licorice root contains bitter compounds that reduce inflammation, decrease the thickness and increase the production of mucosal fluids and relieve muscle spasms. In addition, licorice stimulates adrenal function, reduces the urge to cough, is mildly laxative and enhances immune response. It has been used to treat coughs, colds, arthritis, asthma, peptic ulcers, Addison's disease, dropsy and atherosclerosis.

Coptis root contains bitter astringent alkaloids similar to those found in goldenseal. These compounds normalize liver and spleen function by increasing the production of digestive fluids and enzymes, particularly bile. These compounds are antiseptic, constrict peripheral blood vessels, especially in the uterus, are laxative and relieve pain and inflammation in mucosal tissue. Coptis has been used to treat hepatitis, gastritis, colitis, ulcers, menorrhagia, postpartum hemorrhages, dysmennorrhea, diabetes, infections, hemorrhoids, eczema, obesity and fevers.

Dong Quai root contains aromatic compounds that relieve smooth muscle spasms especially in the uterus, have a sedative effect and increase the production of digestive fluids. It also contains bitter compounds that regulate glycogen production in the liver, reduce pain and inflammation, increase blood flow, especially to the heart, lower blood cholesterol, normalize uterine contractions and are antiseptic. Dong quai is an excellent herbal source of iron, magnesium and niacin. It has been used to treat anemia, abdominal pains, dysmenorrhea, amenorrhea, arthritis, coronary heart disease, atherosclerosis, angina pectoris, indigestion and headaches.

Peony root contains bitter compounds that are sedative, antiseptic and relieve pains. These compounds also lower blood pressure and decrease capillary permeability. It has been used to treat arthralgia, gastric pains, inflammatory skin conditions and dysmenorrhea.

Chrysanthemum flower contains aromatic compounds that promote sweating, reduce fevers and inflammation, lower blood pressure and increase coronary circulation. It has been used to treat atherosclerosis, angina pains, hypertension, colds and headaches.

Arctium fruit contains bitter compounds that shrink inflamed tissue, are antiseptic, increase the flow of urine, lower blood pressure and are laxative. It has been used to treat colds, coughs, bronchitis, tonsillitis and measles.

Vitex fruit contains aromatic compounds that promote sweating, relieve pain and reduce fevers. It also contains bitter compounds that have a sedative effect. Vitex has been used to treat colds, headaches, eye inflammations, arthritis and joint pains.

Gardenia fruit contains bitter compounds that increase the production of bile. These compounds also lower blood pressure, are sedative, reduce fevers and are antiseptic. It has been used to treat fevers, insomnia, hepatitis and constipation.

White Willow Combination

Composition

White Willow   Valerian
Wild Lettuce   Capsicum

Properties

Analgesic   Sedative
Anti-inflammatory   Astringent
Antispasmodic

General Description

White Willow combination is used to alleviate pain due to nervous and muscular tension. This formula is most commonly used as a palliative remedy for minor afflictions of the nervous, respiratory and musculoskeletal systems.

Chinese herbalists would describe this combination as a fire reducing formula. It also reduces the wood and earth elements while enhancing the water and metal elements.

White Willow combination has been used to treat **nervous tension, muscle tension, menstrual cramps, vertigo, coughs, colds, influenza, headaches** and **hysteria.**

Imbalances indicating the use of this formula are commonly noted in the stress acupressure point located on the forehead and by the presence of muscular pains. Imbalances are often noted in the nerve wreath surrounding both pupils. Use caution in cases of inflammatory conditions of the gastrointestinal tract, especially ulcers and gastritis.

This formula is commonly used in conjunction with the vitamin C family, vitamin B-6, l-glutamine, l-tryptophan, dl-phenylalanine, zinc and manganese.

Individual Components

White Willow bark contains bitter compounds (salicylates) which are well known for their anti-inflammatory effects on connective tissues. These compounds relieve pain and reduce fevers. White willow also contains astringent compounds which shrink inflamed tissues. It is an excellent herbal source of magnesium. White willow has been used to treat rheumatism, arthritis, joint pains, fevers, headaches, influenza and earaches.

Wild Lettuce leaf contains bitter compounds that have a mild sedative effect, relieve smooth muscle spasms

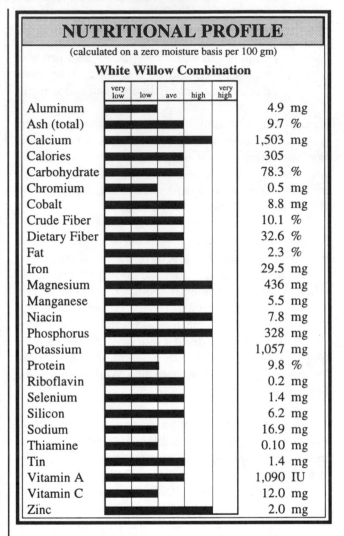

NUTRITIONAL PROFILE
(calculated on a zero moisture basis per 100 gm)
White Willow Combination

	very low	low	ave	high	very high		
Aluminum						4.9	mg
Ash (total)						9.7	%
Calcium						1,503	mg
Calories						305	
Carbohydrate						78.3	%
Chromium						0.5	mg
Cobalt						8.8	mg
Crude Fiber						10.1	%
Dietary Fiber						32.6	%
Fat						2.3	%
Iron						29.5	mg
Magnesium						436	mg
Manganese						5.5	mg
Niacin						7.8	mg
Phosphorus						328	mg
Potassium						1,057	mg
Protein						9.8	%
Riboflavin						0.2	mg
Selenium						1.4	mg
Silicon						6.2	mg
Sodium						16.9	mg
Thiamine						0.10	mg
Tin						1.4	mg
Vitamin A						1,090	IU
Vitamin C						12.0	mg
Zinc						2.0	mg

and relieve pains. It has been used to treat insomnia, cramps, urinary tract infections, bronchitis and as a galactogogue.

Valerian root contains aromatic compounds that have a sedative effect and act to decrease anxiety and aggression. These compounds also relieve smooth muscle spasms, lower blood pressure and improve sleep quality in cases of insomnia. The herb is relatively inactive in normal sleepers. Valerian is the very best herbal source of calcium and an excellent herbal source of magnesium. It has been used to treat nervousness, anxiety, insomnia, stomach cramps, muscle spasms, hysteria and convulsions.

Capsicum fruit contains aromatic resins that increase blood circulation, promote sweating, increase the production of digestive fluids and reduce muscle spasms. It has been used to treat flatulence, colic, ulcers, rheumatic arthritis, cold hands and feet and dropsy.

White Willow and Valerian Combination

Composition

White Willow	Ginger
Black Cohosh	Hops
Capsicum	Wood Betony
Valerian	Devil's Claw

Properties

Analgesic	Antispasmodic
Anti-inflammatory	Nervine
Astringent	

General Description

White Willow and Valerian Combination is used to relieve pain and inflammation in muscles and joints. This combination of herbs is particularly directed to the connective tissues of the structural system. The formula also works to calm the mind, relieves muscle cramps and shrinks inflamed tissues in the digestive and reproductive systems.

Chinese herbalists would describe this combination as a fire reducing formula. It also reduces the wood and earth elements while enhancing the water and metal elements.

White Willow and Valerian combination has traditionally been used to treat **rheumatism, arthritis, menstrual cramping, insomnia, hysteria, headaches** and **fevers.**

Imbalances indicating the use of this formula are commonly noted in painful areas of joints, over stressed muscles, and in the stress acupressure point located on the forehead. Imbalances are often noted in the nerve wreath surrounding both pupils. Use caution in cases of inflammatory conditions of the gastrointestinal tract, especially ulcers and gastritis.

This formula is commonly used in conjunction with the vitamin C family, vitamin B-6, l-glutamine, l-tryptophan, dl-phenylalanine, zinc and manganese.

Individual Components

White Willow bark contains bitter compounds (salicylates) which are well known for their anti-inflammatory effects on connective tissues. These compounds relieve

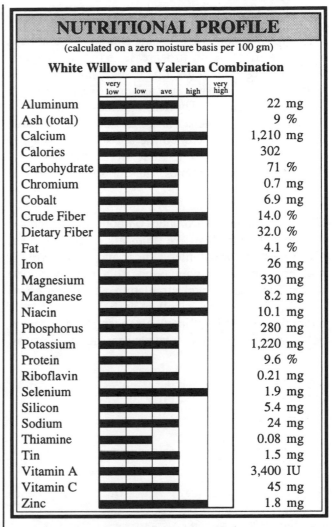

NUTRITIONAL PROFILE
(calculated on a zero moisture basis per 100 gm)
White Willow and Valerian Combination

	very low	low	ave	high	very high	
Aluminum						22 mg
Ash (total)						9 %
Calcium						1,210 mg
Calories						302
Carbohydrate						71 %
Chromium						0.7 mg
Cobalt						6.9 mg
Crude Fiber						14.0 %
Dietary Fiber						32.0 %
Fat						4.1 %
Iron						26 mg
Magnesium						330 mg
Manganese						8.2 mg
Niacin						10.1 mg
Phosphorus						280 mg
Potassium						1,220 mg
Protein						9.6 %
Riboflavin						0.21 mg
Selenium						1.9 mg
Silicon						5.4 mg
Sodium						24 mg
Thiamine						0.08 mg
Tin						1.5 mg
Vitamin A						3,400 IU
Vitamin C						45 mg
Zinc						1.8 mg

pain and reduce fevers. White willow also contains astringent compounds which shrink inflamed tissues. It is an excellent herbal source of magnesium. White willow has been used to treat rheumatism, arthritis, joint pains, fevers, headaches, influenza and earaches.

Black Cohosh root contains bitter compounds that relieve smooth muscle spasms, reduce blood pressure and dilate peripheral blood vessels. It also contains astringent compounds that shrink inflamed tissue. Black cohosh has been employed in most inflammatory conditions associated with spasms or tension. It is an excellent herbal source of iron and vitamin A. Black cohosh has been used to treat menstrual cramps, nervous tension, anxiety, dysmenorrhea, hysteria, menopause, fevers and headaches.

Capsicum fruit contains aromatic resins that increase blood circulation, promote sweating, increase the production of digestive fluids and reduce muscle spasms. It has been used to treat flatulence, colic, ulcers, rheumatic arthritis, cold hands and feet and dropsy.

Valerian root contains aromatic compounds that have a sedative effect, acting to decrease anxiety and aggression. These compounds also relieve smooth muscle spasms, lower blood pressure and improve sleep quality in cases of insomnia. The herb is relatively inactive in normal sleepers. Valerian is the very best herbal source of calcium and an excellent herbal source of magnesium. It has been used to treat nervousness, anxiety, insomnia, stomach cramps, muscle spasms, hysteria and convulsions.

Ginger root contains aromatic compounds that increase the production of digestive fluids and enzymes, lower blood pressure, lower blood sugar and cholesterol. It also contains bitter compounds that reduce muscle spasms, increase blood circulation and dilate blood vessels. Ginger is an excellent herbal source of trace minerals especially silicon, magnesium and manganese. It has been used to treat nausea, motion sickness, flatulence, colds, coughs, indigestion, fevers, vomiting, diarrhea, chronic bronchitis and cold hands and feet.

Hops flowers contain bitter compounds that have a sedative effect and relieve smooth muscle spasms, increase the flow of urine and are antiseptic. Hops is an excellent herbal source of niacin. It has been used to treat insomnia, painful urination, urinary tract infections, spastic colon and anxiety.

Wood Betony contains bitter compounds that relieve muscle spasms, increase the flow of urine and dilate peripheral blood vessels. It has been used to treat arthritis, rheumatism, jaundice, epilepsy, fevers, headaches and muscle twitching.

Devil's Claw herb contains bitter compounds that reduce inflammation in muscles and joints. These compounds have a mild pain relieving effect and reduce uric acid and cholesterol levels in the blood. It is an excellent herbal source of iron and magnesium. Devil's claw has been used to treat rheumatism, arthritis, lumbago and gout.

Eucommia and Achyranthes Combination

Composition

Eucommia	Hoelen
Achyranthes	Dipsacus
Lycium fruit	Cistanche
Rehmannia	Dong Quai
Morinda	Ginseng
Dioscorea	Atractylodes
Drynaria	Astragalus
Ligustrum	Epimedium
Cornus	Succinum

Properties

Stimulant
Astringent
Adaptogen

General Description

Eucommia and Achyranthes combination is a tonic formula used to enhance the body's response to stress and aging. The formula works to strengthen and rejuvenate the structure of the body, particularly the bones, connective tissue and sexual organs. The herbs increase blood circulation, shrink inflamed tissues in the urogenital system and increase calcium absorption.

Chinese herbalists would describe this herbal combination as a water enhancing formula. It also enhances the wood and metal elements while reducing the earth and fire elements.

Eucommia and Achyranthes combination has traditionally been used to treat **impotence, frequent urination, adrenal exhaustion, osteoporosis, backache, lumbago, fatigue, low sex drive, anemia, insomnia, arthritis, greying of hair, poor memory, paranoia, heavy legs** and **spine disorders.**

Imbalances indicating the use of this formula are commonly noted in the reproductive gland acupressure point located over the navel. Imbalances are often noted at the 3:30 position of the left iris. Use caution in cases of chronic constipation.

This formula is commonly used in conjunction with the vitamin C family, pantothenic acid, the complex of B vitamins and zinc.

Individual Components

Eucommia bark contains bitter compounds that reduce blood pressure, relieve muscle spasms, especially in the uterus, and calm the mind. It also contains mucilaginous compounds that absorb toxins from the bowel, lower cholesterol absorption and enhance the production of mucosal fluids, especially in the urinary system. Eucommia has been used to treat backaches, dysuria, impotence, muscular weaknesses, osteoporosis and to prevent miscarriage.

Achyranthes root contains bitter compounds that increase the production of urine, relieve pains, lower blood pressure and decrease peristalsis. These compounds increase the contraction of the uterus and promote menstruation. It also contains mucilaginous compounds that sooth inflamed tissue and increase the production of mucosal fluids. Achyranthes has been used to treat amenorrhea, backaches, hypertension, muscle aches and dysuria.

Lycium fruit contains bitter compounds that lower blood sugar, promote the regeneration of liver cells and lower blood cholesterol. It has been used to treat atherosclerosis, backaches, impotence, vertigo, poor eyesight and diabetes.

Rehmennia root contains astringent compounds that stop bleeding and reduce inflammation, especially in the digestive system. The herb also contains bitter compounds that reduce capillary fragility. It has been used to treat ulcers, menorrhagia, thirst, diabetes, constipation, anemia and infertility.

Morinda root contains bitter compounds that reduce inflammation, increase the flow of urine, lower blood pressure and are laxative. It also contains mucilaginous compounds that absorb toxins from the bowel and increase the production of mucosal fluids. Morinda has been used to treat arthritis, constipation, impotence, backaches, joint aches, osteoporosis and memory loss.

Dioscorea root contains mucilaginous compounds that decrease the thickness and increase the production of mucosal fluids, enhance the efficiency of healing and increase the production of digestive fluids. It has been used to treat lack of appetite, diarrhea, asthma, dry coughs, nocturnal emissions, frequent urination, diabetes and inflammatory skin conditions.

Drynaria root contains bitter compounds that increase blood circulation and strengthen connective tissue by reducing capillary fragility. It has been used to treat varicose veins, arthritis, backaches, joint pains, broken bones, osteoporosis and cold hands and feet.

Ligustrum fruit contains bitter compounds that are cardiotonic, relieve pains, increase the flow of urine and are laxative. In addition, these compounds are antiseptic, increase immune response by stimulating the production of white blood cells and reduce inflammation in the eye. Ligustrum has been used to treat lumbago, constipation, cataracts, retinitis, pneumonia, bronchitis, urinary tract infections, gastroenteritis, colds, flu and dysmenorrhea.

Cornus fruit contains astringent compounds that shrink inflamed tissue, reduce menstrual flow and are antiseptic. It also contains bitter compounds that increase the flow of urine, lower blood pressure and increase immune response. Cornus has been used to treat backaches, dysuria, impotence, uterine bleeding, menorrhagia and vertigo.

Hoelen herb contains bitter compounds that increase the flow of urine, decrease blood sugar and have a sedative effect. It has been used to treat edema, dropsy, diarrhea, insomnia, frequent urination and heart palpitations.

Dipsacus root contains bitter compounds that shrink inflamed tissue, relieve pains, and reduce hemorrhaging. It has been used to treat joint pains, arthritis, rheumatism, to prevent miscarriages, uterine bleeding and backaches.

Cistanche herb contains bitter compounds that enhance the production of urine, rejuvenate renal function and have a mild laxative effect. It has been used to treat impotence, frequent urination and chronic constipation.

Dong Quai root contains aromatic compounds that relieve smooth muscle spasms especially in the uterus, have a sedative effect and increase the production of digestive fluids. It also contains bitter compounds that regulate glycogen production in the liver, reduce pain and inflammation, increase blood flow, especially to the heart, lower blood cholesterol, normalize uterine contractions and are antiseptic. Dong quai is an excellent herbal source of iron, magnesium and niacin. It has been used to treat anemia, abdominal pains, dysmenorrhea, amenorrhea, arthritis, coronary heart disease, atherosclerosis, angina pectoris, indigestion and headaches.

Siberian Ginseng root contains bitter compounds that help the body respond more quickly to stress. These compounds increase the production of DNA, RNA and proteins essential to all life processes. They stimulate the adrenal, pancreas and pituitary glands to lower blood sugar and reduce inflammation. Ginseng also increases the production of digestive fluids and is a mild sedative. It has been used to treat anemia, impotence, insomnia, diarrhea, fatigue, debility, weak digestion and failing memory.

Atractylodes root contains aromatic compounds that are antiseptic, increase the production of digestive fluids and enzymes, increase blood pressure, are laxative, stimulate liver function and increase the flow of urine. It has been used to treat dyspepsia, flatulence, loss of appetite, nausea, indigestion, rheumatic arthritis and night blindness.

Astragalus root contains bitter compounds that increase the flow of urine, are antiseptic, increase the production of digestive fluids including bile, and relieve muscle spasms. Astragalus also contains mucilaginous compounds that enhance immune response, increasing the production of lymphocytes and macrophages. The herb also increases heart action and lowers blood pressure and blood sugar. It has been used to treat fatigue, debility, urinary tract infections, edema, nephritis, ulcers, prolapse of organs and night sweats.

Epimedium herb contains bitter compounds that are antiseptic, lower blood pressure, relieve inflammation, increase the flow of urine and decrease the thickness while increasing the production of mucosal fluids. It has been used to treat impotence, lumbago, arthritis, hypertension and bronchitis.

Succinum resin contains aromatic compounds that increase the flow of urine and increase blood circulation. These compounds also relieve pains, are antiseptic and have a sedative effect. Succinum has been used to treat insomnia, heart palpitations, epilepsy, urinary tract infections, kidney stones, amenorrhea and coronary heart disease.

Horsetail and Gelatin Combination

Composition

Dulse
Horsetail
Sage
Gelatin
Rosemary

Properties

Nutritive
Diuretic
Bulk laxative

General Description

Horsetail and Gelatin combination supplements nutrients essential to the protective tissues of the body, particularly the hair, skin and nails. This formula is an excellent herbal source of minerals whose bioavailability is enhanced by the concentrated protein content of the gelatin. The herbs also work to increase the flow of urine and absorb toxins from the bowel.

Chinese herbalists would describe this herbal combination as a metal enhancing formula. It also enhances the fire and earth elements while reducing the water and wood elements.

Horsetail and Gelatin combination has traditionally been used to treat **skin rashes, acne, splitting nails, night sweats, dry throat and mouth, nocturnal emissions, lymphatic inflammations, dry coughs** and **weakened lungs.**

Imbalances indicating the use of this formula are commonly noted in the thymus acupressure point located in the hollow of the neck. Imbalances are often noted by the presence of a "lymphatic rosary" surrounding each iris. Use caution in cases of extremely dry skin and during lactation.

This formula is commonly used in conjunction with vitamin A, zinc, parthenium root and the vitamin C family.

Individual Components

Dulse herb contains mucilaginous compounds that enhance the detoxifying and eliminative functions of the digestive system. These compounds absorb toxins

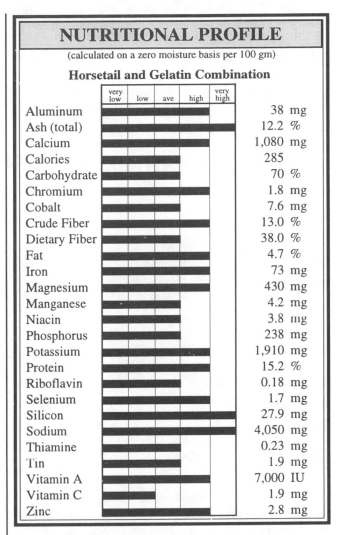

NUTRITIONAL PROFILE
(calculated on a zero moisture basis per 100 gm)

Horsetail and Gelatin Combination

	very low	low	ave	high	very high		
Aluminum						38	mg
Ash (total)						12.2	%
Calcium						1,080	mg
Calories						285	
Carbohydrate						70	%
Chromium						1.8	mg
Cobalt						7.6	mg
Crude Fiber						13.0	%
Dietary Fiber						38.0	%
Fat						4.7	%
Iron						73	mg
Magnesium						430	mg
Manganese						4.2	mg
Niacin						3.8	mg
Phosphorus						238	mg
Potassium						1,910	mg
Protein						15.2	%
Riboflavin						0.18	mg
Selenium						1.7	mg
Silicon						27.9	mg
Sodium						4,050	mg
Thiamine						0.23	mg
Tin						1.9	mg
Vitamin A						7,000	IU
Vitamin C						1.9	mg
Zinc						2.8	mg

from the bowel and provide bulk to the stool. Dulse is an excellent herbal source of calcium, sodium and iodine. Iodine is essential to normal thyroid function. It is used to increase the metabolic rate and strengthen connective tissues including the hair, skin and nails. Dulse has been used to treat enlarged glands, debility, fatigue, eczema, psoriasis and dry coughs.

Horsetail herb contains bitter compounds that increase the production of urine and shrink inflamed mucosal tissue, particularly the prostate. Horsetail is most noted for its trace mineral profile since it is an excellent herbal source of bioavailable silicon, calcium, magnesium, chromium, iron, manganese and potassium. It has been used to treat prostatitis, osteoporosis, enuresis, urinary tract infections and muscle cramps.

Sage leaf contains aromatic compounds that increase the production of digestive fluids, are antiseptic and are powerful antioxidants. It also contains astringent compounds that shrink inflamed tissues and decrease perspiration. Sage has been used to treat dyspepsia, sore throats, night sweats, headaches, colds and influenza.

Gelatin provides a concentrated source of protein which, when digested, contributes free amino acids to the digestive broth. The amino acids can then combine with minerals to form mineral chelates that are easily absorbed by the small intestine. Amino acids also provide the body with the building blocks to manufacture proteins on a cellular level.

Rosemary leaf contains aromatic compounds that have a sedative effect and relieve depression. These compounds also increase the production of digestive fluids and are antiseptic. Rosemary has been used to treat menstrual disorders, dyspepsia, depression, flatulence, influenza, dropsy and nervous exhaustion.

Marshmallow and Plantain Combination

Composition

Alfalfa	Plantain
Marshmallow	Horsetail
Slippery Elm	Wheat grass
Oatstraw	

Properties

Carminative
Antispasmodic
Sedative

General Description

Marshmallow and Plantain combination is a sedative formula. The herbs work to improve the efficiency of digestion and mineral absorption, reduce pain in the extremities, arrest spasms and calm hysteria associated with calcium deficiency.

Chinese herbalists would describe this herbal combination as a fire reducing formula. It also reduces the earth element while enhancing the water, wood and metal elements.

Marshmallow and Plantain combination has traditionally been used to treat **muscle spasms, hysteria, insomnia, night sweats, skin eruptions, weak digestion** and **osteoporosis.**

Imbalances indicating the use of this formula are commonly noted in the calcium deficiency acupressure point located just above the left clavicle on the proximal end. Imbalances are often noted at the 4 o'clock posiiton of the right iris. Use caution in cases of severe lung congestion and edema.

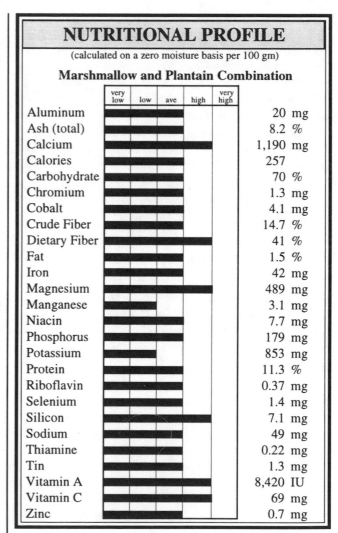

NUTRITIONAL PROFILE

(calculated on a zero moisture basis per 100 gm)

Marshmallow and Plantain Combination

	very low	low	ave	high	very high	
Aluminum						20 mg
Ash (total)						8.2 %
Calcium						1,190 mg
Calories						257
Carbohydrate						70 %
Chromium						1.3 mg
Cobalt						4.1 mg
Crude Fiber						14.7 %
Dietary Fiber						41 %
Fat						1.5 %
Iron						42 mg
Magnesium						489 mg
Manganese						3.1 mg
Niacin						7.7 mg
Phosphorus						179 mg
Potassium						853 mg
Protein						11.3 %
Riboflavin						0.37 mg
Selenium						1.4 mg
Silicon						7.1 mg
Sodium						49 mg
Thiamine						0.22 mg
Tin						1.3 mg
Vitamin A						8,420 IU
Vitamin C						69 mg
Zinc						0.7 mg

This formula is commonly used in conjunction with calcium, magnesium, phosphorus, Vitamin D, iron, manganese, lobelia and comfrey.

Individual Components

Alfalfa herb contains bitter compounds that enhance the efficiency of digestion by increasing appetite and the assimilation of nutrients. These compounds also lower blood pressure and balance oestogenic hormones. Alfalfa is an excellent herbal source of nutrients, including vitamin A, vitamin C, niacin and vitamin B-2. The herb has been used to treat debility, anorexia, arthritis, weak digestion, hypertension and gout.

Marshmallow root contains mucilaginous compounds that decrease the thickness while increasing the production of mucosal fluids, soothe inflamed tissue, heal wounds and increase the flow of urine. It is an excellent herbal source of trace minerals, especially chromium, iron, magnesium and selenium. Marshmallow has been used to treat allergies, gastritis, gastric ulcers, enteritis, coughs, cystitis and hay fever.

Slippery Elm bark contains mucilaginous compounds that decrease the thickness while increasing the production of mucosal fluids. These compounds sooth inflamed tissues, decrease bowel transit time and absorb toxins from the bowel. It also contains astringent compounds that shrink inflamed tissues. Slippery elm has been used to treat asthma, bronchitis, colitis, coughs, weak digestion and inflammatory bowel disease.

Oatstraw stem contains mucilaginous compounds as well as crude fiber that encourage normal bowel function. These compounds reduce bowel transit time, absorb toxins and enhance the efficiency of digestion. Oatstraw is an excellent herbal source of magnesium. The herb has been used to treat hysteria, calcium deficiency, nervous disorders, urinary tract infection and osteoporosis.

Plantain seed contains mucilaginous compounds that absorb toxins from the bowel, soothe inflamed tissues and promote normal bowel function. Plantain has been used to treat chronic constipation, colitis, dysentery, coughs, ulcers and diarrhea.

Horsetail herb contains bitter compounds that increase the production of urine and shrink inflamed mucosal tissue, particularly the prostate. Horsetail is most noted for its trace mineral profile since it is an excellent herbal source of bioavailable silicon, calcium, magnesium, chromium, iron, manganese and potassium. It has been used to treat prostatitis, osteoporosis, enuresis, urinary tract infections and muscle cramps.

Wheat grass is the young shoots of wheat. It contains bitter compounds that enhance digestion. It is an excellent herbal source of trace nutrients and enzymes, especially superoxide dismutase, a natural antioxidant. Wheatgrass has been used to treat general debility, fatigue, arthritis and to enhance immune response.

Chapter 12

The Urinary System

The urinary system is made up of the kidneys, bladder, ureters and urethra. Its prime functions are to maintain proper fluid balance in the body, remove toxins from the blood and eliminate them as urine. Imbalances in the urinary system often affect the glandular and circulatory systems, particularly the reproductive organs, adrenal glands and the major blood vessels. The names for the herbal combinations are chosen based on the properties of the key herbs in the formula.

Therapies for Relieving Excess Conditions

The majority of imbalances seen in the urinary system are "excess" conditions. Excessive concentrations of toxins filtered from the blood cause irritations in the mucosa of the urinary tract. This results in inflammation, pain and blockages in the form of kidney stones or scarring.

Excess conditions in the urinary system are often marked by patterns of minor aches, pains and ailments including: burning, urination, backache, sciatic nerve pains, weariness, dizziness upon standing, heavy feeling in legs, apathy, aloofness, unusual fear, pain in lower abdomen, scanty urine, diarrhea and edema. If left unchecked, these ailments may develop into illnesses including: urinary tract infections, kidney stones, peritonitis, nephritis, urethritis, cystitis, prostatitis, gonorrhea and syphilis.

Early herbal therapies for these conditions consisted of single herbs like juniper berry which increases the flow of urine to speed the removal of toxins from the urinary system. Juniper berry is not simply a diuretic however, and with time and experience, herbalists recognized and recorded in their herbals the several properties of juniper berry. The British Herbal Pharmacopeia lists juniper as a diuretic, antiseptic, carminative, stomachic and antirheumatic.

These lists of empirical properties of an herb are the key to understanding herbal combinations. Herbalists have found that they can enhance a particular property of a single herb by adding herbs that complement and support a given property. Conversely, the herbalist is also able to minimize the effects of unwanted property by adding herbs that counteract and balance that property.

Therapies for Supplementing Deficient Conditions

Weaknesses in the urinary system are characterized by chronic inflammation and infections. Herbalists use mucilaginous herbs which work by reflex action to decrease the thickness and increase the production of protective fluid in the mucosa of the urinary tract.

Weakened conditions of the urinary system are often associated with patterns of minor aches, pains and ailments including: frequent urination, fatigue, passive attitude, weakness in legs, lumbago, backaches, unusual fear, thirst, greying hair, constipation, insomnia, weak digestion, tinnitus and memory loss. If left unchecked, these ailments may development into illnesses including: osteoporosis, nephritis, chronic urinary tract infections, kidney stones, arthritis, renal failure and diabetes.

Early herbal therapies for these conditions consisted of single herbs such as marshmallow root which soothes the digestive tract and by a reflex action decreases the thickness and increases the production of protective fluid by the mucosa of the urinary tract. Marshmallow is not simply a demulcent and expectorant however, and with time and experience, herbalists recognized and recorded in their herbals the several properties of marshmallow. The British Herbal Pharmacopoeia lists marshmallow as a demulcent, diuretic, emollient and vulnerary.

These empirical properties of an herb are the key to understanding herbal combinations. Herbalists have found that they could enhance a particular property of a single herb by adding herbs that compliment and support that property. Conversely, the herbalist is also able to minimize an unwanted property by adding herbs that counteract and balance that property.

Therapies for Relieving Excess Conditions

Alisma and Hoelen Combination

Composition

Alisma	Atractylodes
Hoelen	Pinellia
Stephania	Areca Seed
Astragalus	Magnolia bark
Morus bark	Chaenomeles
Citrus	Cinnamon twig
Ginger	Akebia
Polyporus	Licorice

Properties

Diuretic	Analgesic
Antiseptic	Carminative
Anti-inflammatory	Stimulant

General Description

Alisma and Hoelen combination is a diuretic formula used to relieve water retention, particularly in the legs and chest. The herbs work to increase the flow of urine, relieve pain and inflammation and fight urinary tract infections. In addition, the herbs soothe and moisten inflamed tissues, increase blood flow and reduce lymphatic congestion.

Chinese herbalists describe this herbal combination as a water reducing formula. It also reduces the wood and metal elements while enhancing the fire and earth elements.

Alisma and Hoelen combination has been used to treat **urinary tract infections, joint pains, nephritis, colitis, edema, diarrhea, indigestion, scanty urine, arthritis, mastitis, bloating, hypertension, obesity, prostatitis, apathy, dizziness** and **fatigue.**

Imbalances indicating the use of this formula are commonly noted in the kidney acupressure point located in the small of the back over each kidney. Imbalances are often noted at the 6:30 position of the left iris and at the 5:30 position of the right iris. Use caution in cases of renal bleeding.

This formula is commonly used in conjunction with vitamin A, lobelia, zinc, potassium, fruit juices, watermelon seed, juniper berry, uva ursi and watercress.

Individual Components

Alisma root contains bitter compounds that increase the flow of urine, reduce blood pressure, lower blood sugar and cholesterol and are antiseptic. It has been used to treat edema, nephritis, diarrhea, cholesterolemia and urinary tract infections.

Hoelen herb contains bitter compounds that increase the flow of urine, decrease blood sugar and have a sedative effect. It has been used to treat edema, dropsy, diarrhea, insomnia, frequent urination and heart palpitations.

Stephania root contains bitter compounds that increase the flow of urine and relieve pains. It has been used to treat rheumatic arthritis, edema and frequent urination.

Astragalus root contains bitter compounds that increase the flow of urine, are antiseptic, increase the production of digestive fluids, including bile, and relieve muscle spasms. Astragalus also contains mucilaginous compounds that enhance immune response, increasing the production of lymphocytes and macrophages. The herb also increases heart action and lowers blood pressure and blood sugar. It has been used to treat fatigue, debility, urinary tract infections, edema, nephritis, ulcers, prolapse of organs and night sweats.

Morus bark contains bitter compounds that increase the flow of urine, reduce blood pressure, decrease the thickness while increasing the production of mucosal fluids, reduce muscle spasms and have a sedative effect. It has been used to treat coughs, colds, asthma, hypertension and edema.

Citrus peel contains aromatic compounds that are antiseptic, reduce muscle spasms and decrease the thickness while increasing the production of mucosal fluids. It also contains bitter compounds that are anti-inflammatory, reduce muscle spasms, increase the production of digestive fluid and increase blood circulation. Citrus peel has been used to treat coughs, colds, flu, fevers and bronchitis.

Ginger root contains aromatic compounds that increase the production of digestive fluids and enzymes, lower blood pressure, lower blood sugar and cholesterol. It also contains bitter compounds that reduce muscle spasms, increase blood circulation and dilate blood vessels. Ginger is an excellent herbal source of silicon, magnesium and manganese. It has been used to treat nausea, motion sickness, flatulence, colds, coughs, indigestion, fevers, vomiting, diarrhea, chronic bronchitis and cold hands and feet.

Polyporus herb contains bitter compounds that increase the production of urine, lower blood pressure and are antiseptic. It has been used to treat frequent urination, dropsy, edema and nephritis.

Atractylodes root contains aromatic compounds that are antiseptic, increase the production of digestive fluids and enzymes, increase blood pressure, are laxative, stimulate liver function and increase the flow of urine. It has been used to treat dyspepsia, flatulence, loss of appetite, nausea, indigestion, rheumatic arthritis and night blindness.

Pinellia root contains bitter compounds that decrease the thickness while increasing the production of mucosal fluids, relieve muscle spasms, increase the production of digestive fluids and absorb toxins. Pinellia root must by processed with alum or ginger root before ingestion since it is toxic. It has been used to treat morning sickness, nausea, vomiting, respiratory congestion, ulcers and blood poisoning.

Areca seed contains bitter compounds that kill worms and parasites, increase peristalsis and promote sweating. It also contains astringent compounds that are antiseptic and shrink inflamed tissues. It is a harsh herb and caution should be exercised to avoid overdose. Areca seed has been used to treat constipation, worms, intestinal parasites and edema.

Magnolia bark contains bitter compounds that relieve muscle cramps, are antiseptic, and have sedative properties. It has been used to treat gastritis, coughs, asthma, diarrhea, vomiting and flatulence.

Chaenomeles fruit contains bitter compounds that relieve muscle spasms and increase the production of digestive fluids. It has been used to treat rheumatism, rheumatic arthritis, leg cramps, vomiting, diarrhea and dyspepsia.

Cinnamon twig contains aromatic compounds that promote sweating, increase blood circulation, increase the production of digestive fluids, relieve smooth muscle spasms, increase the flow of urine and are antiseptic. The herb is a general stimulant to the digestive respiratory, urinary and circulatory systems. It has been used to treat colds, edema, dysuria, arthritis, amenorrhea, angina pain and dyspepsia.

Akebia herb contains bitter compounds that increase the flow of urine, increase menstrual flow and reduce inflammation. It has been used to treat urinary tract infections, edema, amenorrhea and rheumatic arthritis.

Licorice root contains bitter compounds that reduce inflammation, decrease the thickness and increase the production of mucosal fluids and relieve muscle spasms. In addition, licorice stimulates adrenal function, reduces the urge to cough, is mildly laxative and enhances immune response. It has been used to treat coughs, colds, arthritis, asthma, peptic ulcers, Addison's disease, dropsy and atherosclerosis.

Cedar Berry Combination

Composition

Cedar berry
Burdock
Chaparral
Goldenseal
Siberian Ginseng

Properties

Carminative
Diuretic
Anti-inflammatory
Hypoglycemic

General Description

Cedar berry combination enhances the function of the glandular system, particularly the pancreas and liver. The herbs increase the production of digestive enzymes, especially pancreatin and bile. The herbs also increase the production of urine, balance blood sugar levels, reduce inflammation and increase the production of mucosal fluid.

Chinese herbalists would describe this herbal combination as an earth enhancing formula. It also enhances the water and metal elements, while reducing the fire and wood elements.

Cedar berry combination has traditionally been used to treat **pancreatitis, hypoglycemia, flatulence** and **nausea.**

Imbalances indicating the use of this formula are commonly noted in the pancreas acupressure point located approximately four inches below and three inches to the left of the sternum. Imbalances are often noted at the 7 o'clock position of the right iris. Use caution in cases of renal failure.

This formula is commonly used in conjunction with chromium, the vitamin C family , the complex of B vitamins, vitamin A and vitamin E.

Individual Components

Cedar berry contains aromatic compounds that increase the flow of urine, increase the production of digestive fluids and enzymes, relieve pain and are antiseptic. It has been used to treat pancreatitis, cystitis, rheumatism, gout, urinary tract infection and hypoglycemia.

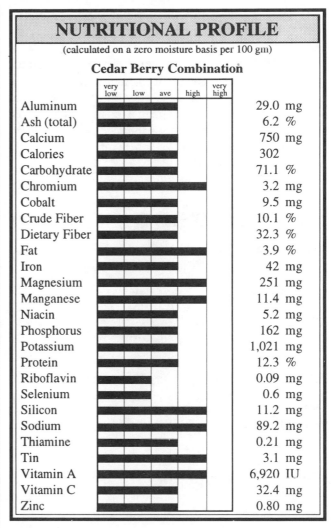

NUTRITIONAL PROFILE
(calculated on a zero moisture basis per 100 gm)

Cedar Berry Combination

	very low	low	ave	high	very high	
Aluminum						29.0 mg
Ash (total)						6.2 %
Calcium						750 mg
Calories						302
Carbohydrate						71.1 %
Chromium						3.2 mg
Cobalt						9.5 mg
Crude Fiber						10.1 %
Dietary Fiber						32.3 %
Fat						3.9 %
Iron						42 mg
Magnesium						251 mg
Manganese						11.4 mg
Niacin						5.2 mg
Phosphorus						162 mg
Potassium						1,021 mg
Protein						12.3 %
Riboflavin						0.09 mg
Selenium						0.6 mg
Silicon						11.2 mg
Sodium						89.2 mg
Thiamine						0.21 mg
Tin						3.1 mg
Vitamin A						6,920 IU
Vitamin C						32.4 mg
Zinc						0.80 mg

Burdock root contains mucilaginous compounds that decrease the thickness while increasing the production of mucosal fluids, soothe inflamed tissues and absorb toxins from the bowel. It also contains aromatic compounds that have an antiseptic effect and increase the flow of urine. The herb is an excellent herbal source of chromium, iron, magnesium, phosphorus, potassium, silicon and zinc. Burdock has been used to treat arthritis, allergies, eczema, bronchitis, urinary tract infections, gout and rheumatism.

Chaparral contains bitter compounds that are antiseptic and increase immune response (antioxidant). It also contains aromatic compounds that increase the flow of urine and decrease the thickness while increasing the production of mucosal fluids. Chaparral is an excellent herbal source of vitamin A and vitamin C. It has been used to treat arthritis, blood diseases, allergies and inflammatory skin conditions.

Goldenseal root contains bitter, astringent alkaloids that normalize liver and spleen function by increasing the production of digestive fluids and enzymes, particularly bile. These compounds are antiseptic, constrict peripheral bloods vessels especially in the uterus, are laxative and relieve pain and inflammation in mucosal tissue. Goldenseal is an excellent herbal source of trace minerals including cobalt, iron, magnesium, manganese, silicon and zinc. It is also an excellent herbal source of vitamin C. It has been used to treat hepatitis, gastritis, colitis, ulcers, menorrhagia, postpartum hemorrhages, dysmenorrhea, diabetes, infections, hemorrhoids, eczema, obesity and fevers.

Siberian Ginseng root contains bitter compounds that help the body respond more quickly to stress. These compounds increase the production of DNA, RNA and proteins essential to all life processes. They also stimulate the adrenal, pancreas, and pituitary glands to lower blood sugar and reduce inflammation. Ginseng also increases the production of digestive fluids and is a mild sedative. It has been used to treat anemia, impotence, insomnia, diarrhea, fatigue, debility, weak digestion and failing memory.

Ginseng and Parsley Combination

Composition

Capsicum	Siberian Ginseng
Goldenseal	Uva Ursi
Ginger	Marshmallow
Parsley	Eupatorium

Properties

Diuretic	Vulnerary
Anti-inflammatory	Stimulant
Antiseptic	

General Description

Ginseng and Parsley combination is a male corrective formula. The herbs in this combination work to reduce inflammation and swelling in the urinary system, especially the prostate and kidneys, and to prevent the formation and growth of kidney stones. This is accomplished by the combined action of the herbs which provide anti-inflammatory, diuretic, antiseptic and astringent properties directed specifically at the urinary system.

Chinese herbalists would describe this herbal combination as a water reducing formula. It also reduces the earth and wood elements while enhancing the fire and metal elements.

Ginseng and Parsley combination has traditionally been used to treat **prostatitis, kidney stones, impotence, urinary tract infections, edema, joint pains, arthritis, nephritis, colitis** and **diarrhea.**

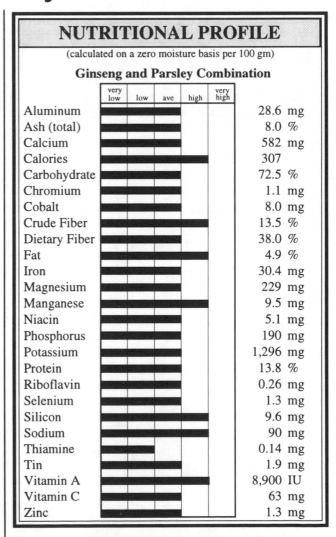

NUTRITIONAL PROFILE

(calculated on a zero moisture basis per 100 gm)

Ginseng and Parsley Combination

	very low	low	ave	high	very high		
Aluminum						28.6	mg
Ash (total)						8.0	%
Calcium						582	mg
Calories						307	
Carbohydrate						72.5	%
Chromium						1.1	mg
Cobalt						8.0	mg
Crude Fiber						13.5	%
Dietary Fiber						38.0	%
Fat						4.9	%
Iron						30.4	mg
Magnesium						229	mg
Manganese						9.5	mg
Niacin						5.1	mg
Phosphorus						190	mg
Potassium						1,296	mg
Protein						13.8	%
Riboflavin						0.26	mg
Selenium						1.3	mg
Silicon						9.6	mg
Sodium						90	mg
Thiamine						0.14	mg
Tin						1.9	mg
Vitamin A						8,900	IU
Vitamin C						63	mg
Zinc						1.3	mg

Imbalances indicating the use of this formula are commonly noted in the prostate acupressure point located at the top of the right hip bone along the inside of the inguinal ligament. Imbalances are often noted at the 5 o'clock position of each iris.

This formula is commonly used in conjunction with vitamin A, and complex of B vitamins, saw palmetto, pumpkin, almonds, vitamin C, zinc and bee pollen.

Individual Components

Capsicum fruit contains aromatic resins that increase blood circulation, promote sweating, increase the production of digestive fluids and reduce muscle spasms. It has been used to treat flatulence, colic, ulcers, rheumatic arthritis, cold hands and feet and dropsy.

Goldenseal root contains bitter astringent alkaloids that normalize liver and spleen functions by increasing the production of digestive fluids and enzymes, particularly bile. The compounds are antiseptic, constrict peripheral blood vessels, especially in the uterus, are laxative and relieve pain and inflammation in mucosal tissue. Goldenseal is an excellent herbal source of trace minerals including cobalt, iron, magnesium, manganese, silicon and zinc. It is also an excellent herbal source of Vitamin C. It has been used to treat hepatitis, gastritis, colitis, ulcers, menorrhagia, postpartum hemorrhage, dysmenorrhea, diabetes, infections, hemorrhoids, eczema, obesity and fevers.

Ginger root contains aromatic compounds that increase the production of digestive fluids and enzymes, lower blood pressure, lower blood sugar and cholesterol. It also contains bitter compounds that reduce muscle spasms, increase blood circulation and dilate blood vessels. Ginger is an excellent herbal source of trace minerals especially silicon, magnesium and manganese. It has been used to treat nausea, motion sickness, flatulence, colds, coughs, indigestion, fevers, vomiting, diarrhea, chronic bronchitis and cold hands and feet.

Parsley herb contains aromatic compounds that decrease the thickness and increase the production of mucosal fluids, increase the production of digestive fluids and increase menstrual and urine flow. It also contains bitter compounds that reduce muscle spasms and pains, reduce blood pressure and are antiseptic. Parsley is an excellent herbal source of trace minerals, especially the electrolyte minerals including sodium, potassium, calcium and magnesium. It is also an excellent herbal source of vitamin A, vitamin C and chlorophyllins. Parsley has been used to treat urinary tract infections, amenorrhea, dysmenorrhea, dyspepsia, bronchitis, allergies, arthritis, asthma, flatulence, dysuria and nephritis.

Siberian Ginseng root contains bitter compounds that help the body respond more quickly to stress. These compounds increase the production of DNA, RNA and proteins essential to all life processes. They stimulate the adrenal, pancreas, and pituitary glands to lower blood sugar and reduce inflammation. Ginseng also increases the production of digestive fluids and is a mild sedative. It has been used to treat anemia, impotence, insomnia, diarrhea, fatigue, debility, weak digestion and failing memory.

Uva ursi fruit contains bitter compounds that are antiseptic and increase the flow of urine. It also contains astringent compounds that shrink inflamed tissue. It has been used to treat urinary tract infections, kidney stones, cystitis, nephritis, hemorrhoids and diarrhea.

Marshmallow root contains mucilaginous compounds that decrease the thickness while increasing the production of mucosal fluids, soothe inflamed tissue, heal wounds and increase the flow of urine. It is an excellent herbal source of trace minerals, especially chromium, iron, magnesium and selenium. Marshmallow has been used to treat allergies, gastritis, gastric ulcers, enteritis, coughs, cystitis and hay fever.

Eupatorium herb contains bitter compounds that increase the flow of urine and are antiseptic. Eupatorium has been used to treat gout, edema, lumbago, urinary tract infections, rheumatism and kidney stones.

Uva Ursi Combination

Composition

Juniper   Dandelion
Parsley   Chamomile
Uva Ursi

Properties

Analgesic   Antispasmodic
Anti-inflammatory   Nervine
Astringent

General Description

Uva Ursi combination is used to treat infection and inflammation in the urinary system. The herbs in this formula are antiseptic, reduce inflammation and smooth muscle spasms. The formula increases the production of urine which helps prevent kidney stone formation.

Chinese herbalists would describe this combination as a water reducing formula. It also reduces the wood and metal elements while enhancing the earth and fire elements.

Uva Ursi combination has traditionally been used to treat **urinary tract infections, nephritis, cystitis, urethritis, uterine bleeding, gonorrhea, insomnia, edema, dysuria, dizziness, fatigue, joint pains, hypertension** and **tinnitis.**

Imbalances indicating the use of this formula are commonly noted in the kidney acupressure point located in the small of the back over each kidney. Imbalances are also common in the bladder acupressure point located just above the pubic bone. Imbalances are often noted at the 6:30 position of the left iris and at the 5:30 position of the right iris. Use caution in cases of kidney stones.

This formula is commonly used in conjunction with vitamin A, hydrangea, marshmallow, lobelia, zinc, potassium, fruit juices, watermelon seed, celery seed and watercress.

Individual Components

Juniper berry contains aromatic compounds that increase the flow of urine, increase the production of

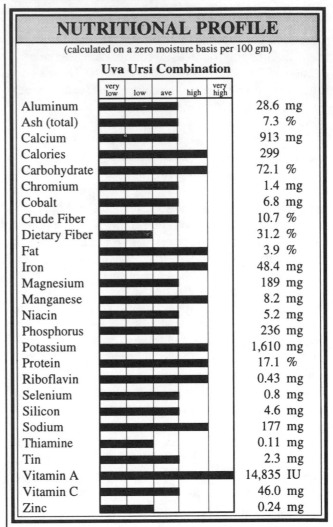

NUTRITIONAL PROFILE
(calculated on a zero moisture basis per 100 gm)

Uva Ursi Combination

	very low	low	ave	high	very high	
Aluminum						28.6 mg
Ash (total)						7.3 %
Calcium						913 mg
Calories						299
Carbohydrate						72.1 %
Chromium						1.4 mg
Cobalt						6.8 mg
Crude Fiber						10.7 %
Dietary Fiber						31.2 %
Fat						3.9 %
Iron						48.4 mg
Magnesium						189 mg
Manganese						8.2 mg
Niacin						5.2 mg
Phosphorus						236 mg
Potassium						1,610 mg
Protein						17.1 %
Riboflavin						0.43 mg
Selenium						0.8 mg
Silicon						4.6 mg
Sodium						177 mg
Thiamine						0.11 mg
Tin						2.3 mg
Vitamin A						14,835 IU
Vitamin C						46.0 mg
Zinc						0.24 mg

digestive fluids, relieve pain and are antiseptic. The herb has been used to treat cystitis, flatulence, burning urination, dysuria, urinary tract infections, kidney stones, rheumatism, gout and edema.

Parsley herb contains aromatic compounds that decrease the thickness and increase the production of mucosal fluids, increase the production of digestive fluids and increase menstrual and urine flow. It contains bitter compounds that reduce muscle spasms and pains, reduce blood pressure and are antiseptic. Parsley is an excellent herbal source of trace minerals, especially the electrolyte minerals including sodium, potassium, calcium and magnesium. It is also an excellent herbal source of vitamin A, vitamin C and chlorophyllins. Parsley has been used to treat urinary tract infections, amenorrhea, dysmenorrhea, dyspepsia, bronchitis, allergies, arthritis, asthma, flatulence, dysuria and nephritis.

Uva Ursi fruit contains bitter compounds that are antiseptic and increase the flow of urine. It also contains astringent compounds that shrink inflamed tissue. It has been used to treat urinary tract infections, kidney stones, cystitis, nephritis, hemorrhoids and diarrhea.

Dandelion root contains bitter compounds that enhance the efficiency of the body's eliminative and detoxifying functions. These compounds help restore normal liver function, increase the production of digestive fluids and enzymes, particularly bile, increase the flow of urine and have a laxative effect. Dandelion is an excellent herbal source of sodium, iron and vitamin A. It has been used to treat jaundice, gallstones, dyspepsia, constipation, inflammatory skin conditions, frequent urination, hepatitis, gout and rheumatism.

Chamomile flowers contain aromatic compounds that increase the production of digestive fluids, reduce muscle spasms and pains, reduce inflammation and are antiseptic. In addition, these compounds have a sedative effect. Chamomile is one of the best herbal sources of niacin, magnesium and essential fatty acids. It has been used to treat dyspepsia, flatulence, nausea, vomiting, dysmenorrhea, bronchitis, urinary tract infections, insomnia, headaches and menstrual cramps.

Appendix

Determinations for this study were made using a Spectraspan V multi-element optical emission spectrometer, which has a focal lentgh of 0.75 and employs a direct current argon plasma jet as the source of spectrochemical excitation. All analyses used a 25mmx 200 mm high entrance slit and a 100 mm wide x 200 mm high exit slit. All samples were analyzed using 2-30 second integration periods. The operation conditions were as follows:

Element	Analytical Wavelength
Calcium	315.887
Sodium	589.592
Potassium	679.896
Aluminum	308.215
Silicon	251.611
Arsenic	193.696
Cobalt	340.512
Iron	259.940
Mercury	253.652
Magnesium	280.270
Lead	283.306
Selenium	196.026
Zinc	206.200
Phosphorus	214.914
Copper	340.512
Manganese	257.610

Samples were in the form of 40-60 mest, dry powders. Commerical preparation included: Botanical identification while whole compared against herbarium standards (microscopy, etc.), washing with purified water to remove dirt, air drying on trays or racks to prevent spoilage, milling and screening to reduce particle size.

Sample Preparation: A 1.0 gram portion of each plant was added to 20 ml of concentrated nitric acid (Mallincrodt. A.R. Grade) and 8 ml of percholric acid (Mallincrodt. A.R. Grade). The mixture was boiled until dense, white fumes appeared. The resulting solution was diluted to 100 ml with deionized, distilled water.

Analytical standards were provided by Spex Industries, Inc. A high standard was prepared consisting of:

Element	mg/ml
Aluminum	80
Lead	80
Selenium	20
Silicon	20
Mercury	20
Manganese	20
Arsenic	20
Cobalt	20
Calcium	1000
Sodium	1000
Potassium	300
Zinc	500
Phosphorus	500
Magnesium	300
Iron	200
Copper	120

One to one, one to ten, one to one hundred and one to one thousand dilution of this standard were made to account for deviations from linearity in detector response caused by the wide variation in analytic concentration (up to four orders of magnitude).

Note: The mineral concentrations reported in this study are average values from lot samples of the 1983, 1984 and 1985 harvests. This compensates in part for the seasonal variations that occur in natural products.

VITAMIN ANALYSIS

Determinations for this study were made using a Beckman Model 334 Gradient Liquid Chromatograph (HPLC). Experimental procedures for HPLC analysis using ion pairing reagents and a gradient solvent elution are described by Jenkins and Wehr.

Fresh samples of the 1983 and 1984 harvests were obtained and analyzed to compensate for the effects of seasonal variations in the herbs. The samples were kept in a freezer until analysis to ensure reliable results.

Sample Preparation: 50 grams of fresh herb was placed in 100 grams of a 0.25 hydrocloric acid solution and digested for 30 minutes in an autoclave. The mixture is cooled and incubated with amylases (Taka diastase) and papain over night at 37° C to break down starches and proteins. Protein residues were then precipitated with trichloroacetic acid filtered and analyzed using the HPLC method described above.

PROTEIN ANALYSIS

Determinations for this study used the Kjeldahl determination for nitrogen described in the **USP** 21st Edition, page 1207, Method 1:

Protein = 6.25 x nitrogen content

TOTAL FAT ANALYSIS

Determinations for this study used the method described in the **USP** 21st Edition, page 1214.

CRUDE, FIBER, WATER, TOTAL ASH

Determinations for this study used the method described in the **USP** 21st Edition, page 1213.

DIETARY FIBER

Determinations for this study were made by exhausting 10 gm air dried herb with ether then digesting in 100 gm of 0.25N HCl for 30 minutes in an autoclave, followed by incubation with amylase [Taka diastase (to solubilize starch)], and filtering off the residue. The dried residue was weighed and the previously determined amount of protein was subtracted from the residue amount to give the final dietary fiber content.

TOTAL CARBOHYDRATES

Determinations for this study were made by calculating the difference of the sum of the fat, protein and ash from the whole.

Glossary

Acidophilus	Lactobacillus acidophilus bacteria, also called "friendly colonic flora"
Alterative	(See blood purifier)
Analgesic	A substance that relieves pain
Antacid	A substance that neutralizes stomach acid
Antidiarrheal	A substance that combats and arrests diarrhea (See tannins)
Anthelminthic	(See vermifuge)
Antiasthmatic	A substance that relieves the symptoms of asthma, (antispasmodic)
Antibiotic	A substance that inhibits the growth of or destroys microbes (i.e. bacteria, viruses, yeasts, amoebas)
Antipyretic	A substance that counteracts fever
Antiseptic	A substance that inhibits or destroys microbes topically
Antispasmodic	A substance that prevents or relaxes muscles spasms
Aperitive	A substance that stimulates the appetite
Aphrodisiac	A substance that increases sexual appetite or activity
Astringent	A substance that has a constricting or binding effect (See tannins, antidiarrheal)
Bentonite	Volcanic clay used in nutrition for its absorptive properties
Carminative	A substance that relieves gas and gripping (severe pain in the bowel)
Chlorophyll	The "green" matter in plants; used in nutrition to absorb toxins and as a vulnerary
Cholagogue	A substance that stimulates the release of bile from the gallbladder
Cod Liver Oil	Natural oils from cod fish which contain essential fatty acids and vitamins A and D
Demulcent	A substance that soothes tissue
Diaphoretic	A substance that induces sweating
Diuretic	A substance that increases the flow of urine
Emetic	A substance that causes vomiting
Emmenagogue	A substance that facilitates and regularizes menstrual flow
Emollient	A substance that reduces inflammations and irritations
Evening Primrose Oil	The seed oil of Evening Primrose, rich in gamma linolenic acid
Expectorant	A substance that stimulates the expulsion of mucous from the lungs and throat

Febrifuge	(See antipyretic)
Galactogogue	A substance that increases milk production
Hemolytic	A substance which destroys red blood cells
Hemostat	A substance that arrests the flow of blood
Hypertensive	Used to increase blood pressure
Hypoglycemant	A substance that causes a reduction in blood sugar level
Hypotensive	Used to reduce blood pressure
Laxative	A substance that stimulates bowel movements
Lithotriptic	A substance that helps eliminate kidney stones
Montmorillonite	Lake clays used in nutrition as a source of trace minerals
Mydriatic	A substance that enlarges the pupil
Nervine	A substance that calms nervous tension
Oxytocic	A substance that stimulates uterine contractions to induce and assist labor in childbirth
Oestrogenic	A substance affecting female sexual functions
Parasiticide	A substance that kills parasites
Purgative	(See laxative)
Rubefacient	A substance that reddens the skin
Sedative	A substance that quiets the nervous system
Sialagogue	A substance that stimulates the flow of saliva to aid digestion
Spasmolytic	(See antispasmodic)
Stimulant	A substance that increases body energy, especially by increasing blood circulation
Stomachic	A gastric stimulant (See carminative)
Synergistic	The simultaneous action of two or more substances whose combined effect is greater than the sum of each working alone
Tonic	A substance that builds or increases the functions of a system of the body
Vasoconstrictor	A substance that constricts blood vessels
Vasodilator	A substance that dilates blood vessels
Vermifuge	A substance that destroys worms
Vesicant	A substance that causes the skin to blister
Vulnerary	A substance that promotes the healing of wounds

Bibliography

1. American Ethnology, Bureau of. *American Indian Medicines*. Washington, D.C.: Smithsonian Institute, 1957.

2. American Pharmaceutical Association. *Handbook of Nonprescription Drugs*. 5th ed. A.Ph.A. Washington, D.C., 1977.

3. Andrews, T. *A Bibliography on Herbs, Herbal Medicine, "Natural" Foods and Unconventional Medical Treatment*. Littleton, Colorado: Libraries Unlimited, 1982.

4. Arber, A. *Herbals, Their Origin and Evolution*. Cambridge University Press, 1938.

5. Bailey, L.H. *Hortus Second*. New York: The Macmillan Company, 1942.

6. Barnhart, E.R., *Physicians Desk Reference*. Oradell, New Jersey: Medical Economics Company, 1985.

7. Bensky, D., A. Gamble, T. Kaptchuk. *Chinese Herbal Medicine Materia Medica*. Seattle, Washington: Eastland Press, 1986.

8. Blair, Thomas S. *Botanic Drugs*. Cincinnati: Theraputic Digest, 1917.

9. British Herbal Medicine Association. *British Herbal Pharmacopoeia*. London, 1983.

10. Brooklyn Botanic Garden. *Dye Plants and Dyeing*. Brooklyn Botanic Garden Handbook No. 46, 1964.

11. Carter, Kate B. *Pioneer Home Cures of Common Diseases*. Salt Lakc City: Daughters of Utah Pioneers, 1958.

12. Carter, Kate B. *Pioneer Medicines*. Salt Lake City: Daughters of Utah Pioneers, 1958.

13. Culpeper, Nicholas. *Culpeper's Complete Herbal*. London: W. Foulsham & Co., undated.

14. Devon, T.K. and A.I. Scott. *Handbook of Naturally Occurring Compounds*, Vol. 1. Acetogenins, Shikimates, and Carbohydrates. Academic. New York, 1975.

15. Devon, T.K. and A.I. Scott. *Handbook of Naturally Occurring Compounds*. Vol 2. Terpenes. Academic. New York, 1972.

16. Dioscorides. *The Greek Herbal*. Oxford: Oxford University Press, 1934.

17. Duke, J.A. *Crop Chemistry and Folk Medicine*, 1975. pp. 83-117 in V.D. Runeckles, ed., *Advances in Phytochemistry*, Vol. 9. New York: Plenum Press 309 pp.

18. Duke, J.A., E.S. Ayensu. *Medicinal Plants of China*. Vols. 1 and 2. Algona, Michigian: Reference Publications Inc., 1985.

19. FAO. *Food Composition Tables for Use in Africa*. Rome: Food and Agriculture Association, 1968.

20. FAO. *Food Composition Tables for the Near East*. Rome: Food and Agriculture Association, 1982.

21. Fernald, M.D., ed. and rev. *Gray's Manual of Botany*, 8th edition. Boston: American Book Company, 1950.

22. Fogarty, J.E. International Center for Advanced Study in the Health Sciences (FOGARTY). *A Barefoot Doctor's Manual*. Department of Health, Education, and Welfare Publication No.(NIH) 75-695. National Institutes of Health. Washington, D.C. (Translation of Chinese text), 1974.

23. *Food Chemicals Codex*. 2nd ed. National Academy of Sciences. Washington, D.C., 1972.

24. Furia, T.E., ed. *Handbook of Food Additives*. 2nd ed. Cleveland, Ohio: CRC Press, 1975.

25. Gopalan, C., B.V.R. Sastri, S.C.B. Subramanian. *Nutritive Value of Indian Food*. 1977.

26. Grieve, Mrs. M. *A Modern Herbal*. New York: Dover Publications, Harcourt Brace, 1931.

27. Guenther, E. *The Essential Oils*. 1948. 6 vols. Van Nostrand.

28. Harriman, Sarah. *The Book of Ginseng*. New York: Pyramid Books, 1973.

29. Harrop, R., ed. *Encyclopedia of Herbs*. Secaucus Avenue, New Jersey: Chartwell Books, 1977.

30. Hartwell, J.L. 1967-71. *Plants Used Against Cancer: A Survey*. Lloydia 30-34, 11 installments. Issued in One Volume by Quarterman Publications. Lawrence, Massachusetts, 1982.

31. Hocking, G.M. *A Dictionary of Terms in Pharmognosy and Economic Botany*. Thomas. Springfield, Illinois, 1955.

32. *Hortus Third: A Concise Dictionary of Plants Cultivated in the United States and Canada*. L.H. Bailey Hortorium Staff. Cornell University, New York: The MacMillian Company, 1976.

33. Hsu, H., C. Hsu. *Commonly Used Chinese Herb Formulas with Illustrations*. Oriental Healing Arts Institute. Los Angeles, California, 1980.

34. Isler, O. et al., Eds. *Carotenoids* . New York: Halsted (Wiley), 1971.

35. Jenkins, Charles, "An HPLC Method for the Separation and Quantitation of Water-Soluble Vitamins in Vitamin-Mineral Formulations," *Pharm. Tech.*, March 1982.

36. Johnson, Edward L., Robert Stevenson. *Basic Liquid Chromatography*.   Palo Alto, California: Variation Association, 1978.

37. Kreig, M.B. *Green Medicine. The Search for Plants that Heal*. Skokie, Illinois: Rand McNally, 1964.

38. Krochmal, A. and C. Krochmal. *A Guide to the Medicinal Plants of the United States*. New York: Quadrangle/The New York Times Book Company, 1975.

39. Krochmal, Arnold. *Guide to Medicinal Plants of Appalachia*. Washington, D.C.: U.S. Agricultural Handbook. Government Printing Office, 1968.

40. Laveille, J., M. Zabik, and K. Morgan. *Nutrients in Food*. 1983.

41. Leenheer, Andre P., Lamber, E. Willy, DeRuyter, and G.M. Marcel. *Modern Chromatographic Analysis of the Vitamins*. New York: Marcel Dekker Inc., 1985.

42. Leung, A.Y. *Encyclopedia of Common Natural Ingredients*. New York: Wiley-Interscience, John Wiley & Sons, 1980.

43. Lewis, W.H. and Elvin-Lewis, M.P.F. *Medical Botany*. New York: John Wiley & Sons, 1977.

44. Leyel, Mrs. C.F. *Green Medicine*. New York: Faber and Faber, 1952.

45. Lighthall, J.I. *The Indian Folk Medicine Guide*. New York: Popular Library, undated.

46. Lucas, Richard. *Nature's Medicines*. London: Parker, 1966.

47. Marquis Academy Media. *Source Book on Food and Nutrition*. 2nd ed. Chicago, Illinois, 1980.

48. Marsh, A.C. et al. *Composition of Foods, Spice and Herbs. Raw, Processed, Prepared*. Agriculture Handbook No. 8-2. Agricultural Research Service, U.S. Department of Agriculture. Washington, D.C., 1977.

49. Martindale: *The Extra Pharmacopoeia*. London: The Pharmaceutical Press, 1977.

50. Merck & Co. *The Merck Index*. 9th ed. Rahway, New York: Merck & Company, 1976.

51. Merck & Co. *Merck's 1907 Index*. Rahway, New York: Merck & Company, 1907.

52. Millspaugh, Charles F. *Medicinal Plants*. Philadelphia: John C. Yorston, 1892.

53. Millspaugh, C.F., *American Medicinal Plants*. New York: Dover Publications, 1974.

54. Morton, J.F., *Major Medicinal Plants: Botany, Culture, and Uses*. Springfield, Illinois: Thomas, 1977.

55. National Academy of Science. *Diet Nutrition and Cancer*. Washington, D.C., 1982.

56. National Academy of Science. *Recommended Daily Allowances*. Washington, D.C., 1980

57. Oriental Healing Arts Institute of the United States. *The Chemical Constituents of Oriental Herbs*. Los Angeles, California, 1982.

58. Pennington, E., and J. Church. *Food Values of Portions Commonly Used*. 13th ed. Harper & Row, 1980.

59. Prevention Editor. "Understanding Vitamins and Minerals," Emmaus, Pennsylvania: Rodale Press, 1985.

60. Raffauf, R.F. *A Handbook of Alkaloid and Alkaloid Containing Plants*. New York: Wiley-Interscience, John Wiley & Sons, 1970.

61. *Remington's Pharmaceutical Sciences*. 15th ed. Eaton, Pennsylvania: Mack, 1975.

62. Schauenburg, P. and F. Paris. *Guide to Medicinal Plants*, Keats Publishing, Guilford Surrey, 1977.

63. Scully, Virginia. *A Treasury of American Indian Herbs: Their Lore and Their Use for Food, Drugs, and Medicine*. New York: Crown Publishers, 1970.

64. *Standard Methods for the Examination of Water and Waste Water*, 15th ed. Washington, D.C., 1980.

65. Swain, T. (ed.) *Plants in the Development of Modern Medicine*. Cambridge, Massachusetts, Harvard University Press, 1972.

66. *The Dispensatory of the United States of America*. 14th ed. Philadelphia: Lipponcott, 1870.

67. *The Dispensatory of the United States of America*. 23rd ed. (USD 23rd) Philadelphia: Lippincott, 1943.

68. Trease, G.E. and W.C. Evans. *Pharmacognosy*. 11th ed. London: Bailliere Tindall, 1978.

69. Tyler, V.E. et al. *Pharmacognosy*. 7th ed. Philadelphia: Lea & Febiger, 1976.

70. Tyler, V.E. *The Honest Herbal*. Philadelphia: George F. Stickey Company, 1982.

71. *United States Pharmacopeia*. 21st revision Easton, Pennsylvania: Mack Publishing, 1985.

72. Uphof, J.C.T. *Dictionary of Economic Plants*. New York: J. Cramer. Stechert-Hafner, 1968.

73. Vandemark, F.L., "Automated Multivitamin Analysis by Liquid Chromatography," Pitt. Conf. Anal. Chem. Appl. Spect., March 1980.

74. Watt, B.K. and A.L. Merrill. "Composition of Foods, Raw, Processed, Prepared." *Agriculture Handbook No. 8*. USDA, Washington, D.C.

75. Watt, J.M. and Breyer-Brandwijk, M.G. *The Medicinal and Poisonous Plants of Southern and Eastern Africa*. 2nd Ed. Edinburgh and London: E. & S. Livingsone, Ltd., 1962.

76. Wehr, C. Timothy, "Separation of Fat Soluble Vitamins in Pharmaceutical Preparations," Unpublished Varian Technical Bulletin, February 1980.

77. Willaman, J.J. and B.G. Schubert. *Alkaloid-Bearing Plants and Their Contained Alkaloids.*. U.S. Department of Agriculture Technical Bulletin 1234. Washington, D.C., 1961.

78. Williams, L.O. *Drug and Condiment Plants*. USDA, Ag. Handbook 172, Washington, 1960.

79. Williams, Sidney, *Official Methods of Analysis*. Association of the Official Analytical Chemists. 14th ed. 1984.

80. Wren, R.W., Ed. *Potter's New Cyclopedia of Medicinal Herbs and Preparations*. New York: Harper and Row, 1972.

81. Youngken, H.W. *Textbook of Pharmacognosy*. Philadelphia: Blakiston Company, 1948.

Index

Menstrual cramps 137, 276, 298, 299
Mental disorders 173
Mentha piperita. *See* Peppermint
Migraines 167
Milk ipecac. *See* Milk Thistle
Milk Thistle 123
Minerals 161
Morning sickness 190, 223
Motion sickness 99
Mountain balm. *See* Yerba Santa
Mucilaginous herbs 11
Mullein 124
Muscle aches 281
Muscle cramps 227
Muscle spasms 108, 155, 172, 304
Muscle tension 269
Myrica cerifera. *See* Bayberry
Myricaceae 44
Myrtaceae 162

N

Nails, chipping 296
Nails, splitting 303
Narrow dock. *See* Yellow Dock
Nasal congestion 292
Nausea 137, 266, 281
Nepeta cataria. *See* Catnip
Nephritis 125, 307, 312
Nerve tonic 104, 185
Nervine 67, 109, 155
Nervine herbs 8
Nervous conditions 65, 100, 173, 272, 276, 298
Nervous stomach 109
Nettle 125, 126
Neuritis 40
Neurosis 278
Niacin 22
Night sweats 150, 236, 304
Ninsin. *See* Ginseng, Panax
Nocturnal emissions 303
Nosebleed 170
Nutritient 159
Nutritive Herbs 11

O

Oatgrass 127
Obesity 197, 202, 243
Orange root. *See* Golden Seal
Oscillatoriaceae 161
Osteoporosis 301, 304

P

Pain 134, 170, 188
Palmae 153

Panax ginseng. *See* Ginseng, Panax
Pancreas 90
Pancreatitis 238, 309
Pannag. *See* Ginseng, Panax
Papaya 130
Papilionaceae 34
Pappoose root. *See* Blue Cohosh
Paranoia 270
Parasites 203
Parsley 131, 132
Parthenium 133
Parthenium integrifolia. *See* Parthenium
Passiflora incarnata. *See* Passionflower
Passifloraceae 134
Passionflower 134
Pau D' Arco 135, 136
Pedaliaceae 80
Peppermint 137, 138
Peridontal disease 46
Pernicious anemia 82. *See also* Anemia
Petroselinum crispum. *See* Parsley
Pewterwort. *See* Horsetail
Phenylalanine 25
Phlebitis 60
Phosphorous 23
Pin heads. *See* Chamomile
Pinaceae 115
Pipperidge bush. *See* Barberry
Plantaginaceae 139, 142
Plantago major. *See* Plantain
Plantago psyllium. *See* Psyllium
Plantain 139
Pneumonia 289
Poke week. *See* Lobelia
Pollen 140, 141
Polygonaceae 176
Polyps 44
Postpartum conditions 221, 225, 231, 273, 278
Potassium 24
Premenstrual syndrome 56, 278, 296
Prostate 153, 165, 241
Prostatic hypertrophy 115
Prostatitis 217, 236, 307, 310
Protein 25, 161
Psoriasis 115, 151, 176
Psyllium 142, 143
Purple coneflower. *See* Echinacea
Pyrethrum. *See* Feverfew

Q

Quay. *See* Sarsaparilla
Quercus alba. *See* White Oak
Quill. *See* Sarsaparilla

R

Radiation 128
Ranunculaceae 47, 102
Rapid pulse 107
Rattleroot. *See* Black Cohosh
Red berry. *See* Ginseng, Panax
Red Clover 144
Red Raspberry 145, 146
Respiratory allergies 292
Respiratory conditions 61, 72, 84, 85, 86, 122, 160, 178, 288, 293
Restlessness 226
Rhamnaceae 63
Rhamnus purshiana. *See* Cascara Sagrada
Rheumatism 34, 136, 178, 179, 246
Rheumatism root. *See* Wild yam
Riboflavin 26–27
Ripple grass. *See* Plantain
Rosa canina. *See* Rosehips
Rosaceae 107, 145, 147
Rosehips 147
Rubus idaeus. *See* Red Raspberry
Rumex Crispus. *See* Yellow Dock
Ruscus aculeatus. *See* Butcher's Broom

S

Safflower 148
Sage 149, 150
Salicaeae 170
Salix alba. *See* White Willow
Salvia officinalis. *See* Sage
Saponin containing herbs 11
Sarsaparilla 151, 152
Satin flower. *See* Chickweed
Saw Palmetto 153
Saxifragaceae 114
Scabwort. *See* Elecampane
Scarlet fever 48
Scarwort. *See* Chickweed
Schizandra 154
Schizandra chinensis. *See* Schizandra
Schizandraceae 154
Scrophulariaceae 88, 124
Scullcap 155
Scutellaria lateriflora. *See* Scullcap
Sedative 109, 121, 155, 163
Seizures 68
Selenium 27
Seminal emission 48
Senna 156, 157
Serenoa repens. *See* Saw Palmetto
Serpyllum. *See* Thyme
Setwell. *See* Valerian
Seven barks. *See* Hydrangea

ALSO AVAILABLE:

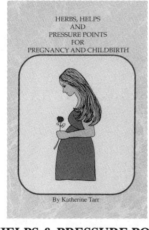

THE ABC HERBAL
By Steven Horne

★ Herbs Used for Children's Conditions
★ Home Remedies
★ Common Sense Approach to Health
★ How to Make Herbal Preparations

Retail Price: $ 7.95 (96 pages)

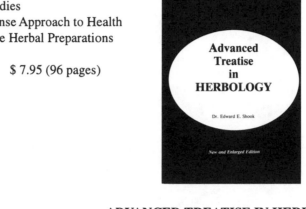

ADVANCED TREATISE IN HERBOLOGY
By Dr. Edward E. Shook

★ All-time Classic
★ Study Course Format
★ Includes Remedies
★ Gives Valuable Insight to Herbal Combinations
★ New and Enlarged Edition

Retail Price: $12.95 (359 pages)

HERBS, HELPS & PRESSURE POINTS FOR PREGNANCY & CHILDBIRTH
By Katherine Tarr

★ Information for a Healthy Pregnancy
★ Recommendations for a Safe Childbirth
★ Helps for Newborn Problems
★ Focuses on, but is not limited to, Home Birth

Retail Price: $ 7.95 (96 pages)

**THE WENDELL W. WHITMAN CO.
NUTRITIONAL RESOURCES INC.**
302 E. Winona Avenue
Warsaw, IN 46580
1-800-421-2401
0-700-AUTHORS

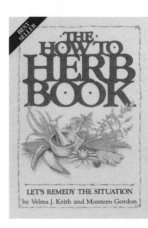

THE HOW TO HERB BOOK
By Velma Keith and Monteen Gordon

★ Historical Herbal Information
★ Sources of Vitamins
★ Sources of Minerals
★ Ailment Classifications and Remedies
★ Single Herb Profiles
★ Combination Herb Profiles

Retail Price: $11.95 English (256 pages)
                     $12.95 Spanish (255 pages)